THE
REIKI
SOURCEBOOK

Reviews

"A balanced, respectful and up-to-date overview of Reiki history and practice, both in Japan and the West. A MUST for any good practitioner and teacher." James Wells, Reiki Master

"One of the few Reiki books I can recommend: a complete guide to Reiki in its many guises, with the latest information about original Reiki from various sources, presented in a neutral and open way. Excellent." Reiki Evolution eZine

"Will satisfy anyone from novice to master. I highly recommend it." Pamir Kiciman, Oasis Reiki Institute

"The definitive manual for teacher, student and general reader alike." Book News

"The most complete work ever done on Reiki. The depth of the research is inspiring. Deserves its name." A to Zen magazine

"A comprehensive and professional guide, a must read for all Reiki followers." The Art of Healing

"A wonderful book." William Lee Rand, author of Reiki the Healing Touch

"An incredible job of researching and pulling the pieces together into a well-organised book." Kathleen Milner, author of Reiki and Other ways of Touch Healing

"You will find EVERYTHING you would like to know about Reiki in this book, which will be highly appreciated and treasured by all Reiki people." Hyakuten Inamoto, Japanese Reiki Master and founder of Komyo Reiki

"It captures everything a Reiki practitioner will ever need to know about the ancient art. This book is hailed by most Reiki professionals as the best guide to Reiki. For an average reader, it's also highly enjoyable and a good way to learn to understand Buddhism, therapy and healing." Michelle Bakar, Beauty

"Sold all around the world, it is hitting the top of the online charts in Reiki." Natural Life

"Well written, an excellent guide. It is easy to see why this book as been heralded around the world as "the Reiki book". Wellbeing

"The most comprehensive book on the system of Reiki ever produced, this book will become an invaluable asset for Reiki novices, students and teachers alike. An incredibly informative and practical book." Nature and Health

"A Reiki practitioners encyclopedia. A credit to the authors' integrity, desire for Reiki to be unravelled, and passion for this most amazing healing modality. Annym

"The most comprehensive book on the system of Reiki ever written." newmetrotimes

"This book will satisfy anyone from novice to Master. I highly recommend it. Pamir Kiciman

"I am so thrilled that a Reiki book of this calibre has finally been published! A masterpiece, an essential handbook." Healing Energy

"Of all the Reiki books on the market, this is a must have. It has absolutely everything in it." Sky

THE
REIKI
SOURCEBOOK

BRONWEN and FRANS STIENE
Founders of the International House of Reiki
Sydney, Australia

info@reiki.net.au
www.reiki.net.au

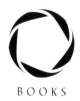

BOOKS

Winchester, U.K.
New York, U.S.A

Copyright © 2003 O Books
46A West Street, Alresford, Hants SO24 9AU, U.K.
Tel: +44 (0) 1962 736880 Fax: +44 (0) 1962 736881
E-mail: office@johnhunt-publishing.com
www.o-books.net

U.S. office:
240 West 35th Street, Suite 500
New York, NY10001
E-mail: obooks@aol.com

Text: © 2003 Bronwen and Frans Stiene

Design: Jim Weaver Design
Illustrations: Lolly Ellena Rados

ISBN 1 903816 55 6

Reprinted 2004, 2005

A CIP catalogue record for this book is available
from the British Library.

Printed by Oriental Press, Dubai, U.A.E.

Table of Contents

Preface

To collate all of the information that you are about to read has not been an easy task. We experienced a multitude of setbacks. On top of the list was our lack of understanding of the Japanese culture (you can stop that knowing laughter now). It's true, the culture is renowned as being notoriously difficult for foreigners to comprehend and, well – we can vouch for that. In times of need, determination and faith were our only assets.

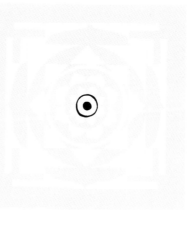

We were determined that this book would be written. The confusion that we experienced as fledgling Reiki Masters in 1998 encouraged us to seek out the truths and fictions that surrounded Mikao Usui's early teachings and the system of Reiki in the West. This was for our own benefit and for those who are interested in or involved in the system of Reiki as it stands today. We tackled Japanese customs learning that information is only given when the right question is asked. We fell down when we didn't understand that a Japanese lack of enthusiasm actually meant 'NO!' We never wish to hear the words, 'think laterally' again and are glad that we continued asking and shaking the tree till some information fell from its branches. This is an ongoing task and we hope to zealously continue researching in the future.

There was also our faith that this book would be fleshed out from a Japanese perspective and thankfully along came some very patient friends. Our thanks go to Hyakuten Inamoto who allowed us to ask a lot of difficult cultural and historical questions by simply saying, 'shoot!' Hyakuten Inamoto also gave generously of his time and his knowledge to expertly translate Mikao Usui's memorial stone and the Meiji Emperor's *waka* (poetry) at our request. Other aspects of the Japanese language left us dumbfounded until we came across our translator, Anne Radovic, whose love of the intricacies of the Japanese culture and language was a blessing.

Some aspects of this book were easy. The perfect illustrations were designed and drawn up by a truly spiritual Australian artist and Reiki practitioner, Lolly Ellena Rados. Thanks to Michiko Honda for her calligraphy work too.

The writing in itself was a clarification and joy for us as eternally self-learning human beings.

Our teachers, fellow Reiki practitioners and friends who provided us with a great deal of information and support – we sincerely thank. To name a few we would have to begin with Light and Adonea (our Usui Reiki Ryôhô teachers), whose personal dedication to researching Reiki is always an inspiration; Robert Fueston who openheartedly shared his research, encouraging us with his generosity of spirit; Viviana Puebla, another big-hearted and supportive Reiki practitioner and Maurizio Floris for his enthusiastic and honest editing.

Thanks also go to Chris Marsh, Andrew Bowling, Dave King, Frank Arjava Petter, Hiroshi Doi, William Lee Rand, Vincent Amador, Rick Rivard, Patrick McCarthy, Seiji Tabatake, Tokiko Minamida and Andrew Gordon, for their personal information, exhaustive research and/or informative books and websites.

There are too many people whom we questioned (and quite possibly annoyed) in our quest for answers. Thanks for your patience Tokushin, Reverend Jion Proser, Exie Lockett, Miek Skoss, Stanley Pranin, Daniel Lee and Seikou Terashima and anyone else we may have forgotten to mention.

Thanks to Nevill Drury, our agent, for his simple faith in us, and *The Reiki Sourcebook*. Thanks too, to John Hunt and his team for making the publishing of this book a pleasure.

We would never have begun this journey without the support of our friends and families, especially our mothers – Elaine Voll and Henny Stiene. Thank you. Our fathers who are no longer with us, especially Jan Stiene who we know would have loved to be researching alongside us. The most special thanks of all goes to our precious daughter, Bella – for simply bringing us joy.

And thank you to those too who wished not to have their names mentioned.

There is one more important thank you – to Mikao Usui and those who practice his teachings, in whatever form, everywhere.

There is a common saying in Japanese that we think is highly appropriate at this point in the book. We hope it expresses our desire to achieve great things for Mikao Usui's teachings by bringing information together in one easily accessible tome. We do not wish to harm anyone or anything and would like to apologize in advance for any inconsistencies, or mistakes that may be found within the text. To the best of our knowledge, we have accurately portrayed the information that we have read or received.

Let us begin the book by writing:

mangaichi ayamariga arimashitara goyousha kudasai

Please forgive us if we've made a mistake

Do not believe in anything (simply) because you have heard it.
Do not believe in traditions because they have been handed
down for many generations.
Do not believe in anything because it is spoken and rumored
by many.
Do not believe in anything (simply) because it is found written
in your religious books.
Do not believe in anything merely on the authority of your
teachers and elders.
But after observation and analysis, when you find that
anything agrees with reason and is conducive to the good and
benefit of one and all then accept it and live up to it.

Guatama Buddha
Anguttara Nikaya Vol I, pp. 188–193, R.T.S. Ed.

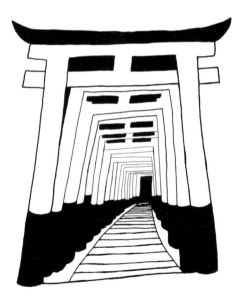

Introduction

The system of Reiki is changing.

You may wonder why? Why should the teachings that were started in the early 1900s by a Japanese man called Mikao Usui need to change? Perhaps because they have already been changed – many, many times. Mikao Usui's teachings have constantly been altered and adapted to suit the people who have practiced them and the worlds they live in.

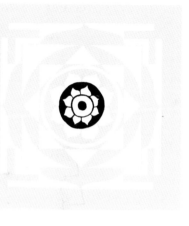

The real change that is taking place with these teachings today is that practitioners are returning to its origins. In this cyclical return to the roots of the system of Reiki, we encounter the many diversions that have taken place over the last 100 years.

The Reiki Sourcebook has been written to guide you through this journey. It aims to be a complete resource for all aspiring Reiki practitioners throughout the world, including Japan.

To begin the book we look at what is understood by the word Reiki. Translated it means 'spiritual energy', yet at the same time it also represents the system of Mikao Usui's teachings in their modern form. Following this brief explanation is detailed information about the teachings today, for the benefit of those who are interested in or are currently practicing the system of Reiki.

We then move on to a deeper look into Mikao Usui's teachings and a concise history of Reiki as seen through the eyes of its numerous practitioners. To create a clear understanding for the reader of what is to come there is a Reiki Timeline and Lineage Chart. Many of the historical notes included are the results of our own research, which took us, naturally, to Japan. There we met with traditional Japanese Reiki practitioners and viewed some of the sites that are relevant to Reiki's history, such as Mikao Usui's gravesite and memorial stone, *kurama yama* (Mt Kurama) and *hiei zan* (Mt Hiei). There are also major contributions in this sourcebook from many Reiki practitioners the world over. To them we are extremely thankful for aiding us in our attempt to create a book that is the ultimate in Reiki knowledge.

Included in *The Reiki Sourcebook* are the names of branches, schools and associations that have stemmed from Mikao Usui's teachings. Major Reiki techniques from both the East and West are explained. Reiki terminology is available in an extensive glossary and there is much more.

The system of Reiki continues to change.

There will always be more information to add to this journey. Mikao Usui's teachings are a practice in motion, which means that in each moment we capture a picture perfect shot of its truth. But there are many of these moments and therefore many truths. It all depends on what sort of camera you use, when you use it and from which angle it is photographed. We have tried to capture as many sides of this wonderful technique for you in this practical, comprehensive and intriguing book.

There is a truth to these teachings that can't be negated no matter which branch you may associate yourself with. This truth can be described as belonging to the energy of the universe, or that of the earth and the heavens, the yin and the yang, the soul connection or simply the spiritual or healing energy. No matter which language you choose to describe these teachings there will always be the sense of what that truth is: Reiki is far greater than us as individuals. Our desires and needs are impotent when faced with Reiki – it renders them powerless. Our intent opens us up to accept Reiki through us. It washes us, and others, clear. No life force is unaffected by Reiki.

We practice these teachings so that we may heal inside and out, let go and be One with the universe, reconnect with the path of our inevitable enlightenment and help others. To experience this we need to know that it is also our personal awareness of Reiki that creates an even more effective technique.

Controversy abounds concerning individual teaching methods and yet we all take this energy into our lives with the intent to evolve and heal. Reiki is far greater than our concerns of time, money and power. As humans, we are challenged by ourselves every step of the way. Reiki is our magical tool, proffering us strength, calm and light. We must take what we can with gratitude and work on ourselves, knowing that we can do this. We are empowered and the world can only become a more beautiful place through this knowing and the practice of Mikao Usui's teachings.

This versatile, free-flowing method is perfect for our times in that it is ultimately simple. Children can learn about Reiki, it's switched on with a thought and the practice of it can take place in bed or on the bus. This simplicity makes it accessible to our 'busy, busy' lifestyles that 'don't have time for spirituality'. Conversely, the complexity of understanding Reiki is beyond the ability of our rational and technical twenty-first-century mind. The challenge for us then is to just let go and to see what we will discover. Letting go is not as easy as it sounds. If we can learn to let go and resist controlling ourselves, our situations and others we might find a peaceful beauty of contentment in our lives; one that, in turn, might result in world peace.

The intent of *The Reiki Sourcebook* is to link together information that has been spread far and wide by time and circumstances. By capturing the results of this systematic global research, it aims to share the information and to promote and stimulate discussion in the global Reiki community. It is not necessarily about 'new' information but the bringing together of histories and anecdotes to create a cohesive understanding of what has happened to and been said about the teachings during the past 100 years.

It is hoped that this will be a valuable resource for anyone interested in the history of Mikao Usui, his teachings, Reiki and related practices. It is also for beginners or those who feel lost and confused by the myriad of choices that are presented to them as Reiki in today's society.

This is an attempt to create unity rather than dissension – unity for all who work with this wondrous energy. Do not be distracted by the human frailties you will encounter within these pages, just remember that it is human strength that initially formed the teaching's solid base. If we can see where we came from – we can see clearer where we are heading.

Respect is a word that must be remembered and practiced by all when dealing with such a pure and beautiful energy. Correspondingly, we have attempted to retain this respect for the sacredness of the teachings by not baring the traditional mantras and symbols or attunement processes to the general public. The research information in this book is not just about what is taught but, most importantly, where these teachings originated. We respect that methods often involve the student completing certain energetic levels before being handed specific information.

Verification of historical material about Mikao Usui and his teachings is a continuing struggle. In the West, Hawayo Takata taught her history of Reiki. Her historical anecdotes, though entertaining, have unfortunately appeared to be unreliable. In the aftermath of her death in 1980, Western eyes turned to Japan for answers and discovered a country quietly practicing Mikao Usui's teachings. This was a great surprise, as it had been understood by Western practitioners that the system of Reiki was 'dead' in Japan.

Information is gradually seeping through to the West. This is the result of Westerners contacting Japanese people and studying with them. Cultural and linguistic differences have made this far more difficult than it might sound. The result is that the information coming out of Japan is only doing so through limited channels – those who have the contacts and the language.

To truly verify much of this 'new' information it is necessary to see notes or photos or preferably to talk to these original Japanese sources. The few Westerners, who have become the middle people, are protective of their information and are not willing to show (or cannot show) authenticating material. The question this lays at our feet is, 'is it the truth?' Without doubting the integrity of those supplying this information, we must always ask questions. Recently, there was the case of Men Chhos Reiki (also known as Medicine Dharma Reiki and Universal Healing Reiki) that claimed to have 'true' and 'original' teachings as well as notes from Mikao Usui – at least one complete book was even written about it. Not one piece of this information was verifiable after years of questioning by its students. Senior students eventually walked out – disillusioned after all the support (financial and emotional) they had given the founder of the branch. This is not just heartbreaking for the students who were searching for the truth but for all those that the teachings have confused. To try to prevent this happening again verification must be called for.

There is another society in Japan called the Usui Reiki Ryôhô Gakkai. It is not open to Westerners but has at least one member, Hiroshi Doi, who talks about the origins of Mikao Usui's teachings. Members of this society are even asked not to disclose that they are members. It is therefore a welcome surprise to receive his information. The downside to this is that Hiroshi Doi's information is not always complete as he is restricted in what he may or may not say. It has even been suggested that some of the information Hiroshi Doi offers is a smoke screen to protect traditional information.

From these examples, you can see that verification is an important issue when dealing with the history of Mikao Usui's life and teachings. Naturally, it is also most important to follow our heart and place trust in its inner sense.

To present objective viewpoints, information from all sources has been used and footnoted (where available) in *The Reiki Sourcebook*. Information that is knowingly incorrect or untruthful has not deliberately been included as fact.

It is good to remember that Mikao Usui's teachings cannot be learnt from a book. The information that has been gathered here is not an alternative to seeking out a teacher.

How to read this book:

- An asterix (*) before the name of a technique indicates that it can be found in Part III – Reiki Techniques.
- Japanese words are italicized. The *kanji* plus the translation or description of the word can be found in the Reiki Glossary in the Appendix.
- The Reiki Glossary in the Appendix includes descriptions of people, places, techniques, branches and associated material concerned with Mikao Usui's early teachings and the system of Reiki.

This is a useful tool for understanding any unfamiliar terminology in *The Reiki Sourcebook*.

- The use of upper case is a Western notion and not a Japanese one. When printing Japanese words the authors have taken the liberty of using capitals for people's names and places (in the Western custom) for added clarity.
- This book may be used solely as a reference material for Reiki practitioners or as a comprehensive manual for beginners that can be read from cover to cover.
- We would advise all Reiki practitioners to take note of Part II – Reiki History as this information has changed dramatically over the last few years.

The contents of this book are for general information only. The authors do not endorse the methodology, techniques or philosophy of individual modalities detailed herein, and accept no liability for the use or misuse of any practice or exercise in this book.

We invite those who possess vital information about Mikao Usui's teachings or other relevant research knowledge to share it via *The Reiki Sourcebook* so that this awareness can flow back into the Reiki community.

Japanese Pronunciation:

a is similar to the *a* in father
i is similar to the *ea* in eat
u is similar to the *oo* in look
e is similar to the *e* in egg
o is similar to the *o* in go

(From *An Introduction to Modern Japanese* by Osamu and Nobuko Mizutani.)

Part I

Approaching Reiki

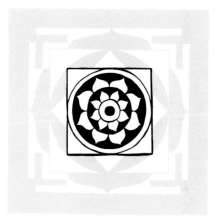

If you've picked up *The Reiki Sourcebook* with no prior knowledge of Reiki then this is where you should begin...
Many people have heard the word Reiki but have no idea of what it actually is. Is it a religion, a massage procedure or could it even be dangerous? 'No,' is the answer to all three questions. It is neither a belief system nor a physically manipulative technique and it is completely safe. The system of Reiki is a method of working with energy that allows the body to clear itself leaving you feeling lighter, healthier and happier.

Discussed in Part I are the origins of the word Reiki. Reiki represents both the name of the system that is practiced in the West today and the concept of spiritual energy. Sound information about the workings of this system from a Western perspective are looked at in depth from both the client's and the student's viewpoint. There are many beliefs about Reiki and this section hopes to clarify what is and what is not a part of the modern practice of Reiki.

Teachings that are more traditional exist in Japan but have only recently begun to be known to the general public. These teachings may differ in content and focus but are not, yet, widespread.

1   Reiki, the Word

Meaning of Reiki

Reiki, the word, is Japanese. It is written with two Japanese *kanji*, 霊気, meaning 'spiritual energy'.

霊 is *rei* – (lit. Japanese) spiritual or sacred
気 is *ki* – (lit. Japanese) energy

Previously these 2 *kanji* have been translated as 'Universal Energy' (or Universal Life Force Energy) in the West. This is obviously a translation of the second *kanji*, 'ki', only. *Ki* is naturally the energy of everything including heaven and earth, the entire universe.

The first *kanji*, 'rei', may have been left out of English translations due to the fact that the term 'spiritual' was not the focus of the Western practice in the twentieth century.

To pronounce the word, Reiki, in Japanese it is necessary to forego any preconceptions about language. The first sound in 'rei' is neither an 'R' nor an 'L', as some Westerners believe. In Japanese the sound is in fact somewhere in between the two letters. The Japanese language has no correlation with English or its pronunciations.

The first time that the government initiated a standardized system and romaji[1] were introduced was in 1885. The *kanji* for 'rei' is officially spelt with an 'R' when translating into English and is therefore pronounced with an 'R' (even though the Japanese pronunciation might sound similar to what is understood as an 'L' in English).

[1] *Romaji* are the English Letters used to translate *kanji*.

Reiki, a System or an Energy?

The word 'Reiki' is used in the West to also represent a healing system. Mikao Usui, the founder of Reiki, did not call his teachings by this name. 'Reiki' appeared written in conjunction with his teachings but this was merely to point out that the teachings worked with spiritual energy. Generally, his teachings were called 'Usui dô' meaning 'the way of Usui', and his healings were known as 'Usui teate' translated to mean 'Usui hands-on healing'.

'Reiki' the word can be found in the branches of schools that developed from Mikao Usui's teachings. Both the Usui Reiki Ryôhô Gakkai (Society of the Usui Spiritual Energy Healing method) and *Hayashi Reiki Kenkyû Kai* (Hayashi's Spiritual Energy Research Society) use the word 'Reiki' to signify 'spiritual energy' but neither actually called the system, Reiki.

Hawayo Takata was the first student of these teachings in the West. Chûjirô Hayashi, her teacher, came with her to Hawaii to help her set up her practice. At his farewell dinner he presented her with a westernized certificate. This official gesture ensured that she was seen as a legal teacher and practitioner in the Japanese system. The certificate states in English that she was a 'Master of the Usui Reiki System of Drugless Healing'. Once again the term 'Reiki' is used to mean spiritual energy rather than any complete system. Included in the certificate though are other statements that appear to refer to 'Reiki' as a form of energy as well as a 'system'. This was 1938 and was the first time that there was any inconsistency in the use of the term 'Reiki'. This was probably due to the difficulty of translating Japanese into English. From that point on the word 'Reiki' jointly represented the system based on Mikao Usui's teachings as well as 'Universal Life Force Energy'.

The downside of using 'Reiki' to mean a system is that people are unsure as to what particular practices fall under that name. All the systems named Reiki today claim to use spiritual energy in their practice. There appears to be no other definition to the system than that. This leaves the door wide open for individual discrepancies.[2]

---

[2] For more information about the various branches of Reiki see page 171.

Many traditional Japanese teachers call the system 'Ryôhô' which means 'healing method' or 'Reiki Ryôhô' which means 'spiritual energy healing method'. The word 'Reiki' to the Japanese is considered to be quite spooky. 'Rei' means not only spiritual or sacred but can also represent the spirit of dead people. For this reason in modern Japan today the kanji for Reiki is not used. Instead, the word Reiki is written in *katakana* as this writing system is phonetic and holds no meaning.

The Reiki Sourcebook attempts to clearly define whether it is discussing the modern system of Reiki, Mikao Usui's original teachings or 'spiritual energy' when using the word 'Reiki'.

Today, people even talk about 'Reikiing' something. This particular use of the word is a new addition to its many interpretations.

Origins of the Word Reiki

Kanji are made up of both pictographs[3] and ideographs.[4]

In China, *kanji* originated in the Yellow River area about 2000 BC. During the third and fourth century AD it was brought across from China and Korea to Japan. Until this time Japan had only ever used the spoken language. The Chinese characters were used phonetically to represent similar sounding Japanese syllables, the actual meaning of the characters were ignored.

In between AD 710 and 1185 the symbols underwent a further simplification. This is what is called *hiragana* today. *Hiragana* is used to write the inflectional endings of the conceptual words that are written in *kanji*. It also is used for all types of native words not written in *kanji*. This was an attempt to cut down on the amount of *kanji* needed to express a multi-syllabic Japanese word.

Katakana was developed a little later and became phonetic shorthand based on Chinese characters. It was used by students who, while listening to classic Buddhist lectures, would make notations on the pronunciations or meanings of unfamiliar characters, and sometimes wrote commentaries between the lines of certain passages. *Katakana* is used chiefly for words of foreign origin. This

---

[3] Pictographs are pictures that represent ideas.
[4] Ideographs are symbols (*kanji*) that represent the sounds that form its name.

style made reading and writing much less complicated, creating a higher literacy rate amongst the Japanese people.

In Chinese, the same two *kanji* used to represent Reiki are pronounced differently but have a similar meaning. In Chinese, Reiki is called *Ling chi.*

> Ling chi is the subtlest and most highly refined of all the energies in the human system and the product of the most advanced stages of practice, whereby the ordinary energies of the body are transformed into pure spiritual vitality. This type of highly refined energy enhances spiritual awareness, improves all cerebral functions, and constitutes the basic fuel for the highest level of spiritual work.
>
> (Excerpt from *Chi-gung: Harnessing the Power of the Universe* by Daniel Reid.)

There are two methods of pronouncing Japanese *kanji*. The first is *kun yomi*. Here Chinese *kanji* are used to express Japanese words that have a similar meaning to the original Chinese word. When a Japanese word's sound uses *kanji* this is then called a *kun yomi* reading. The second is *on yomi*. Here the Chinese reading and meaning are attached to the *kanji*.

Kanji on its own generally uses *kun yomi* readings and *kanji* in compounds (more than one *kanji*) often uses *on yomi* readings. There has been such a great deal of change in the Japanese language that most modern *kanji* have two or three *kun yomi* and *on yomi* readings. This allows the language to express many varied concepts and expressions in contrast to Chinese where each character has only one reading.

By the twentieth century there were around 50,000 *kanji* in use in Japan but after World War II the Japanese Ministry of Education began simplifying the language. To be able to read a newspaper at that time the reader would have needed to know about 4000 *kanji*. In 1946 the number of *kanji* used in official publications was limited to 1850. A Japanese person of average education would be familiar with about 3000 *kanji*.

Styles of *Kanji*

There are also different styles of calligraphy. Here are three modern styles and one older style. The older style would have been in use at the time Mikao Usui developed his teachings.

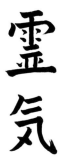

1) *Kaisho* modern, standard style. This style is similar to the printed style of *kanji*, and is taught in schools.

2) *Gyôsho* modern, semi cursive style. A simplification of the standard style, allowing it to be written in a more flowing and faster manner.

3) *Sôsho* modern, cursive style. This is a kind of simplified shorthand that is drawn according to aesthetic standards.

4) *Kaisho* old, standard style. This is the standard style written before World War II and was how Reiki was drawn during Mikao Usui's lifetime.

How to Draw *Kanji*

In the system of Reiki, two of the four symbols that are practiced are in fact *kanji*. These are Symbol 3 and Symbol 4. To draw these symbols correctly it is valuable to understand the basic brushstroke technique for calligraphy. *Kanji* have an exact order in which the strokes must be drawn.

Intent is clearer and stronger when there is the assurance that one is working in a correct and certain manner. There is also an added beauty to something that is drawn with accuracy and care.

The guidelines, as set out by the Japanese Ministry of Education in 1958, are summarized below. Some modern branches of Reiki have created their own *kanji*-like symbols or altered existing ones. It is possible to verify the symbols by comparing the order and directions of the brushstrokes with the official Japanese calligraphic guidelines.

Stroke direction

Horizontal strokes are written from left to right.

Vertical or slanting strokes are written from top to bottom.

Strokes can change direction several times; they run from top left to bottom left or right.

Stroke order (the rules are given in order of importance)

From top to bottom.

From left to right.

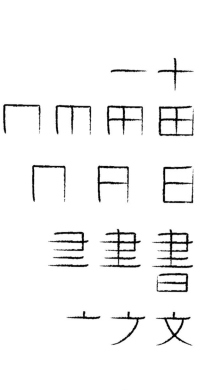

Middle strokes are written first and then left and right strokes if the left and right strokes do not exceed two strokes each.

The horizontal stroke usually precedes vertical stroke.

In some circumstances the vertical stroke precedes the horizontal stroke.

Outside strokes comes first – except the bottom stroke, which comes last.

Vertical strokes through the center are drawn last.

The upper right to lower left diagonal strokes precede the upper left to lower right strokes.

Horizontal strokes, which go through the middle of the kanji, are written last.

2 Treatments

Ki is the basic unit of the universe.
It is the infinite gathering of infinitely small particles.
Everything is ultimately composed of Ki.

If you pursue this concept to the depth of human consciousness, you will understand the universal mind which governs all creation, loving and protecting all life ...

Everything originates from the Ki of the universe.

(Excerpt from the *Book of Ki* by Koichi Tohei.)

A treatment may be experienced when a colleague, who has studied the system of Reiki, places his/her hand on your aching shoulder muscle. Before you realize it the pain has miraculously melted away.

Or, even better, it may be a luxurious, full one-hour Reiki treatment. You lie on a professional practitioner's massage table with relaxing music and soft lighting as your mind and body float off.

Reiki treatments come in all shapes and sizes and, no matter what the conditions, will always work. This is the magic of Reiki.

Reiki's Path

Reiki re-aligns one with one's true path, source and spirit.

It must be conceived that everything has energy or *ki* in it – even a piece of paper or a plant, every item in the room, the building itself, the city, the country, the world, the universe and on and on. Gradually, comprehension dawns that there is an unlimited amount of energy. This energy may seem invisible, or elusive but it is, instead, all-encompassing. It is this energy that makes not just humans, but worlds, function. It is the fuel that drives humans and gives ultimate structure and purpose in life. This is Reiki.

Occasionally, humans get a bit of dirt in the fuel line or a better way to explain it is perhaps by envisaging a free-flowing river. This beautiful river is like energy flowing easily down through the body. Occasionally a pebble, or even a rock, will fall into that river making the flow of the water a little more difficult. These pebbles are human worries, fear, anger, and each pebble builds on top of the other. Soon there is only a trickle of water running in that once beautiful free-flowing river. And so it is with energy in the human body. At this point physical pain may be experienced.

During a Reiki treatment the pure flow of energy is re-aligned within the body. It washes down, clearing obstructions and strengthening the flow of energy. This signifies a connection to the understanding of one's purpose on earth and the easiest, most successful way of achieving it.

The Procedure

The client lies or sits and the practitioner's hands are placed on or just above the body. It is unnecessary for the client to remove any clothing and no private parts of the body need ever be touched. *There is no place for sexual contact or inference within the system of Reiki.*

A professional practitioner is someone who has generally completed at least the second level of a Reiki course. Ideally, a professional Reiki practitioner should have counselling skills, first-aid skills, business skills and knowledge of physiology and anatomy. There is more to a professional practice than just placing the hands on the body. Most countries have Reiki associations that practitioners can become members of. These associations will have set standards of practice and ethics that practitioners must abide by or consequently lose their membership.

Quiet during a treatment is an asset for both the practitioner and the client. The practitioner reaches a meditative state quite quickly and the client eventually lets go of the busy mind and tense physicality.

This sense of utter relaxation is, in fact, a healing state. It is often likened to being in the womb. There is consciousness yet the client feels separate and safe from all outside influence. It is also in this state that the client may glean spiritual guidance.

The practitioner has the intent that Reiki will move through the practitioner's body, out through the hands and into the client's body. The hands do not manipulate the Reiki they are just the vessel for the Reiki to flow through. Hand positions can be held roughly from one minute to half an hour or longer – depending on what the practitioner can sense in the body.

A general rule of thumb is that as long as the practitioner can sense something vibrating, moving, heating up, tingling (or whatever the energetic interpretation is) then one stays there. The client can generally feel 'something' happening too.

Sensing Ki

These sensations are the side effects of clearing the energy in the body. They also serve to remind that Reiki really does work. Descriptions of the effects of sensing energy might be twitching or involuntary movement; the seeing of colours or a visual journey while the eyes are closed; the gaining of an intuitive knowledge or understanding. No matter whether something is sensed or not the Reiki is still working.

Expected Outcomes

To hold expectations of what will happen in a treatment will only lead to disillusion. Although the practitioner and the client may think that they know what is needed – the non-conscious self may decide otherwise. Energy is drawn into the client's body by whichever area feels that it needs the energy. This may be an emotional, physical, mental or even spiritual area.

The system of Reiki is not a manipulative one. Energy knows it's true path. Reiki is not different from one's own energy; there is no disconnection. There is a continuous flow of energy without beginning or end. A client simply draws on more of the same energy, building personal resources and clearing the meridians – balancing the body at all levels. A client will only draw the amount of energy that is needed or desired. Therefore if the client consciously or subconsciously does not want to draw on the energy then there will be little or no effect. This means that the client is continuously in control of what is happening with the Reiki even if it is in a non-conscious manner.

The beauty of this is that the client no longer works with the rational mind but allows the true self to do the healing. This cannot harm and always holds the client's highest good in mind. When people begin to bring fear into the system then it is their own personal issues that are involved. Remember – Reiki is the energy that makes the universe function in all its perfection. Specific results are therefore impossible to rely on, though in the long term changes will occur – they may just not be the ones that are expected.

An example of this is where one practitioner regularly treated her father in the hope that it would improve his worsening diabetes. After one month they both believed there had been no improvement until her father realised that he was hearing better!

By letting go of making conscious decisions the pressure is taken off to perform, the ego is sent on vacation and the practitioner and client can get to work on what is integral to one's well being.

Intent

The practitioner does not need to work hard to make Reiki work. The intent is there once the thought to place the hands on the body takes place. It is this intent which sparks the movement of energy. *Ki*, or energy, follows the mind.

As far as Reiki is concerned, if the practitioner intends to use Reiki in the manner one was taught, then that is what will happen. If a practitioner intends to treat a client with Reiki then that person will receive a Reiki treatment.

If a practitioner tries to overly concentrate and force the energy to work then interference is taking place and the energy does not flow smoothly.

Respect

Every practitioner knows of someone who would benefit from a Reiki treatment. This person, though, may not be a willing participant in a Reiki treatment. It is important that the client (or friend or family member) is not being pushed into receiving the treatment. A practitioner cannot heal – that is the client's responsibility. A practitioner must always respect the wishes of those around them. Respect is one of the five precepts of Reiki[1] and ensures that true practitioners never judge others.

Remember that life is continually changing. So, a client may not want a treatment one day and yet happily accepts one another.

Chronic or Acute

All illnesses can be treated with Reiki. As mentioned earlier – it is not possible to predict an outcome when using Reiki. Some practitioners will use other methods that are not Reiki to define the energetic information received. The Reiki itself will work away on what it feels is necessary at the time. This might be a physical problem, an emotional imbalance, a busy mind or the sense of a lack of connection to life.

A good example is of a client who has experienced a chronic illness over many years and is near to death. A practitioner cannot predict or calculate whether there will be recovery or how long recovery might take. Instead, the practitioner lets the Reiki do what is needed; it may be to emotionally settle the person, to relieve pain or to offer spiritual insight. The client and doctors may not expect recovery but a Reiki practitioner is always open to the possibility of a miracle. Depression, insomnia and fear-based illnesses and other non-physical illnesses can also benefit from Reiki.

Reiki works with acute problems that may arise too. As a first-aid tool, it offers pain relief while attempting to return the body to its most natural state. Stress is a word that is familiar in all sectors of the community today. When stressed the immune system weakens leaving humans prone to ill health. Reiki brings about calm and thus

---

[1] For more information about the 5 precepts see page 66.

deals effectively with stress. Reiki brings about clarity of thought and decision-making with ease.

Not only does Reiki help illness but it also enhances whatever it is used on – bringing everything back to its most natural state.

Contraindications

There are no contraindications with Reiki. Reiki is simply about clearing and enhancing energy according to the needs of the body. To bring the body back into balance is all that can occur and this cannot be harmful.

Listening to the body is in fact the most sensible thing anyone can do for good health and the system of Reiki promotes that.

Clearing

After a treatment, it is advisable to drink lots of water to continue the clearing that was initiated by the Reiki. The client may also find that the body reacts to the Reiki in a 'negative' way. Some symptoms may be slightly exaggerated. This is, in fact, a very positive sign indicating that the Reiki is moving things in the body. If this is the case, it is good to receive more Reiki to follow up on the work already done.

One Treatment or More

Practitioners often suggest three initial treatments if the client wishes to work on a specific issue. This might be of an emotional, physical, mental or spiritual nature. If, after three treatments, the symptoms are still apparent treatments may be continued. Practitioners should work within time frames as it gives the client the chance to work toward recovery by a certain date. Unlimited Reiki treatments may mean unlimited ill health for some.

Reiki treatments are also an excellent tool for relaxation and can be experienced in the same manner as, for example, a one-off Swedish massage – for pure enjoyment. Don't forget that Reiki will always be working on something even if the client is not consciously aware of it.

Animals, Plants and the Rest

Animals, plants and other 'things' can also draw on Reiki. Science tells us that everything has energy in it. Whether it is a human, a cat, a coffee mug or a thought form. When Reiki is drawn in, it clears and enhances the existing energy. This is beneficial to all things.

For animals, it is practiced in much the same way as on humans. Of course, an animal cannot be asked if it wants Reiki. Be assured that an animal will signal if it does or doesn't want the Reiki. Generally, animals are attracted to energy and will attempt to get into whatever position is best to draw the Reiki's maximum benefits. If it just walks (or runs) away, an attempt later might be more successful. The animal may then feel less nervous about this new experience.

Plant life flourishes with Reiki. Treating the seeds is just the first step. As the plant grows, the hands are placed above the leaves or wrapped around the pot. A trick to using Reiki in a house filled with potted plants is to first use Reiki on the bucket of water. This can then be used for watering the plants.

Food and drink can be enhanced energetically with Reiki too. Imagine eating food that is energetically heightened? Many people say it immediately tastes better. Its energetic vibration is lifted and therefore improves any elements that may be less than fresh or have stayed too long on the shelf or in the freezer. Each day that a piece of fruit or vegetable is away from its plant it is fast losing nutrients and goodness.

The same goes for allopathic[2] medicines or herbal remedies. By lifting the vibration level of allopathic medicines, the side effects have less impact. Herbal remedies become more effective with spiritual energy.

Stones, crystals and other natural elements can often be felt to draw great amounts of energy. Reiki does not take away from their own natural abilities – it just enhances them.

People have also been known to use Reiki on computers, batteries, wallets and the list goes on.

All that limits us is our own imagination.

[2] Allopathy: That system of medical practice that aims to combat disease by the use of remedies which produce effects different from those produced by the special disease treated. Webster Dictionary, 1913.

3   Courses

The process of healing a personal illness is, in fact, a rite of passage, designed by yourself as one of the greatest learning tools you will ever encounter

(Excerpt from *Light Emerging* by
Barbara Ann Brennan.)

Treating the self is the most important aspect of Mikao Usui's teachings.

Learning to treat one's self is actively taking our health into our own hands. Self-responsibility changes how a life situation is viewed. We are no longer victims to our circumstances but choose to live optimally at every level. Life becomes easier as stress dissolves and perceptions alter. The immune system strengthens and illness takes a backseat in life. Most importantly the connection to our true spiritual nature is re-established.

Feeling strong in ourselves also gives us the ability to help those around us. Reiki courses teach not only how to heal oneself but to help others too.

Before beginning to work with Reiki, the student will need to find an appropriate teacher.

Teachers

Some lineages of the system of Reiki will say that they are the only ones who can really use Reiki or that 'their Reiki' is better than that of others. This elitist attitude is generally used to promote insecurities in the minds of students so that they join or remain with the teacher.

There are definitely different styles of systems of Reiki and according to the amount of practice undertaken by the teacher different levels of energy. As with anything in this life – the more one practices, the better one becomes. One teacher explains this by writing that *people* are 'higher vibrations' while systems are not.

Don't be fooled by teachers who say they no longer need to work on themselves. Enlightenment is not so easily come by.

What is the difference between a Reiki Master, a Reiki Master/ Teacher, a Reiki Teacher, Level 3b or *shinpiden?* These are names used by different branches to show that the individual has the ability to perform attunements on students. This is the minimal requirement to becoming a 'Reiki Master'. The title might not necessarily mean that this individual can guide students on their spiritual path or even understand the concept of Reiki. Some branches may only teach the attunement to their teacher students while others may offer an extensive training. This does not indicate that the more levels one takes the more advantageous it is; added levels may not teach the essence of becoming a professional Reiki teacher but simply focus on add-ons to the system.

Students must find out what Reiki and teaching qualifications the teacher has and if they teach a style of Reiki that feels right for them.

Associations are where Reiki practitioners and teachers are open to scrutiny by their peers. The codes of practice and ethics in these associations often assure a certain level of conduct on behalf of the teacher. Associations can be contacted for a list of teachers in specific areas. Generally teachers who are members of an association will also advertise the fact. Some associations are open to all branches of Reiki (to a sensible limit) while others will only accept members from one specific branch.

There are some things students must be aware of (or beware of!) when looking for a teacher. Some teachers may say that everything they teach is a secret – this is once again a method to keep the sheep in the flock. This is not to say that there isn't an appropriate time for students to learn different skills according to their abilities. Humans learn step by step. An example is where a child who has just learnt to add and subtract will not be able to understand an algebraic equation. Secrecy as a technique to keep knowledge intact is only as trustworthy as the trustworthiness of its students. Humans are fallible and such an excuse for keeping secrets is a weak one. Secrecy and the forbidding of discussion with outsiders tend toward sect-like activities and misuse of power. Neither of these have any place in the system of Reiki. Teachings should never be secret because someone does not wish to divulge them.

They may be secret or sacred for two main reasons. The first is that knowledge must be received in sequential steps. It is useless to learn step 3 before completing steps 1 and 2. Second, things that cannot be commonly spoken, like 'secret' or 'sacred' mantras and symbols, have more psychological 'power'.

These can be effective triggers to invoke much deeper and profound states of mind. The Jewish culture is renowned for having achieved this when the name of Yahweh was made unspeakable.

Many roads can be taken. Students need to be discerning and to choose the road that is appropriate for them.

Students must also ask themselves, 'Under which conditions do I learn best?'

Course Length

Reiki courses are taught in a variety of ways depending on their origin of lineage[1] and the specific teacher's cultural and personal beliefs. Research shows that Mikao Usui developed his teachings over a long period of time.

The system of Reiki can be learnt in one hour, one day, two days, three weeks or over the rest of one's life. This depends upon how much students wish to learn and in what style of course they are interested. Working with Reiki is extremely simple and this can create problems for people. By learning about Reiki in too short a course it is difficult to grasp its uniqueness and complexity. It is tempting to think that Reiki is too simple to have an impact and then disregard it. This is part of the true nature of Reiki. Scratch its surface and it take us deeper and deeper into spiritual, emotional and intellectual issues.

Completing Levels 1 and 2 together in a weekend (some even include Level 3 in this 'package') is pointless and leaves students feeling powerful (temporarily) without actually becoming empowered.

[1] For more information about lineages see the Reiki Lineage Chart page 41.

The focus here is on achieving levels rather than working with the energy. Reiki is about energy – it is not about pieces of paper with letters on them.

There may also be misunderstandings as to the function of the attunement[2] process. Yes, attunements lift energy levels but it is the practice that makes a great practitioner. In some more traditional styles of Mikao Usui's teachings the attunement process or *reiju* is exactly the same for all levels. The body must first adjust to the energy; it can only take in so much at one time. When an individual receives attunements over a couple of days the body's energy cannot differentiate between having received a Reiki Level 1, 2 or 3 certificate. Reiki is not about certification – it is about personal practice.

In the West, an approximate length of time for a Level 1 course is a minimum of 14 hours and for Level 2 is a minimum of seven hours. Ongoing practice either alone or with a group is imperative.

Course Costs

Costs will vary for Reiki courses. Some courses are plain cheap and others exclusively expensive. Human nature may tell us that expensive means better but that is not always true. In the West, Hawayo Takata introduced a system where she asked her students to charge set prices, including US$10,000 to become a Reiki Master. Very few teachers charge these prices today and there is also no guarantee that what is taught for that price is any better than other courses that are offered.

Students need to find out what they are paying for. Is there a manual, experienced teachers, a suitable venue, post-course support and practice evenings for students?

Course Contents

The system of Reiki as it is taught today can roughly be broken up into Western or Japanese methods. There are differences between the two and it is the Western method that has swept across the planet over the last couple of decades.

---

[2] Attunement is the Western term for the Japanese word *reiju*. There are many versions of attunements and *reiju* in both the West and Japan. Traditional *reiju* are performed without symbols and mantras and the ritual does not change with each level. For more information about *reiju* and attunements see page 97.

There are three levels to the Western system of Reiki. A basic level course (generally called Level 1) in Western Reiki will teach one how to practice healing the self and the basics about helping others. Students will also receive between one and four attunements (four being most common). Level 2 is where students learn three mantras and three symbols that aid the student in focusing the energy. Students receive between one and three attunements at this level. Level 3 is occasionally broken up into two sub-levels and has one attunement. The first sub-level focuses on personal development generally using non-traditional add-ons and teaches one mantra and one symbol. The second sub-level teaches the student how to perform the attunement on others.

There are infinite varieties of Reiki courses in the West depending on the teacher's own interests, motivations or beliefs. Therefore the number of levels and what is taught within them can vary quite extensively.

In the West there are a number of elements that are essential to a Reiki course today (there are differences between these and Mikao Usui's initial teachings).

Here these elements are listed and then explained in detail individually:

- Attunements
- The physical practice on the self/others for the purpose of healing
- The spiritual and mental connection using the five precepts
- Four Mantras and four symbols
- Techniques

There are many other variables to the system of Reiki. This is due to the manner in which individual teachers work, continual adjustments are always being made.

Attunements

'Initiation' is, first and foremost, a means calculated to induce the novice to discover for himself certain facts that are not directly revealed to him but which, by the aid of symbolical rites, he will eventually perceive himself… It is not intended to enlighten the novice but rather to lead him to become conscious of what has hitherto been hidden from him because his mental eye has not been capable of perceiving it.

(Excerpt from *Initiations and Initiates in Tibet* by Alexandra David-Neel.)

Attunements are integral to Mikao Usui's teachings. To practice the system of Reiki, students must first receive attunements. Methods differ but the purpose is the same: to strengthen the students' connection with spiritual energy and to raise their personal energy levels.

An attunement is where a teacher completes a physical ritual around a seated student. The student generally has his/her eyes closed and might concentrate on breathing or another form of meditation. There have been many variations on this. Some teachers touch the body and others do not. Some move around the front of the body and the back, some claim to even 'attune' the feet. An attunement is relatively short – a couple of minutes – but it is pleasant for the student to sit and enjoy the sense of energy in the body.

Attunements were initially called *reiju* in Japan and when the system moved to the West they were called initiations, empowerments or attunements.

Without an attunement it is not Reiki, the system, which is being practiced. Many people practice similar techniques but do not use attunements and therefore do not practice what is called the system of Reiki. This is not to say that whatever they practice is better or worse than this system.

There have been many claims made about the effect of an attunement. In the West it is habitual to rationalize each thought and movement. Here the hunt for the perfect explanation of 'what an attunement does' is ongoing. Some traditional Japanese Reiki schools explain the attunement with the words 'more practice'. In other words, 'if you keep practicing then you will discover the answer for yourself'. Something as profound as an attunement cannot be analyzed on the human level merely experienced.

In essence the purpose of an attunement is:

- A sense of reconnection to one's true self.
- A clearing of the meridians allowing the student to conduct more energy through the body.

No matter which branch of Reiki students find themselves in, there appear to be no right or wrong attunements. Many roads are taken within the boundaries of the system of Reiki.

Though attunements may vary from branch to branch they all seem to work to some degree – provided there is a perceptible basic core of the ritual coupled with clarity of intent.

There are different set-ups that teachers will use when performing attunements on students. Most teachers perform the complete attunement on one student at a time. Some may even go so far as to take each student into a separate room, once again performing the complete attunement on the back and front in one go.[3]

If students are in a very large group people may make noise etc... creating distractions and it is necessary to wait a long time before receiving the attunement. If it is a large group some teachers walk down the front row of students completing only the front section of the ritual and then walk down the back of the row, completing only the back section. The attunement ends with the person they began with. It has been suggested that this method creates an incomplete energetic connection between the teacher and student.

Whether one is alone in a room or with a group of other students the attunement will still work.

Students may also receive as many attunements as they wish – in fact, the more the better. In Japan these are repeated on a weekly or monthly basis and are not aligned to receiving new levels of certification. They do not appear to change the ritual for separate levels either. In the West the attunements have a different focus and work toward achieving a new level with each new attunement. The attunement is also altered for each level. This system is less aligned to the traditional belief that a student will only ever take in the amount of energy from an attunement that is needed (or desired) by the student at that particular time. At no point does an attunement rely on

---

[3] There are NO sexual connotations or suggestions in the system of Reiki whatsoever. If a teacher acts suggestively or inappropriately it is imperative that the student notify the appropriate authorities immediately.

the 'power' of the teacher. It is true that the more work that a teacher does on him/herself the more energy that can flow through the body. This gives the student the opportunity to draw more energy – but the student can only draw as much energy as is needed or desired.

Teachers have been known to announce that the first level attunement works on the physical level while the second level attunement works on the emotional level and so on. These are examples of Western mystification where the teacher pretends to control the attunement process with their 'power'. An individual will draw the energy in wherever the body decides, whether it be physical, mental, emotional or spiritual. This is not for the teacher to decide.

As an attunement is a powerful clearing of the body's meridians it is impossible to undo this or 'wipe it out'. Each attunement received takes the student a step further to re-aligning oneself with the natural function of the body – once again either mentally, physically, emotionally or spiritually.

For this reason it is also impossible to 'make' an attunement last for a limited period of time. Some crafty individuals have been known to say that a free 'sample' attunement will only last for four (or five or six or seven…) days. Students believe they are given something wonderful and then it is taken away again. If students did not know any better and wanted to continue receiving the benefits of Reiki they would then need to pay (maybe again) to do a course with the teacher. Apart from the fact that an attunement cannot 'wear out' within a pre-arranged time (energy doesn't wear a watch!) there is also a major misconception about Reiki here.

Attunements are beneficial and integral to the system of Reiki but it is the personal practice that brings the student blessings – not the 'power' of the teacher. Once again, if fear is used as a method of getting students and clients then this is not the way of the system of Reiki but the way of an individual's ego.

Practice

> Attunement is just a beginning and the real ability is to develop on your own [with personal practice].
>
> (Excerpt from *Modern Reiki Method for Healing* by Hiroshi Doi.)

The attunement is just the first step to changing a student's life – yet even more important is the practice. Remember the system of Reiki is about self-empowerment. The more work a student does on himself the clearer the meridians will become and the healthier and calmer life will be.

During a course a system will be taught to students enabling them to feel confident in practicing the hand positions and techniques by themselves at home. A seminar is very nice to sit and listen to but it is the personal experience that is enriching. For this reason it is integral to this concept that the course allows time for experiential work. Within the course it is most beneficial if the student is given the opportunity to work with Reiki on different people – this broadens the experience immediately and helps build confidence.

There is often talk about a cleansing process when learning Reiki. This is initiated by working with Reiki. There is truth in this but then life, itself, is one great cleansing process. Humans are continually working through things, whether it's a tiny revelation about an issue or a massive change that throws life into disarray. These are cleansings where the old moves out and the new takes over. Reiki definitely aids this process but it is certainly not unique to it.

Today some teach that there is a three-week cleansing process after completing a Reiki course. Though this is a recent Western addition to Reiki it certainly has had its share of esoteric interpretations. Basically the popularity of the three-week cleansing process concept can be put down to the fact that it is successful – it achieves its aim. That aim is to get people practicing. Some smart individual knew that human nature technically takes 21 days to break a habit and therefore also takes 21 days to *make* a habit. After practicing Reiki for three weeks students don't want to stop practicing – it feels too good!

Working with Reiki does increase the effect of the cleansing process and often students will have quite immediate results (life turned into disarray!) a day or two after beginning their practice. The key is to keep practicing, allowing the energy to keep moving.

Practicing the system of Reiki actually entails using hand positions on the self and others; understanding and integrating the five precepts; using mantras and symbols and working with the techniques.

Hand Positions[4]

> Everyone needs to be touched, stroked, cuddled, fondled, and held. Without this tactile stimulation, children and adults do not grow in a healthy way. Their emotional selves grow gnarled, crooked, bent, and deformed. They can be smoothed, straightened, and supported by touch.
>
> (Excerpt from *Time In: A handbook for child and youth care professionals* by Michael Burns.)

Hand positions are specific places on the body where students are taught to place their hands. This is for the purpose of assisting the energy to move through the body, clearing and strengthening the spiritual and energetic connection.

In the West, students practice this on themselves and on others. A one-hour Reiki treatment is made up of a practitioner placing hands on (or off) the body of the client. The energy moves down through the practitioner and is drawn by the client into the body. This is the same concept when practiced on one's self.

Some teachers' instructions about hand positions are very exact while others work solely intuitively. There is no right or wrong though it is useful to have some guidelines to follow as a beginner. Guidelines initially build confidence to a point where students can eventually break away from them.

The Five Precepts[5]

> For today only:
> Do not anger
> Do not worry
> Be humble
> Be honest in your work
> Be compassionate to yourself and others

This is a simple translation of the five precepts that are associated

---

[4] For historical information about hand positions see page 77.
[5] For the traditional Japanese version and an in-depth discussion of these precepts see page 66. The precepts are also known in the West as affirmations.

with the teachings of Reiki. They were introduced by Mikao Usui and are universal teachings. These precepts should be kept in mind throughout each day. This is the beginning of the student's spiritual journey.

Mantras and Symbols[6]

… Since the stars have fallen from heaven and our highest symbols have paled, a secret life holds sway in the unconscious. That is why we have a psychology today, and why we speak of the unconscious. All this would be quite superfluous in an age or culture that possessed symbols …

(Excerpt from C. G. Jung – *Psychological reflections, an anthology of his writings 1905 – 1961,* edited by Jolande Jacobi.)

There are only four mantras and four symbols in traditional forms of Reiki.

Here again there has been great change in the use of mantras and symbols since Mikao Usui began his teachings. Their meanings have changed and many new symbols have either been created or taken from other cultures and systems and added to the system of Reiki.

Mantras and symbols have had a certain mysticism attributed to them since their practice in the West. This has even led to the meanings behind the four traditional symbols gaining in significance over the years. At first, they were provided, like training wheels, for students to discard once they had become the appropriate energy. Today they are credited with ideals such as protection, bringing in power, enhancing, manifesting and healing karma. These were never the focus of the mantras and symbols and yet it is true some of these ideals are biproducts of their practice. There is a misunderstanding here about the basic reason for the introduction of mantras and symbols to the teachings.

Initially, Mikao Usui introduced symbols for those who had difficulty invoking the energy – that was all.

---

[6] For more in depth information about the 4 mantras and 4 symbols see page 82.

Techniques[7]

> What I teach is not a technique but a way (dô)...
> The principle of a 'way' is that it is applicable to other aspects
> of a person's life. The true meaning of jûdô is the study and
> practice of mind and body. It is at the same time, the model for
> daily life and work.
>
> (Excerpt from a speech by Jigorô Kanô during the
> Olympics in LA, USA in 1932 at the University of
> Southern California.)

A number of techniques are (or have been) used in Mikao Usui's
early teachings. Only a very few of these made it across the ocean to
America in the late 1930s with Hawayo Takata.

Since that time a great variety of techniques have been added to
the system of Reiki. Many of these techniques have no foundation in
the Japanese culture and the majority have been introduced through
the New Age movement. A good example of this is the chakra system
that is almost taught across the board in the system of Reiki, as we
know it today. Traditionally Japan has used the *hara* center as a
method to stimulate and balance energy in the body, not the chakra
system.[8]

Techniques are included in the system of Reiki for a number of
reasons. They strengthen the connection to the energy, to build one's
own energy, to create focus, and to support a spiritual journey. Some
'new' techniques support these aims while others seem to complicate
the system of Reiki needlessly – giving the teacher more 'power'.

One key reason why 'new' techniques have been added to the
system of Reiki is that there has been limited understanding in the
West of Mikao Usui's original teachings. This lack of understanding
has been exacerbated by the lack of documented materials available.
It does not mean that many of these techniques are not of value (that

[7] Part III of *The Reiki Sourcebook* is dedicated to both Japanese and Western techniques, see page 185

[8] Research indicates that Hawayo Takata did not use the chakra system. She has
been quoted a number of times discussing an energy center of the body that cor-
relates to the *hara* center.

is not necessarily so) although it does mean that they do not belong to the early teachings of Mikao Usui or the system of Reiki.

Next Level

When is it correct to move to the next level in the system of Reiki?

Reiki is not about paperwork or a timetable or any other man-made schedule. It is an energetic practice and therefore can only be experienced energetically.

Some schools of the system of Reiki will provide time limits for when it is appropriate to move on to a new level but for each individual this will be different.

Largely, it will depend upon a student's home situation and the availability of time to practice. A mother with a full-time job and numerous hobbies may have little time to practice. A traveler who has taken 12 months off may have 'all the time in the world'.

Even if these levels are taught close together the student can only adjust so much to the new level of energy in the body.

Reiki is a lifetime practice.

> After practicing for a while, if we feel discouraged or tired because of how far we are from the goal of our spiritual journey, we should look back at our life in the days before we started training and celebrate any progress we have made.
>
> (Excerpt from *The Healing Power of The Mind* by Tulku Thondup.)

Part II
Reiki History

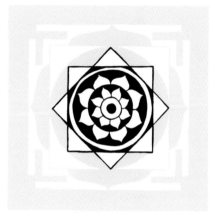

Much of the history of the system of Reiki taught in the West since its arrival in the late 1930s can be relegated to myth or unverifiable facts. Reasons for this are varied:

- Each individual will retell its history according to his/her own experience, situation and agenda.
- The introduction of historical material to the system of Reiki that is unverified and conflicts with recent verifiable (and also questionable) information.
- The difficulty for Westerners in finding out information in Japan, due to the difficulty of translating Japanese (especially pre-1940s Japanese) to English, the remote locality and the unique culture.
- The restrictions placed on traditional Japanese Reiki practitioners (based on cultural mores and Eastern religious mystery teachings) mean that little is passed on to the West. First, a strong connection with the traditional Japanese practitioners needs to be built before any learning can begin.
- At the turn of the century no photocopying machines existed to pass on course notes. Early methods required that students copied what notes there were by hand. Symbols were also copied from the teacher in this manner. Students of Mikao Usui who are said to be alive today do not allow photographs or machine copies to be made of their original notes as they are considered to be sacred.

Fortunately there have recently been some redeeming factors to the system's history in the West. These include the discovery of Mikao Usui's revealing memorial stone in 1994; Japanese teaching manuals; early students who are still alive and the Usui Reiki Ryôhô Gakkai.[1]

Chapter 4 includes a timeline and a lineage chart to aid reader orientation on the history and development of Mikao Usui's teachings. These pages can be utilized as reference points. For more detailed reference

---

[1] The Usui Reiki Ryôhô Gakkai (Society of the Usui Spiritual Energy Healing Method) claims to have been created by Mikao Usui in 1922. The society still exists today, and has its seventh president. It is closed to foreigners and members are asked not to discuss the details of the society with non-members.

information about people, places, events, techniques and branches readers should refer to the extensive Reiki Glossary in the Appendices.

Chapter 5 begins by tracing the life of Mikao Usui through the numerous facts and fictions that have been told and written about him.

Mikao Usui (1865–1926), the founder of the system of Reiki, was born into a world of radical change. The Meiji Emperor (1852–1912) introduced Japan to modernization and industrialization after more than two centuries of national isolation or *sakoku* from the rest of the human race. Even Christianity, which had been banned during this time of isolation with punishment by death, was legalized in 1877. This environment explains certain developments in Mikao Usui's teachings, as does the impact of World War II on the evolution of the system of Reiki in the West.

The actual practice of the teachings is dissected in Chapter 5 and then restored in a logical order, which allows the reader to follow its many digressions. It explores the origins of the five precepts which aid students' spiritual development; the use of *gyosei*[2] as practiced at traditional gatherings; the hand positions, as taught by various Japanese teachers; the practice (and non-practice) of meditations, symbols and mantras; to the practice and variations of *reiju* or attunements in Japan.

The lives and practices of the students that followed in Mikao Usui's footsteps including the Usui Reiki Ryôhô Gakkai and Chûjirô Hayashi are discussed in Chapter 6.

The Reiki system of the West has its own history from the late 1930s and this is presented in Chapter 7. In Hawaii it thrived under the care of a Japanese woman, Hawayo Takata, for many years until her death in 1980. Just over 20 years on from that date and we find the system called Reiki becoming a globally popular alternative therapy with many individual faces.

These 'faces' are reflected in the number of branches of Reiki that have existed and died out and the many others that still exist today. Chapter 8 gives a brief analysis of what requirements (if any) are necessary to become a branch of Reiki and details their commonalities and irregularities.

---

[2] *Gyosei* means *waka*, poetry, written by an Emperor

The world is fascinated with any scientific evidence that proves the existence of Reiki. Though its effects can be readily experienced by all it is often the scientific data that truly amazes us. Chapter 9 summarizes a number of experiments that have taken place in modern times to, amongst other things, measure Reiki's effectiveness.

4   Historical Facts

Lineage Chart

Mikao Usui created the origins of the system that is called Reiki today. As can be seen in Part IV under Reiki Branches there are a great many offshoots from these initial teachings. To give a quick and clear overview of the branches and their influences a Reiki lineage chart has been drawn up. This chart incorporates two methods to simplify the reading of it.

To begin with, Mikao Usui and his teacher students have been named in person (where known). The naming of teachers continues on through the lineages until the teachings reach the West. At this point, instead of following the path of individuals, the major branches are followed and their influence on one another. It is impossible to include the names of all of the students of each lineage leading up to a new branch.

It is mainly the major branches that have been included in the lineage chart. Some of the channeled Reiki branches that are written about in the Reiki Branches section have not been included. This is either because they do not credit Reiki with their branch origins or they are too small.

[Authors' note: Hiroshi Doi, Usui Reiki Ryôhô Gakkai member, states that Kaiji Tomita and Toshihiro Eguchi did not study to the teacher level with Mikao Usui. Mariko Obaasan, Yuri in and Suzuki san have yet to be verified as teacher students of Mikao Usui.]

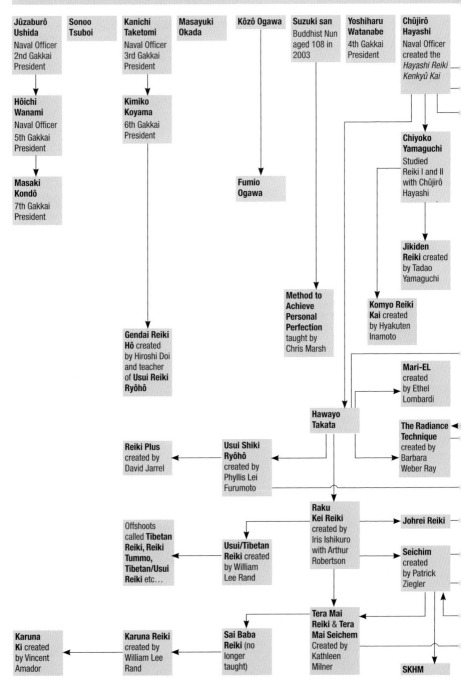

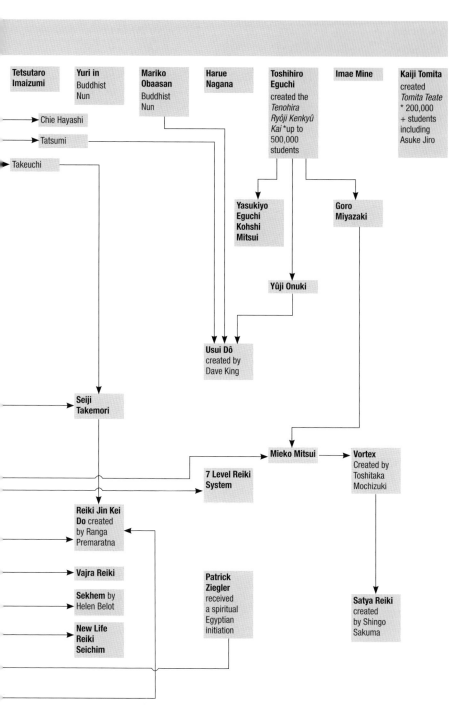

Timeline

Reiki Events		Japanese Events

800 Japanese Buddhist precepts are written that are the base for Mikao Usui's precepts (SS) **— 800**

1865 15 August, Mikao Usui is born in Taniai mura, Yamagata gun, Gifu ken (MUMS) **— 1865 —** 1865 Japan opens its ports etc… after a self-imposed exile of over 200 years

1880 Chûjirô Hayashi is born (CY)

1889 Mikao Usui receives *menkyo kaiden* in martial arts (SS)

1887 Chie Hayashi is born

1895 Suzuki san is born, cousin of Mikao Usui's wife (SS)

1896 Yuri in, Tendai nun and student of Mikao Usui is born (DK)

1897 Mariko Obaasan (Buddhist name is Tenon in) Tendai nun and student of Mikao Usui is born (DK)

1868 Meiji Emperor moves the capital from Kyôto to Edo, now named Tôkyô

1870 Commoners are permitted to take surnames

1871 *Samurai* are ordered to cut off their topknots

1871 First Japanese-language daily newspaper, *Yokohama Mainichi Shimbun*, begins publication

1871 An 18-month tour to study the social systems of the United States and European nations is sponsored by the Japanese government

1872 Compulsory elementary education is established

1872 Army and Navy ministries are established

1874–77 *Samurai* protest movements

1877 Christianity is legalized

1890 Imperial Rescript on Education is written

— 1895 — 1894–95 Sino-Japanese War

1907 US President Theodore Roosevelt bans Japanese from immigrating to the United States

1908 Fuji, Mikao Usui's son is born (MUMS and gravesite)

1909 Jigorô Kanô founder of jûdô becomes the first Japanese member of the International Olympic committee

1910 Korea is made a colony of Japan

1912 6 July, Japans first entry in the Olympic games held in Stockholm, Sweden

1913 Toshiko, Mikao Usui's daughter is born (MUMS and gravesite) **— 1913 —**

1914 *Kenzen no Genri*, written by Bizan Suzuki, includes precepts that are similar to those of Mikao Usui (http://member.nifty.ne.jp/okojo/index.htm)

1914–18 WWI. Japan sides with the 'Allies', seizing German island colonies in the Pacific and German concessions in the Shandong peninsula

Reiki Events		Japanese Events
1915 Suzuki san starts her training with Mikao Usui (SS)	**1915**	
1915 Mikao Usui begins teaching the five precepts (SS)		
1917 Mikao Usui becomes well known as a healer (SS)		1918 High rice prices incite riots throughout Japan
1920 Mariko Obaasan and Yuri in begin their study with Mikao Usui (MO)		1920 Shinpei Goto becomes Mayor of Tokyo
1922 March, Mikao Usui completes his *shûgyô* training, the 21-day meditation on *kurama yama* (MUMS)		
1922 April, Mikao Usui opens his seat of learning in Harajuku, Aoyama, Tokyo (MUMS)	**1922**	1922 First national athletic exhibition in Tokyo where many martial artists are asked to perform
1922 April, Usui Reiki Ryôhô Gakkai is created by Mikao Usui (HD)		
1923 Symbols are introduced in Mikao Usui's teachings (SS)		1923 1 September, the great Kanto earth quake in Tokyo and surrounds
1925 February, Mikao Usui moves his dôjô to a suburban house at Nakano (MUMS)		
1925 Kaiji Tomita studies with Mikao Usui (HD)		
1925 May, Chûjirô Hayashi studies with Mikao Usui (DK)		
1925 November, Jûzaburô Ushida and Kanichi Taketomi study with Mikao Usui (DK)		
1926 16 February, Photo of Mikao Usui and his students and family is taken (Toshitaka Mochizuki's book, *Chô Kantan Iyashi No Te*)		
1926 9 March, Mikao Usui dies of a stroke in Fukuyama in Hiroshima (MUMS)		
1927 February, the Usui Reiki Ryôhô Gakkai erects the memorial stone of Mikao Usui (MUMS)	**1927**	1927 Severe depression (which has been in place since the 1920s) causes many commercial banks to collapse
1927 Tatsumi receives the teacher level from Chûjirô Hayashi (DK)		
1927–28 Toshihiro Eguchi establishes his own center, *Tenohira Ryoji Kenkyû Kai* (Hand Healing Research Center) (HD)		

Reiki Events		Japanese Events
1928 Wasaburo Sugano (Chiyoko Yamaguchi's uncle) studied with Chûjirô Hayashi Level 1 (CY)	**1928**	
1928 Shûô Matsui writes an article about Chûjirô Hayashi, his teacher and the system of Reiki (article www.reiki.net.au)		
1930 Toshihiro Eguchi and Kohshi Mitsui, write a book together called *Te No Hira Ryôji Nyûmon (Introduction To Healing With The Palms)*		
1931 Chûjirô Hayashi names his own clinic *Hayashi Reiki Kenkyû Kai* (Hayashi Spiritual Energy Society) (HD)	**1931**	1931 Manchurian Incident – Japan sent troops into southern Manchuria
1933 Kaiji Tomita, a student of Mikao Usui writes a book called *Reiki To Jinjutsu – Tomita Ryû Teate Ryôhô* (Reiki and Humanitarian Work – Tomita Ryû Hands Healing)		1932 Shanghai Incident – Japan sent troops into Shanghai China.
1935 Hawayo Takata becomes a client of Chûjirô Hayashi (HT)		
1935 23 September, Mikao Usui's daughter Toshiko dies (MUMS and gravesite)		
1937 Hawayo Takata returns to America to begin teaching the system of Reiki. Chûjirô Hayashi and his daughter accompany her and help her to begin her practice (HT)	**1937**	1937–45 Second Sino-Japanese War
1938 21 February, Chûjirô Hayashi awards Hawayo Takata a Master certificate before returning to Japan (HT)		
1938 Chiyoko Yamaguchi studies *shoden* and *okuden* with Chûjirô Hayashi (CY)		1939–45 WWII
1940 10 May, Chûjirô Hayashi commits suicide (CY and HT)	**1940**	
1940 Chie Hayashi, Chûjirô Hayashi's wife becomes the President of his school (HD and CY)		1941 Pearl Harbor is attacked. Many Japanese living in the US are placed in internment camps as a result
1942 Fumio Ogawa joins the Usui Reiki Ryôhô Gakkai (FAP)		
1946 10 July, Mikao Usui's son Fuji dies (MUMS and gravesite)		1945 Atomic bomb dropped on Hiroshima. Another bomb is dropped on Nagasaki days later

Reiki Events	1946	Japanese Events
1946 17 October, Mikao Usui's wife, Sadako Suzuki, dies (MUMS and gravesite)		
1950 Tatseyi Nagao receives the Master Level from Chie Hayashi in Japan (WLR)		1952 End of Allied Occupation of Japan
1975 Advertising Poster for a workshop by Hawayo Takata states; The Only Teacher of the Usui System of Reiki in the World Today		1964 Olympics held in Tokyo
1976 Hawayo Takata teaches her first Reiki Master student, Virginia Samdahl, for US$10,000		
1980 11 December, Hawayo Takata dies of a heart attack	1980	
1982 Hawayo Takata's Master students meet to compare symbols, mantras and attunements		
1983 The Reiki Alliance standardizes symbols and mantras and attunements at their official inaugral meeting at Barbara Brown's house in British Columbia (Carel Anne Farmer, student of Phyllis Lei Furumoto and John Harvey Gray)		
1983 The Reiki Alliance chooses Phyllis Lei Furumoto to become the lineage bearer of their system of Reiki. She receives the 'title of holder' of the 'Office of the Grandmaster' (The Reiki Alliance)		
1985 Mieko Mitsui begins teaching Levels 1 and 2 in Japan		
1991 Frank Arjava Petter and his wife Chetna begin teaching all three levels in Japan (FAP)	1991	
1993 22 October, Hiroshi Doi received *shoden* from the Usui Reiki Ryôhô Gakkai (HD)		
1992 Phyllis Lei Furumoto resigns from The Reiki Alliance		
1995 Toshitaka Mochizuki's book is published, *Iyashi No Te (Healing Hands)*		

Reiki Events		Japanese Events

Reiki Events

1995 Diane Stein's book is published, *Essential Reiki* — **1995**

1997 Yuri in, Tendai nun and student of Mikao Usui, died (DK)

1997 Historic meeting between Phyllis Lee Furumoto and Kimiko Koyama cancelled (HD)

1997 The trademark office rejects Phyllis Lei Furumoto's application to trademark the words Usui Shiki Ryôhô and Usui System in America (WLR) International trademark attempts also fail except in South America

1997 Frank Arjava Petter's first book, *Reiki Fire*, is published

1998 January, Masaki Kondô becomes the seventh President of the Usui Reiki Ryôhô Gakkai

1999 September, Kimiko Koyama, the sixth President of the Usui Reiki Ryôhô Gakkai, dies

1999 Hiroshi Doi teaches a *reiju* at the URRI (Usui Reiki Ryôhô International) in Vancouver

2000 Hiroshi Doi's book is translated into English and called *Modern Reiki Method for Healing* — **2000**

2000 Chris Marsh meets with Suzuki san, a cousin of Mikao Usui

2000 The URRI takes place in Kyôto

2001 Chris Marsh meets another 11 students of Mikao Usui

2001 The URRI takes place in Madrid

2002 The URRI takes place in Toronto

2003 The URRI takes place in Denmark

Japanese Events

1998 Olympic games held in Nagano prefecture

Key to Sources of Information for Timeline

MUMS – Mikao Usui Memorial Stone in Tôkyô.

SS – Suzuki san, a nun and a cousin of Mikao Usui's wife, was born in 1895 and is still alive today. There are also 11 other students of Mikao Usui who are alive. According to Chris Marsh they possess some of Mikao Usui's notes and teachings. He is currently translating this information.

MO – Mariko Obaasan, a 105-year-old nun who studied with Mikao Usui. Information supplied by Dave King.

DK – Dave King.

HD – Hiroshi Doi, member of the Usui Reiki Ryôhô Gakkai.

FAP - Frank Arjava Petter.

CY – Chiyoko Yamaguchi is in her late 80s and was a student of Chûjirô Hayashi.

HT – Hawayo Takata, an American citizen of Japanese descent who brought the system of Reiki to America in 1938.

WLR – William Lee Rand.

5 Mikao Usui's Teachings

Mikao Usui, his Life and Times (1865-1926)

Like stars, mists and candle flames
Mirages, dewdrops and water bubbles
Like dreams, lightning and clouds.
In that way I will view all existence.

(Taken from the notebook of Mikao Usui,
dated 1923.)[1]

The main source of factual history about Mikao Usui, at present, is written in stone – literally. This is the carved memorial stone of Mikao Usui's life at his gravesite at the Pure Land[2] Buddhist Saihôji Temple in Tôkyô.[3] It was placed there by a number of his students, just one year after his death in 1927. The memorial stone is one aspect of Mikao Usui's life as seen through the eyes of his students from the Usui Reiki Ryôhô Gakkai.

Apart from this information there are very few historical facts about Mikao Usui's teachings that can claim authenticity through

---

[1] The quote is an extract from an eighth-century Buddhist prayer /contemplation on the nature of impermanence. It was written in Mikao Usui's notes and may have been translated by him into Japanese. Chris Marsh provided the English translation. According to Chris Marsh, the notes and teachings of Mikao Usui are in the possession of the 108-year-old Suzuki san who is a cousin of Mikao Usui.

[2] Information supplied by Hyakuten Inamoto, Pure Land monk and Reiki Master.

[3] There is a full translation of the Mikao Usui Memorial Stone, translated by Hyakuten Inamoto, on page 339.

verification. That is not to say that there aren't a great many stories told about Mikao Usui and his teachings – there are.

When these teachings were introduced to the West they were adapted to suit the political situation of World War II by Hawayo Takata, a wonderful teller of anecdotes and 'parables'. For 40 years she employed the method of storytelling to teach people about the system she called Reiki and its history. It is difficult today to verify much of this information; however, we do know for certain that some of it is incorrect. Hawayo Takata's anecdotes were perhaps appropriate for her at that particular period in her life and for the world in which she lived. It would be mistaken to downplay the fact that through her strength as a Reiki teacher, her system of Reiki is practiced in every country of the world.

Since the rekindled interest in the teachings of Mikao Usui there have been many theories and histories coming out of the woodwork. Some have been proven false – causing havoc, while others have yet to be verified. It is wiser to believe that which can be verified and at some level is open to perusal by others.

Frank Arjarva Petter, a Reiki Master and researcher, said that he and his wife, Chetna, contacted a relative of Mikao Usui who explained that a female relative had left a clause about Mikao Usui in her will. The clause mysteriously stated that his name should never be spoken again in her house. This may have also added to the lack of information available about Mikao Usui's personal life.

The most straightforward information to be found, as mentioned earlier, is that from Mikao Usui's memorial stone. This was written just one year after his death and therefore leaves little leeway for the historical information to have changed drastically. Unfortunately, the students who wrote this information up are said to not have consulted Mikao Usui's family and therefore may have left out information that would be relevant in a truly comprehensive memorial to Mikao Usui.[4]

Hiroshi Doi is yet another source of historical information. His status as a Usui Reiki Ryôhô Gakkai[5] member means that he has access to historical information that is not available to non-members. Hiroshi Doi has studied many styles of Reiki, Western and Japanese,

---

[4] Information supplied to the authors by Chris Marsh.

as well as numerous energetic and spiritual techniques and does not speak English. The Usui Reiki Ryôhô Gakkai is believed to restrict what he does pass on. This has caused confusion in the past with some information not being as 'original' as initially believed. His teachings are communicated to the West via his translators and/or students.

Frank Arjava Petter and Hyakuten Inamoto have also successfully researched aspects of Mikao Usui's teachings in Japan through their own contacts.

A nun called Suzuki san, the cousin of Mikao Usui's wife and one of his students, is said to still be alive today. She was born in 1895 and is in contact with Chris Marsh. In total, there are 12 students of Mikao Usui who are believed to be aged between 98 and 112. These students have acquired a number of notes and teachings from Mikao Usui. Suzuki san's information has not been taught widely in the greater Reiki community in either Japan or the West. Unfortunately this group of 12 considers the information that they have as sacred and consequently are unwilling to allow it to be photographed or copied (except by hand). This adds a frustrating element when attempting to verify any of the material. On researching these claims it appears to be true that in Japan this is often the case with revered texts. Chris Marsh is currently translating much of this 'sighted only' material for publication.

There is also said to be another living nun called Mariko Obaasan[6] who studied with Mikao Usui. This too is unverified information at present.

To show an objective view, information from most sources has been used and footnoted where possible.

It is good to remember that it is impossible to know the full story behind Mikao Usui, his life and teachings. The remnants that still exist of both can be somewhat pieced together but they will never create a whole. We must satisfy ourselves with the knowledge that can be gained and take advantage of the practices that have been left

---

[5] The Usui Reiki Ryôhô Gakkai claims to have been created by Mikao Usui in April 1922. The society still exists today, and has its seventh president. It is closed to foreigners and members are asked not to discuss the details of the society with non-members.

[6] Obaasan is a term used in Japan for Grandmother or old woman.

for our spiritual development.
To clearly illustrate the history of Mikao Usui direct quotes from his memorial stone have been used. Any historical background has been italicized.

> …the samurai, (who) commonly wanted to be known both as swordsmen and poets … The greatest warriors of feudal Japan were therefore also men of the mind, the spirit and the cultivated senses.
>
> (Excerpt from *A History of Warfare* by John Keegan.)

Born into a *Samurai* Family

Mikao Usui was born on 15 August 1865 in the village of Taniai (now called Miyama cho) in the Yamagata county of the Gifu Prefecture, in Japan.

Japan was just opening up in 1865 after a self-imposed exile which had left it culturally prosperous though far behind the Western world technologically and militarily. Kyôto was the capital of Japan and remained so until 1868 when the advent of the Meiji Restoration moved it to Tôkyô.

Today in Miyamo cho, Mikao Usui's name can be found carved on a large *torii*[7] at the Amataka shrine close to where his home once stood. The three Usui brothers donated the stone *torii* in April 1923. Mikao Usui's brothers, Sanya and Kuniji, grew up to become a physician and a policeman respectively. He also had an older sister called Tsuru.[8] Mikao Usui's father's name was Uzaemon[9] and his mother was from the Kawai family.

Mikao Usui was born into a society based on a class system. There was the privileged class to which he belonged and then there were

---

[7] *Torii* is a shrine gate.

[8] Hiroshi Doi, member of the Usui Reiki Ryôhô Gakkai, received this information from a relative of Mikao Usui.

[9] Information supplied to the authors by Chris Marsh states that his father's name was Uzaemon Tsunetane. Hiroshi Doi and Hyakuten Inamoto have both translated the memorial stone to read that his father's name was Taneuji. Chris Marsh explains that this is a diminutive of a name with the tane suffix. Research shows that it may in fact mean Mr Tane. It has also been suggested that Mikao Usui used a different name for a portion of his lifetime. If this is so, then it is likely to have hampered many research efforts in the past.

the common people. Common people were not even permitted the luxury of surnames until 1870. Mikao Usui's family was *hatamoto samurai* – a high level within the ranks of *samurai*.[10] *The hatamoto were the shôgun's personal guard. During the tokugawa shôgunate (1600–1867), the hatamoto were direct vassals of the shôgun, and their annual revenue was less than 10,000 bushels of rice.*

Due to the major changes that were happening in Japan from the 1860s onwards, the samurai class were no longer required. In 1871, samurai were ordered to cut off their topknots and cast aside their swords. Topknots were considered a symbol of maturity, virility and manhood. These clans were offered positions as public servants instead. This certainly did not satisfy the majority of the samurai clans and for many years there remained struggles between the privileged class and the law.

The memorial stones states that the famous *samurai*, Tsunetane Chiba (1118 to 1201) was Mikao Usui's ancestor. Recently Hiroshi Doi noted that this was incorrect and that it was in fact Toshitane Chiba, a famous *samurai* warlord from the 1500s. In 1551 he conquered the city Usui and thereafter all family members acquired that name. Whether the ancestor was Tsunetane or Toshitane or both is inconsequential, both were from the Chiba clan, as was Mikao Usui.[11]

The Chiba clan was once an influential samurai family in Japan according to Chiba family records. The Usui family crest, otherwise known as the Chiba crest, is designed using a circle with a dot at the top. The circle represents the universe, and the dot (a Japanese representation for a star) represents the North Star. The North Star never moves while the universe must move around it.

Mikao Usui was born a Tendai Buddhist and as a young child studied in a Tendai monastery.[12] In the West, it was once believed that he was born a Christian. Hawayo Takata probably added this information as a reaction to the anti-Japanese sentiment in America during and after World War II. Christianity was actually outlawed in Japan at the time Mikao Usui was born.

---

[10] Teachings of Suzuki san, a living student of Mikao Usui, supplied to the authors by Andrew Bowling's website: www.usuireiki.fsnet.co.uk.

[11] Even if this is a technical fault it does not automatically negate other facts that are inscribed on the memorial stone.

[12] This information was supplied to the authors by Andrew Bowling and Dave King.

From 1639 to 1854, Japan was shut under a policy called sakoku or 'national isolation'. Westerners were forbidden to enter Japan and trade. Only the Dutch and Chinese were excluded. Through the small port of Dejima in Nagasaki the traders became Japan's single link to the West for more than two centuries. This privilege was only extended to contact with Japanese merchants and prostitutes. Any Japanese who dared to venture abroad during this period were executed on their return to prevent any form of 'contamination'.

At present there is little known about Mikao Usui's personal life. What can be told, though, are experiences from other Japanese who were of a comparable age and born under similar conditions.

Three well-known Japanese budô masters[13] lived in the same era as Mikao Usui and are even said to have known of him.[14] Gichin Funakoshi, the founder of modern karate, was born into a samurai family in 1868 (three years after Mikao Usui). Jigorô Kanô, born in 1860, was the son of a wealthy family. Morihei Ueshiba was slightly younger, born in 1883, and belonged, too, to a wealthy and prominent samurai family.

During this period, young children from the privileged class all began their study with the Chinese classics. The classical elements of Japanese culture were still retained in their early training. Traditional Japanese flute playing and the recitation and writing of poetry were just a few hobbies of the well-to-do youth of that time.

Gichin Funakoshi passed his test to enter medical school but due to the fact that he still had his samurai topknot was not accepted as a student of the school. Many gentrified families were unhappy with the changes that were taking place in Japan. They refused to accept the changes around them and consequently joined, what was known as, The Obstinate Party.

---

[13] In Toshitaka Mochizuki's book, *Iyashi No Te*, there is a group photo in which Mikao Usui, friends, family and students are gathered together on 16 January 1926. Dave King claims that his teacher, Mariko Obaasan, has told him that Jigorô Kanô is seen standing at the furthest right hand side of the picture. Though there is a slight resemblance this has been denied by every martial arts source contacted by the authors. This includes respected authorities such as the Kodokan Jûdô Institute in Japan, Stanley Pranin of the Aikidô Journal and Miek Skoss of Koryu Books. Morihei Ueshiba and Gichin Funakoshi are also not in the photo.

[14] Information supplied to the authors by Chris Marsh.

Martial Arts Training

At the age of 12 Mikao Usui began with the practice of a martial art called *aiki jutsu*. He also studied a form of *yagyu ryû* and gained *menkyo kaiden* (the highest license of proficiency) in weaponry and grappling.[15] There are a great many forms of *yagyu ryû* practiced today. The *yagyu ryû* tradition entails both life giving and life taking (*kappo* and *sappo*) and includes exercises such as grappling, *taijutsu* and *katsu*. *Katsu* is a method of infusing life into a person and is mentioned on page 35 of the Chûjirô Hayashi *Ryôhô Shishin*[16] as a method to aid resuscitation.

Family Life[17]

Mikao Usui married Sadako Suzuki and they had two children, a boy and a girl called Fuji and Toshiko. Fuji (1908–46) went on to teach at Tôkyô University and Toshiko lived a short life, dying at the age of 22 in 1935. The entire family's ashes are buried at the gravesite at the Saihôji Temple in Tôkyô.[18]

Mikao Usui had children late in life according to the times he lived in. He was 43 when his first child, Fuji, was born and it was another six years before he had his second child, his daughter Toshiko. Gichin Funakoshi wrote in his autobiography, *Karate dô, My Way of Life*, that he did not marry and have children until he was over 20 'quite an advanced age for marriage' in those days in his area.

Career

From his youth he surpassed his fellows in hard work and endeavor. When he grew up he visited Europe and America, and studied in China.

He was by nature versatile and loved to read books. He engaged himself in history books, medical books, Buddhist

---

[15] Information supplied to the authors by Andrew Bowling's website: www.usuire iki.fsnet.co.uk.

[16] This is the *Healing Method's Guideline* created by Chûjirô Hayashi.

[17] There is little information on the memorial stone about Mikao Usui's family as his students, not family members, wrote it.

[18] Dave King alleges that only some of Mikao Usui's ashes are at this site and the rest are in a secret shrine in Tôkyô. The Japanese practitioners the authors spoke to were unaware of this.

scriptures, Christian scriptures and was well versed in psychology, Taoism, even in the art of divination, incantation, and physiognomy.

(Excerpt from the Mikao Usui Memorial Stone, 1927).

Due to the fact that he traveled greatly through Japan and overseas his career was also varied. At one point he was a private secretary to a politician called Shinpei Goto who, among other positions, was Governor of the Standard of Railways. In 1920 Shinpei Goto became the Mayor of Tôkyô.

Men of Mikao Usui's class were trained well in the arts. Gichin Funakoshi wrote that he went to a 'moon viewing party' when he was a young karateka.[19] This consisted of martial artists, sitting around, chatting about karate and reciting poetry under the moon.

Mikao Usui has shown his leaning toward poetry by his inclusion of 125 *waka*, or poems, into his teachings. In his notes it's claimed that he wrote his own form of *waka* and jotted down poetry written by others that he had enjoyed.[20] Toshitaka Mochizuki wrote in his book, *Iyashi No Te (Healing Hands),* in 1995 that it was quite a common and natural thing to read and recite poetry at that period in time. During Japan's 'national isolation' there had been a great focus on the arts. In a book from 1933,[21] a student of Mikao Usui describes a technique called **hatsurei hô.* Here *waka* is recited silently to one's self in an attempt to become One with the essence of the poem.

Religion

Mikao Usui was never a doctor[22] as professed in the West but did become a lay Tendai priest called a *zaike.*[23] This meant that he could remain in his own home with his family, without having to reside in

---

[19] Karateka is a karate student.

[20] See poem at the beginning of this chapter.

[21] This book was written by Kaiji Tomita and is called *Reiki To Jinjutsu – Tomita Ryû Teate Ryôhô.*

[22] Mikao Usui never studied to become a doctor and there is no documentation of him ever being called by this title. It is likely to be an inaccurate translation by Hawayo Takata when she translated the respectful term of *sensei* into English. For more information about *sensei* see page 137. Mikao Usui's brother was a physician.

[23] Information supplied to the authors by Andrew Bowling's website: www.usuireiki.fsnet.co.uk.

a temple as is commonly expected of priests. At the time that Mikao Usui became a *zaike* he took the Buddhist name or extra name of Gyoho, Gyohan or Gyotse.

Tendai was brought to Japan by Saichô in the early ninth century and names Nagarjuna as its patriarch. Apart from the belief that the Lotus Sutra is Buddha's complete and perfect teaching it also teaches meditation based on esoteric elements like mudras and mandalas.

It's also believed that Mikao Usui included techniques as well as *jumon*[24] in his teachings that are based on Shintô practices.[25]

Shintô (the way of the gods) is the indigenous faith of the Japanese people, and it is as old as the culture itself. The kami, or gods, are the objects of worship in Shintô. It has no founder and no sacred scriptures like the sutras or the bible. Initially, it was so unself-conscious that it also had no name. The term, Shintô came into use after the sixth century when it was necessary to distinguish it from the recently imported Buddhism.

Its origins are of a people who were sensitive to nature's spiritual forces and believed that every rock and pebble could speak. The kami are sacred spirits and can take the form of natural elements like the sun, mountains, trees, rocks, and the wind. They can also be abstract things like fertility, ancestors or protectors of family clans.

It is not unusual for Japanese people to be followers of both Buddhism and Shintôism as the two have come to co-exist and complement each other throughout the years. Shintôism uses its festivals and shrines to celebrate its kami while Buddhism works from within a wealth of religious literature and an elaborate body of doctrine. Buddhism in Japan has actually integrated the Shintô kami by naming them as manifestations of various Buddhas and bodhisattvas.

A Healing Path to Enlightenment

It is impossible to offer a commencement date for Mikao Usui's teachings. He was 35 years old at the turn of the century and, as re-

[24] *Jumon* means spell or incantation and relates to the mantras used in the system of Reiki today.
[25] Shintô priests practice *kenyoku hô* or the dry bath method, a purifying technique according to some Usui Reiki Ryôhô teachers. One Shintô practitioner said that he performed a similar ritual with a group of men from his village where they wore only a red loincloth at the *hekogaki* festival (putting on the loincloth festival).

corded, was proficient in martial arts from his mid-20s. Suzuki san had been aware of Mikao Usui her whole life as she was his wife's cousin. Her formal training with him began in 1915 when she was 20 years old and her relationship with him continued on a less formal basis until his death in 1926.[26] It's understood that Suzuki san and the other 11 living students have preserved a collection of papers including the precepts, *waka*, meditations, and teachings.[27]

In a translated 1928 article[28] a student of Chûjirô Hayashi states that the system was founded decades ago.

For these reasons it is believed the teachings of Mikao Usui began long before 1922 when he opened his official seat of learning and the Usui Reiki Ryôhô Gakkai claims to have been created.

What Mikao Usui taught was called 'Usui dô' – 'the way of Usui', and what he practiced on people would have been called 'Usui teate' – meaning 'Usui hands-on healing'. Early students had never heard of the word Reiki in relation to the entirety of Mikao Usui's teachings. The two *kanji* for Reiki are extremely common in Japan and can be found in a variety of situations unrelated to the word Reiki, as we understand it. It was also often used in conjunction with Mikao Usui's teachings but not as the name of them merely in its literal form meaning 'spiritual energy'. Only once it came to the West was the word 'Reiki' turned into the name for a system.

The aim of these teachings was to provide a method for students to achieve enlightenment. Unlike religion, though, there was no belief system attached.

Though enlightenment was the aim, the healing that was taking place for students was a wonderful 'side effect'. What sets Mikao Usui's teachings apart from other hands-on healing methods is his use of *reiju* or attunement to remind students of their spiritual connection.[29] It seems that all students of Mikao Usui received *reiju* and the five precepts and those with a further interest in the teachings became dedicated students. There does not appear to have been a dis-

---

[26] Information supplied to the authors by Chris Marsh.

[27] Information supplied to the authors by Chris Marsh.

[28] 'A Treatment to Heal Diseases, Hand Healing' by Shûô Matsui in the magazine *Sunday Mainichi*, 4 March, 1928, translated by Amy to be viewed at www.reiki.net.au.

[29] The use of *reiju* though was not totally unheard of at that time – Johrei also uses a *reiju* of some kind.

tinction between clients and students in the beginning though this changed in 1917.[30] People began coming to Mikao Usui for different purposes – some for healing and others for the spiritual teachings. The *reiju* appears to have links to practices from within the more esoteric elements of Tendai called Mikkyô.[31]

Early on in the history of Tendai a close relationship developed between the Tendai monastery complex, hiei zan (Mt Hiei), and the imperial court in Kyôto. As a result, Tendai emphasized great reverence for the emperor and the nation. There are five general areas taught in Tendai. They are the teachings of the Lotus Sutra; esoteric Mikkyô practices; meditation practices; Buddhist precepts; and Pure Land teachings.

Mikao Usui initially gave mantras to students as a device for tapping into specific elements of energy. As each individual learns in his/her own unique manner just one device was impractical to serve the whole of mankind. Meditations too, became integrated into the teachings.[32]

Once the Usui Reiki Ryôhô Gakkai was formed in 1922 the teachings became more formalized. A healing guide, *Ryôhô Shishin*, was created and added to the already existing notes. This became known as the *Reiki Ryôhô Hikkei*.[33] Hand positions were taught to those who found working intuitively difficult. Symbols were also added to the mantra recitations as a helpful tool to evoke specific energy. The introduction of symbols was useful for those whose experiences with spiritual work had previously been limited or those who had difficulty sensing the energy.

Whether mantras, meditations, or mantras and symbols together were practiced it did not matter as all were focused on working with the same energy.

Chûjirô Hayashi, who broke away from the Usui Reiki Ryôhô Gakkai, naturally emerges as the individual who created a structured system of healing that did not principally focus on spiritual development. His teachings are the forerunner to what is known as the system of Reiki in the West. It is suggested that Chûjirô Hayashi

[30] Information supplied to the authors by Chris Marsh.
[31] Mikkyô is an esoteric form of Buddhism and can be translated as 'the secret teaching'. The *reiju* has similarities to the Mikkyô practice called *go shimbô* (Dharma for Protecting the Body).
[32] Information supplied to the authors by Chris Marsh.
[33] For more information about the *Reiki Ryôhô Hikkei* see page 106.

may have created Mikao Usui's healing guide in 1925 on Mikao Usui's behalf. If Mikao Usui himself appeared disinterested in the task, it might support the idea that he was more involved in spiritual growth rather than teaching people to treat others.

Mountains and Divine Inspiration

Now and again, it is necessary to seclude yourself among deep mountains and hidden valleys to restore your link to the source of life. Breathe in and let yourself soar to the ends of the universe; breathe out and bring the cosmos back inside. Next, breathe up all the fecundity and vibrancy of the earth. Finally, blend the breath of heaven and the breath of earth with that of your own, becoming the Breath of Life itself.

(Quote by Morihei Ueshiba from *The Art of Peace* by John Stevens)

As *hiei zan* is the main Tendai complex in Japan, and is very close to Kyôto, it has been surmised that Mikao Usui practiced there as a lay priest. A Tendai meditation practice called *zazen shikan taza*[34] may well have inspired him and his teachings either on *hiei zan* or *kurama yama*.[35] It has been suggested that old sutra copies on *hiei zan* have Mikao Usui's Buddhist name on them of Gyoho or Gyotse.[36]

According to the memorial stone Mikao Usui's teachings were developed, almost miraculously, during a meditation in 1922. The concept of Divine Inspiration is a must for the founder of any Japanese Arts.

One day, he climbed *kurama yama* and after 21 days of a severe discipline without eating, he suddenly felt One Great Reiki over his head and attained enlightenment and he obtained Reiki Ryôhô. Then, he tried it on himself and experimented on his family members. The efficacy was immediate.

(Excerpt from the Mikao Usui Memorial Stone, 1927).

[34] For the complete *zazen shikan taza* meditation see Appendix C page 343.
[35] Information supplied to the authors by Chris Marsh.
[36] Information supplied to the authors by Chris Marsh.

Mount Kurama, or kurama yama as it is called in Japan, (570 meters above sea level) is 12 kilometres due north of the Kyôto Imperial Palace and can be reached in 30 minutes from Kyôto by car or train. The main Kurama Temple was founded in 770 as the guardian of the northern quarter of the capital city (Heiankyo) and is located halfway up the mountain. The temple formerly belonged to the Tendai sect of Buddhism, but since 1949, it has been included in the newly founded kurama kokyo sect as its headquarters.

The legend behind kurama yama is that more than six million years ago Maô son (the great king of the conquerors of evil and the spirit of the earth) descended upon kurama yama from Venus with a great mission – the salvation of mankind.

Since then, Maô son's powerful spirit emanates from kurama yama and governs the development and evolution, not only of mankind but, also, of all living things on Earth.

Maô son, Bishamon ten, and Senju kannon are the symbols of the universal soul, forming a Trinity known as Sonten or the Supreme Deity. These three are the symbols of power, light, and love.[37] Sonten is the creator of the universe, and cultivates the development of everything all over the earth.[38]

Mikao Usui's 21-day practice on *kurama yama* was called *kushu shinren*,[39] (which is a form of *shûgyô*,[40] or discipline or training) according to the memorial stone. *Kurama yama* was also well known for its *yamabushi* or mountain ascetics. These were men who practiced martial arts and also spent time in the mountains for solitude and personal practice. It was a sort of quest where they pitted themselves against the elements in order to seek some sort of revelation or to test their mettle.

Both Hawayo Takata and the memorial stone have stated that Mikao Usui had a strong connection with *kurama yama* and its temple. According to the Kurama Temple, there are no records of his having undertaken any form of ascetic training at the temple itself.

---

[37] Interestingly, some Reiki practitioners have used 'love and light' as a salutation in the West for a number of years. How this came about is unknown and it does not seem to have been a salutation used by Hawayo Takata.

[38] Information supplied by *kurama yama* tourist information pamphlet

[39] On the memorial stone the term *kushu-shinren* is used. Hyakuten Inamoto states that *kushu* literally means painful discipline and *shinren* means difficult training.

[40] *Shûgyô* is also written as *shyu gyo* as seen in some memorial stone translations.

The temple goes on to say that Mikao Usui has 'no special connection to Kurama Temple whatsoever'.[41] The memorial stone was written and erected by students of the Usui Reiki Ryôhô Gakkai. This society was set up one month after Mikao Usui's experience on *kurama yama*. For the Usui Reiki Ryôhô Gakkai, the experience on *kurama yama* defines the society's creation and purpose. Therefore it has been acknowledged in detail on the memorial stone.

The memorial stone's text grants that Mikao Usui was an avaricious learner of anything spiritual from all cultures throughout his whole life. Even from the society's stance he may well have taught before his experience at *kurama yama*. It certainly does not discount earlier anecdotes about Mikao Usui's teachings. His experience at *kurama yama* may have brought him a new understanding of energy and his methods of teaching.

Whether Mikao Usui practiced on *hiei zan* or *kurama yama* is relatively unimportant. His teachings are the focus of modern research. It is true that if he practiced on *hiei zan* or *kurama yama* it is likely that Tendai would have more heavily influenced the teachings than was previously assumed.

Reiki Ryôhô

Sensei thought that it would be far better to offer it widely to the general public and share its benefits than just to improve the well-being of his own family members. In April of the eleventh year of Taisho (AD 1922) he settled in Harajuku, Aoyama, Tokyo and set up the Gakkai to teach Reiki Ryoho and give treatments. Even outside of the building it was full of pairs of shoes of the visitors who had come from far and near.

(Excerpt from the Mikao Usui Memorial Stone, 1927).

Mikao Usui's move to Tôkyô is guessed to have come through his connection with Shinpei Goto who was Mayor of the city. Harajuku became Mikao Usui's first official seat of learning.

---

[41] Letter from Kurama Temple to the authors, 2002. Further research is continuing. Authors' note: research can be painstakingly slow.

This 'Reiki Ryôhô' or 'spiritual energy healing method' that people lined up for was most likely the *reiju*[42] and the spiritual teachings of Mikao Usui. It is believed that Mikao Usui did not need to perform a long ritual when performing *reiju* himself but could just become One with a student by standing near them or touching them. This would be enough for them to strengthen their energy.

In September of the twelfth year (AD 1923) there was a great earthquake and a conflagration broke out. Everywhere there were groans of pains from the wounded. Sensei, feeling pity for them, went out every morning to go around the town, and he cured and saved an innumerable number of people. This is just a broad outline of his relief activities during such an emergency.

(Excerpt from the Mikao Usui Memorial Stone, 1927).

On 1 September 1923, just before noon, an earthquake measuring 8.3 on the Richter scale occurred near the modern industrial cities of Tôkyô and Yokohama, Japan. This was not the largest earthquake to ever hit Japan, but its proximity to Tôkyô and Yokohama and the surrounding areas, with combined populations numbering 2 million, made it one of Japan's most devastating earthquakes. Tôkyô's principle business and industrial districts lay in ruins. There was an estimation of nearly 100,000 deaths with an additional 40,000 missing. Hundreds of thousands were left homeless in the resulting fires.

Gichin Funakoshi was also living in Tôkyô at that time. He wrote in his autobiography, 'We who survived did all we could to succor the injured and the homeless in the days immediately following the terrible disaster... I joined other volunteers to help provide food for the refugees, to clear the rubble and to assist in the task of disposing of the dead bodies.'

This earthquake may well have been the background inspiration for Hawayo Takata's well-known 'beggar story'.[43] There was a great

---

[42] The Japanese word *reiju* is called an attunement in the West. There are many versions of attunements and *reiju* in both the West and Japan. Traditional *reiju* are performed without symbols and mantras and the ritual does not change with each level. For more information about *reiju* and attunements see page 97.

[43] Most Western practitioners know this beggar story as a parable. It teaches practitioners that Reiki must be paid for or it will not be respected. Many teachers dispute this concept today and there exist groups of teachers and practitioners who offer Reiki for free – for more information see Internet Yahoo Group, Grass Roots Reiki. There is an account of the 'beggar story' in *Living Reiki, Takata's Teachings* by Fran Brown.

deal of poverty in Japan at that time due to the depression. After the earthquake Mikao Usui moved his home and *dôjô* to Nakano ku, outside of Tôkyô, in 1925. Selection of this particular house was decided through the art of divination.[44] He was often invited to travel throughout Japan treating people and teaching students. Mikao Usui had over 2000 students in total,[45] about 60 to 70 *okuden* students and 21 teachers students who reached *shinpiden*.[46]

> Sensei's personality was gentle and modest and he never behaved ostentatiously. His physique was large and sturdy. He always wore a contented smile.
>
> (Excerpt from the Mikao Usui Memorial Stone, 1927).

Spiritual Healers

At the turn of the century hands-on-healing or *teate* was very popular in Japan.[47] Toshihiro Eguchi was a friend of Mikao Usui and studied with him in the 1920s.[48] Toshihiro Eguchi created the *Tenohira Ryôji Kenkyû Kai* (Hand Healing Research Center), wrote a number of books and ran a healing community for a number of years.

Law and order had largely broken down in the late 1800s and ronin[49] *roamed the streets. Martial arts practices from all over the country joined togther in the cities and official and more respectable schools were created such as Kodokan Jûdô. There was a definite code of ethics and honour attached to early martial arts practices that often verged on the spiritual. Morihei Ueshiba taught a spiritual martial arts called aikidô, the Art of Peace. This may largely have been due to his involvment with a religion called the Oomoto sect.*

This link between martial arts and spirituality had always been a quest for the samurai. It was also a reflection of the cultural period itself, which held the antithesis of military action and spiritual healing in one hand. Of the many naval personnel in Japan, many were interested in martial

---

[44] Information taken from the Mikao Usui Memorial Stone.
[45] Information taken from the Mikao Usui Memorial Stone.
[46] Information supplied to the authors by Hyakuten Inamoto. The Usui Reiki Ryôhô Gakkai has 11 of these listed by name in their booklet called *shiori*.
[47] For a list of other *teate* groups around that time see Chapter 6: Reiki in Japan.
[48] Dave King states that it was in 1921 and Hiroshi Doi states that Eguchi was involved with the teachings from 1925 to 1927.
[49] A *ronin* is a masterless *samurai*.

arts and intrigued by spiritual healing. This interest was to form a further historical element to the journey of Mikao Usui's teachings.

Shinpei Goto, Mikao Usui's boss, wrote a calligraphic work in the foreword to Gichin Funakoshi's first book in 1922. Gichin Funakoshi also taught Jigorô Kanô for a couple of months. Jigorô Kanô would send his students to either Morihei Ueshiba or Gichin Funakoshi for further study.[50] There are numerous connections between these figures during Mikao Usui's lifetime.

Due to his respected and far-reaching reputation many people from local districts wished to invite him. Sensei, accepting the invitations, went to Kure and then to Hiroshima and Saga, and reached Fukuyama. Unexpectedly he became ill and passed away there. It was 9 March of the fifteenth year of Taisho (AD 1926), aged 62.[51]

(Excerpt from the Mikao Usui Memorial Stone, 1927).

Mikao Usui died of a stroke.

These are truly great teachings for cultivation and discipline that agree with those great teachings of the ancient sages and the wise. Sensei named these teachings Secret Method to Invite Happiness and miraculous Medicine to Cure All Diseases ; notice the outstanding features of the teachings. Furthermore, when it comes to teaching, it should be as easy and common as possible, nothing lofty. Another noted feature is that during sitting in silent meditation with Gassho and reciting the Five Precepts mornings and evenings, the pure and healthy minds can be cultivated and put into practice in one's daily routine. This is the reason why Reiho is easily obtained by anyone.

(Excerpt from the Mikao Usui Memorial Stone, 1927).

Gichin Funakoshi wrote that, 'Times change, the world changes, and obviously the martial arts must change.' Mikao Usui's own teachings

---

[50] *Three Budô Masters*, John Stevens, Kodansha International, 1995.
[51] During Mikao Usui's lifetime the age of a Japanese was counted not on the birthday, but on a New Year's Day without regard to one's actual birthday. Today he is considered to have died at the age of 61.

appeared to have gone through many changes during his lifetime and were set to continue to change…

Reiki Precepts

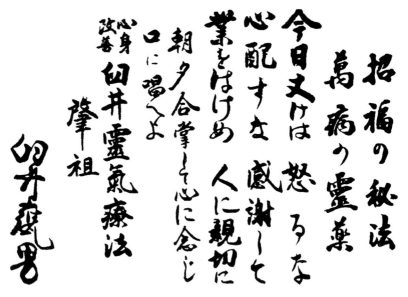

The secret of inviting happiness through many blessings
The spiritual medicine for all illness

For today only:
Do not anger
Do not worry
Be humble
Be honest in your work
Be compassionate to yourself and others

Do gasshô every morning and evening
Keep in your mind and recite[52]

Improve your mind and body

Usui Reiki Ryôhô Founder Mikao Usui

---

[52] This translation was supplied to the authors by Chris Marsh.

What are the Five Precepts?

The five precepts,[53] or *gokai* as they are called in Japan, are guidelines to aid students in their journey toward spiritual development. Mikao Usui taught them from as early as 1915.[54] The Usui Reiki Ryôhô Gakkai perform *gokai sansho*, or the chanting of the five precepts three times, at the end of their regular group meetings. They are also printed in the *Reiki Ryôhô Hikkei*.[55]

The five precepts are the six sentences in the center of the entire poetic teaching found at the beginning of this chapter. The teaching consists of an introduction, the five precepts themselves, directions on how and when to use them and what the result of this practice will be. An old Japanese version of the five precepts was in the top left hand corner of a photo of Mikao Usui that was provided to Frank Arjava Petter by Tsutomu Oishi.[56]

Origins of the Five Precepts

The origins of the precepts are uncertain. The memorial stone states that Mikao Usui requested that his students practice two things:

> Thus, before the teachings, the 'Ikun' (admonition) of the Meiji Emperor should reverently be told and Five Precepts be chanted and kept in mind mornings and evenings.

Here it is likely that there are two different teachings being described – the 'ikun' and the precepts.

[53] A precept is a general rule that helps you decide how you should behave in particular circumstances. (Collins Essential English Dictionary, 1989.)

[54] Information supplied to the authors by Chris Marsh. Dave King states that a Japanese nun told him that Mikao Usui had written the precepts in 1921 on *hiei zan*. He believes the original copy is kept in a private shrine to Mikao Usui.

[55] Information taken from the *Reiki Ryôhô Hikkei (Spritual Energy Healing Method Manual)*, a manual that is given to Usui Reiki Ryôhô Gakkai members in Japan. For more information about the *Reiki Ryôhô Hikkei* see page 106.

[56] There is uncertainty whether these precepts are written in Mikao Usui's handwriting. It was initially believed that this was so by Westerners. Though that was probably because Mikao Usui's name is written in the last sentence – not unlike how signatures are written in the West.

According to the translator of this copy of the memorial stone, Hyakuten Inamoto, '*ikun*' is, in fact, referring to the Meiji Emperor's *waka* (poetry). This would indicate that the precepts are a separate teaching.

Frank Arjava Petter states in his books, *Reiki Fire* and *Reiki – The Legacy of Dr Usui* that the precepts originated from the Meiji Emperor's *Imperial Rescript on Education*[57] It seems that he has linked the two teachings that were written about on the memorial stone together. The Imperial Rescript was written by the Meiji Emperor in 1890 and is an edict that became a fundamental Japanese moral code until the end of World War II. The rescript was treated with quasi-religious reverence and in schools was kept, together with the picture of the Emperor and Empress, in a special safe.[58] There are elements of the five precepts taught by Mikao Usui in this edict but it is certainly not a direct translation. It is only natural that there is some connection as all moral and civic instruction after 1890 was based on the rescript's principles.

Jigorô Kanô, who is believed to have known Mikao Usui, introduced a very similar system of cultural and moral codes to jûdô.[59] Traditional jûdô teachings claim that the purpose of training is the cultivation of the perfection of character. Therefore, in order to perfect the personality students must first learn and understand the *Imperial Rescript on Education* by the Meiji Emperor. These codes, he taught, included filial piety to parents, friendship to the siblings, harmony between husband and wife and trust between friends. It was also necessary to be modest and respectful to others, and to love mankind.

Due to the rescript's nationalistic focus it may have been obligatory for all official schools to teach at that particular stage in history.

---

[57] A rescript is an edict or decree. For more information about the Meiji Emperor see page 76. For two English translations of the rescript (one formal and one less formal) see Appendix D page 349.

[58] It was taken so seriously the story goes that some School Principals committed suicide if they mispronounced a word in reciting the rescript or if it perished in a fire.

[59] Jigorô Kanô, the founder of jûdô, was also a great sportsman, teacher and philospher – he was a member of the International Olympic Committee for 23 years.

Jigorô Kanô's precepts resemble those of Mikao Usui in a broad sense only and appear to be excerpts from the rescript. Mikao Usui's precept of 'do not worry', and the unique concept of 'just for today' are not mentioned. Suzuki san has said that the precepts were taught from as early as 1915 to students. Hiroshi Doi, however, writes that they were officially introduced in April 1922 when Mikao Usui created the Usui Reiki Ryôhô Gakkai.[60] Hiroshi Doi also claims that the book, *Kenzen no Genri*, written by Bizan Suzuki in 1914 may have inspired the writing of them.[61]

A translation of the piece in Bizan Suzuki's book is:

Today do not be angry,
do not worry and be honest,
work hard and be kind to people

Though the exact same *kanji* are not used, this reflects the same five precepts as taught by Mikao Usui. The vital element, 'today', has interestingly taken the same placement in the poem.

Recently, it has also been asserted that the origins of the five precepts actually date back to ninth-century Japanese Buddhist precepts.[62]

Perhaps Suzuki Bisan influenced Mikao Usui (or was it the other way around?) who, in turn, was originally influenced by these early Buddhist teachings.

The five precepts as taught by Mikao Usui, no matter what their history, are universal and valuable to all regardless of religion or creed. They are spiritual teachings rather than religious teachings and all students were asked to practice them in their daily lives.

The precepts have the syllabic regularity of 6-4-6-6-7-8 denoting that they fall into the category of a Japanese poem (this is not *waka*). The word for 'poem' in Japanese is also the word for 'song' and this lack of distinction may verify that the precepts were always sung or chanted.

---

[60] *Modern Reiki Method for Healing*, Hiroshi Doi, Fraser Journal Publishing, 2000.
[61] Information supplied to the authors by website: http://member.nifty.ne.jp/okojo/index.htm.
[62] Information supplied to the authors by Chris Marsh.

The Five Precepts in Detail

Here is a look at some meanings that may lay behind the five precepts from the translation at the beginning of this section:

> The secret of inviting happiness through many blessings
> The spiritual medicine for all illness

This first paragraph introduces the 'secret'. It alludes to spirituality being an instrument to good health. The 'many blessings' may be the benefits of the repeated receiving of the attunement. Mikao Usui and the Usui Reiki Ryôhô Gakkai performed attunements on a regular basis, believing that many attunements lead to enlightenment. After many years of personal practice and the receiving of the attunement it is understood that the practitioner becomes one with the universe. Another viewpoint may see the practitioner being showered with the blessings that the universe has to offer when practicing the teachings.

> For today only:
> Do not anger
> Do not worry
> Be humble
> Be honest in your work
> Be compassionate to yourself and others

For today only is a practical sentence to keep the practitioner's minds focused on the NOW. It is a typical Buddhist stance. By focusing on tomorrow – well, tomorrow never comes. Each moment of life is NOW. If these precepts are practiced NOW then they are being practiced in each and every moment of the practitioner's life.

> If you no longer want to create pain for yourself and others,
> if you no longer want to add to the residue of past pain that
> still lives on in you, then don't create any more time, or at least
> no more than is necessary to deal with the practical aspects
> of your life. How to stop creating time? Realize deeply that
> the present moment is all you ever have. Make the NOW the

primary focus of your life.

(Excerpt from The Power of NOW by Eckhart Tolle.)

Do not anger is a basic Buddhist principle. Anger not only hurts those in the practitioner's vicinity but the practitioner him or her self. It is the antithesis of balance. Once the practitioner is no longer a victim to the senses then focus can energetically be placed on the spiritual path.

> Sometimes people feel that anger is useful because it brings extra energy and boldness. When we encounter difficulties, we may see anger as a protector. But though anger brings us more energy, that energy is essentially a blind one. There is no guarantee that that energy will not become destructive to our own interests. Therefore, hatred and anger are not at all useful.
>
> (Excerpt from the *Power of Compassion* by His Holiness the Dalai Lama.)

Do not worry as this causes stress at all levels. Stress lowers the immune system opening the practitioner up to the possibility of disease. To worry is a lack of faith. Fearfulness is a reaction that does not trust the universe to provide what is best for the practitioner.

> ... Shantideva says:
> If you can solve your problem,
> Then what is the need of worrying?
> If you cannot solve it,
> Then what is the use of worrying? ...
>
> (Excerpt from *The Healing Power of Mind* by Tulku Thondup.)

Be humble and the practitioner will find this humbleness and thankfulness permeating each and every aspect of his or her life. Thoughts will be of a life of abundance rather than want. The importance of material circumstances will no longer be the gauge that existence is based on.

... True happiness relates more to the mind and heart. Happiness that depends mainly on physical pleasure is unstable; one day it's there, the next day it may not be ...

(Excerpt from *The Art of Happiness* by His Holiness the Dalai Lama and Howard C. Cutler.)

Be honest in your work is asking for the practitioner to be truthfully dedicated to spiritual progress by not becoming a 'spiritual materialist'.[63]

... Understanding the energy consequences of our thoughts and beliefs, as well as our actions, may force us to become honest to a new degree. Lying, either to others or to ourselves, should be out of the question. Genuine, complete healing requires honesty with oneself. An inability to be honest obstructs healing as seriously as the inability to forgive. Honesty and forgiveness retrieve our energy – our spirits – from the energy dimension of 'the past.'

(Excerpt from *Anatomy of the spirit* by Carolyn Myss, Ph.D.)

Be compassionate to yourself and others and the practitioner will remember the connection of all things under the universe.

… numberless times in previous lives we have each fulfilled the role of a mother. The feeling of a mother for a child is a classic example of love. For the safety, protection and welfare of her children, a mother is ready to sacrifice her very life.

(Quote by His Holiness the Dalai Lama.)

Mindfulness brings peace to life. This thought reminds human nature that it is compassionate and to understand and experience connectedness. Oneness.

---

[63] A term coined by Chogyam Trungpa that relates to one who gathers spiritual knowledge in the same manner as one who constantly buys the latest shopping trend. It is the gathering of spiritual knowledge to prove how 'spiritual' you really are.

Do gasshô every morning and evening
Keep in your mind and recite

Gasshô is the placing of both palms together in front of the chest. It is a sign of respect for oneself, the action and the energy. This simple act balances both the mind and body. Keep these precepts in the mind throughout the day. They are not just for reading but also for living.

Improve your mind and body
Usui Reiki Ryôhô
Founder Mikao Usui

The last three sentences name the motto, the system and its founder.

Precepts in our Daily Life

It is almost impossible to keep focused on these five precepts 100 per cent of the time. Therefore it must not be considered a 'sin' when the practitioner is unsuccessful in following each one of them. Buddhist thought offers the idea that when a precept is 'broken' focus can be placed on forgiveness and kindness towards oneself. This contemplation brings the practitioner full circle back to the original precepts finding the focus, once more, on compassion and the five precepts.

It is like the precepts. Even though it is almost impossible to observe them, we must have them. Without an aim or the precepts we cannot be good Buddhists, we cannot actualize our way.

(Excerpt from *Crooked Cucumber* by David Chadwick.)
(Quote by Shunryu Suzuki talking about Ian Kishizawa-roshi.)

Waka

> Poetry has its seed in the human heart and blossoms forth in innumerable leaves of words ... it is poetry which, with only a part of its power, moves heaven and earth, pacifies unseen gods and demons, reconciles men and women and calms the hearts of savage warriors.
>
> (Excerpt from the preface of *Kokinshû* (Collection of *Waka* of Ancient and Modern Times) by Ki no Tsurayuki (884–946))

What is *Waka*?

A component of Mikao Usui's teachings were the recitation of *waka* as written by the Meiji Emperor. Once again there is a strong link between the Japanese culture and Mikao Usui's teachings. A certain portion of the Japanese community commonly recited *waka* at the turn of the twentieth century. It was a remnant of the strong cultural base that Japan had built up throughout its 250 years of national isolation.

In the book *Tapenshu*, Gichin Funakoshi's[64] students are asked to ponder the words of a classical poem used by a fierce swordsman Jigenryu:

Spring blossoms.
Autumn moon.
Conditions.
Confrontation.
Swordsmanship.
No conditions.

Mikao Usui, having lived under the reign of the Meiji Emperor must have been highly influenced by his spiritual insight. He asked his students to realize the emperor's teachings and to chant or sing his poetry. The Japanese believed that the monarchy was in fact godly

---

[64] Gichin Funakoshi is the founder of modern karate and is said to have been an acquaintance of Mikao Usui.

and in that context it is easy to see how the emperor could exert such great power over the people.

Mikao Usui placed over 125 *gyosei* from the Meiji Emperor in the *Reiki Ryôhô Hikkei*.[65] His recommendation was that all students recite these *gyosei* as a form of self-development. In this way students would not only be practicing energy enhancement with his meditations and techniques but also mind expansion.

The power of *waka* was evident to him and it is taught today that he even wrote his own *waka*.

A student of Mikao Usui's called Kaiji Tomita wrote a book in 1933 called, *Reiki To Jinjutsu – Tomita Ryû Teate Ryôhô (Reiki and Humanitarian Work - Tomita Ryû Hands Healing)*. In a technique called **hatsurei hô* he asks the students to become one with the Meiji Emperor's *waka*.

The word *waka* is made up of two parts: *wa* meaning 'Japanese' and *ka* meaning 'poem' or 'song'. The word may have been written to distinguish between the poetry written by the Japanese in their own language to differentiate from that which they read and wrote in Chinese.

Origins of *Waka*

In the historical Japanese, *Hotsuma Tsutae* or *The Hotsuma Legends*,[66] there is a legend about the origins of *waka* poetry. Princess *Waka*, or *Wakahime*, was very skilled in writing a particular style of song. She inscribed these songs onto wooden tablets sending them to her lovers. One of her lovers was supposedly moved to distraction by her written love songs. On the strength of her skill and ability this style of song or poetry eventually became recognized as *waka*.

---

[65] Information taken from the *Reiki Ryôhô Hikkei (Spritual Energy Healing Method Manual)*, a manual that is given to Usui Reiki Ryôhô Gakkai members in Japan. For more information about the *Reiki Ryôhô Hikkei* see page 106.

[66] Its first parts, 'Book of Heaven' and 'Book of Earth', were recorded and edited around 660 BC (according to the Nihonshoki calender) by Kushimikatama-Wanihiko. His descendant, Ootataneko, recorded the third part, 'Book of Man', which contains the stories after Emperor Jinmu (660 BC), and offered the complete *Hotsuma Tsutae* to Emperor Keiko (the twelfth emperor) in 126 AD. The origin of the *Hotsuma Tsutae* is controversial. It is guessed to be very old while some researchers challenge the dates written above.

Waka is a short form of poetry that contains 31 syllables. In English it is typically divided into five lines of 5,7,5,7 and 7 syllables. Usually, each line consists of one image or idea and there is no definite linking or wrapping of text between lines. Yet, a true *waka* poet is able to make the five lines magically flow together into one thought. *Waka* was often performed on public occasions at the Imperial court. In fact, many emperors were renowned for their *waka*. It also became an essential skill for noblemen, women and *samurai*. *Waka* were often composed as a kind of finale to every sort of occasion – no experience was complete until one had been written about it. In the fourteenth century, a competition developed where one person would write the first half of a *waka* and another would complete it with the last two 7-syllable stanzas. Up to four people took part in these games with the rules becoming extremely complex ensuring that a courtly standard was preserved.

Waka Today

Today, the *waka* has become outdated and is now known in its modern form as a *tanka*. The best-known poetry outside of Japan is neither the *waka* nor *tanka* but the *haiku*. The *haiku* is said to have also originated from the *waka*. It is shorter still and consists of three lines of 5,7 and 5 syllables and traditionally focuses on nature using descriptive seasonal terms. *Haiku* are popular throughout the world and are written in numerous languages.

Meiji Emperor and *Waka*

The Meiji Emperor ruled Japan from 1867 to 1912 and is said to have written over 100,000 *waka* and his Empress Shôken over 30,000. These *waka* are not only excellent as literary works but also constitute significant teachings to enhance national moral character'.[67] *Waka* written by emperors are called *gyosei* meaning 'created by the emperor'.

---

[67] Information supplied to the authors by website: www.meijijingu.or.jp/english.

He was the first emperor ever to be seen by foreigners. Hiroshi Doi stated at the URRI[68] workshop that when politicians visited the Meiji Emperor they would begin to sweat – not just because they were nervous but because of the great amount of energy he exuded.

Hand Positions

Every position on the body is a possible hand position.

(Excerpt from *Reiki – 108 Questions and Answers* by Paula Horan.)

What is a Hand Position?

Since the beginning of time humans and animals have instinctively used touch – to comfort, support, connect, rejuvenate and heal. It is not 100 years old or even 5000 years old – it is as old as our living planet.

From the beginning, as a baby, humans have drawn on the energy of those around them while being held, cuddled and fed. Premature babies are known to gain weight faster when touched and held.[69] As humans grow older the power of touch remains integral to their well-being. In everyday life it continues to express intention in an energetic manner. By reaching out humans transfer energy from one person to another; the comforting pat on the shoulder; the compassionate look; welcoming, open arms or the healing kiss on a child's sore finger.

Natural, intuitive actions that are used to connect on an energetic level – this is the concept behind hand positions.

Mikao Usui is believed to have taught students to place their hands on or near the body, to pat, stroke, gaze at and blow on the body[70] – all with the intention that the body would restore its balance. This

---

[68] Usui Reiki Ryôhô International is an organization that promotes traditional Japanese Reiki teachers and their teachings through workshops that are held annually in different countries throughout the world.

[69] Field, T.M., S.M. Schanberg, et al. 1986. Tactile/kinesthetic stimulation effects on preterm neonates. *Pediatrics* 77: pp. 654-58.

[70] Information taken from the *Reiki Ryôhô Hikkei (Spritual Energy Healing Method Manual)*, a manual that is given to Usui Reiki Ryôhô Gakkai members in Japan. For more information about the *Reiki Ryôhô Hikkei* see page 106.

physical action brings awareness to a natural skill and with practice, a stronger connection to this innate healing ability.

It is probable that Mikao Usui never used set hand positions himself. More likely he would have simply performed an attunement. He would do this by being either near or touching the recipient. For him the ability to become One with the energy of others was his form of healing.

Hand positions were created later in his life, in the same manner as the symbols and mantras, to be training wheels for those who could not yet accomplish Mikao Usui's energetic prowess. When experiencing difficulty in intuiting where the hands should be placed on the body hand positions were taught as a useful tool.

The Origins of Treating Others

There are a number of versions of set hand positions for treating others that have been used in Mikao Usui's teachings at one time or another. Mikao Usui apparently taught five hand positions around the 1920s. These were centered solely on the head. The rest of the treatment for the body was intuited, if treated at all.[71]

Similar head positions were also written up in the healing guide of the *Reiki Ryôhô Hikkei*, used by the Usui Reiki Ryôhô Gakkai and Chûjirô Hayashi's own healing guide, *Ryôhô Shishin*. Toshihiro Eguchi, a well-known healer around the time of Mikao Usui, used a similar set of hand positions in his manuals. He studied with Mikao Usui and was a good friend of his.[72]

Frank Arjava Petter in his book, *The Original Reiki Handbook of Dr Mikao Usui*, states that Mikao Usui mainly used his left hand when treating people.

All head positions focus on the mind because once it is calm and balanced the rest of the body naturally returns to its original state. The first four positions appear to balance the energy. By the time the fifth and last position is reached, on top of the crown, the mind is relaxed and the energy is easily drawn down and into the whole body. The crown is also our connecting point to spirit. Working on the crown strengthens this spiritual connection. In the *Reiki Ryôhô*

---

[71] Information supplied to the authors by Andrew Bowling's website: www.usui reiki.fsnet.co.uk.
[72] Information supplied to the authors by Chris Marsh.

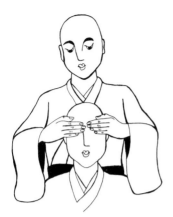

Zentô bu – Forehead

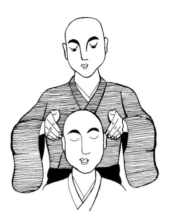

Sokutô bu – Both temples

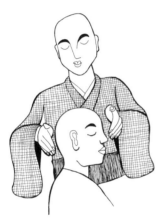

Kôtô bu – Back of your head
and forehead

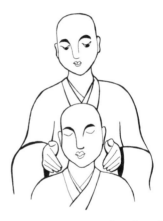

Enzui bu – Either side of neck

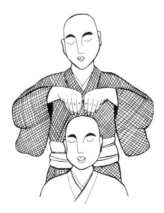

Tôchô bu –
Crown on top
of head

Hikkei it states that if the spirit is healthy and connected to the truth, the body will naturally become healthy. These positions can be performed while the recipient is seated. The hands are held in place for as long as the energy is felt flowing – this could take a couple of minutes or up to half an hour. Some versions of this method rest the hands physically on the person while others hold them 2 to 3 inches (5 to 8 cm) off the body.

Once the practitioner has finished the five positions the hands are moved to the part of the body where an imbalance is sensed.

Apart from these head positions the *Reiki Ryôhô Hikkei* also contains over 20 pages of specific hand positions for certain illnesses. It is thought that Chûjirô Hayashi may have compiled this list. As he was a doctor he would have been a good choice to write up this technical part of the manual. Chûjirô Hayashi's own healing guide, *Ryôhô Shishin*, which he gave out later in life, contained almost identical hand positions for treating specific illnesses.

It is uncertain when Chûjirô Hayashi first used a healing guide. Hawayo Takata possessed a copy of this manual and she was taught between 1936 and 1938.[73]

The reason for creating specific and detailed hand positions is probably because Chûjirô Hayashi was more interested in the technicalities of hands-on healing because of his medical background. At that time there were a number of groups working who were experimenting with similar ideas.

Alongside the creation of Chûjirô Hayashi's hand position method was the development of his official clinic called the *Hayashi Reiki Kenkyû Kai* or Hayashi Spiritual Energy Research Society. Clients paid money for treatments and there existed a system where students would complete an internship that included working as volunteers at the clinic. Fran Brown states that Chûjirô Hayashi never changed the system but simply brought it inside the clinic.[74]

When Hawayo Takata first came to him as a patient he had a clinic

[73] In his book, *Hand to Hand*, John Harvey Gray wrote that Hawayo Takata received the manual from Chûjirô Hayashi in 1941. This is unlikely as Chûjirô Hayashi died in 1940. Hawayo Takata was in Japan in 1940 when Chûjirô Hayashi committed suicide and may have received it at that time. She had already completed an internship, received his blessing and certificate to teach in 1938.

[74] *Living Reiki – Takata's Teachings*, Fran Brown, Life Rhythm, 1992.

that had eight beds with two practitioners working at each bed. One practitioner would begin at the abdomen or *hara* and the other would begin at the head. Neither of the healing guides mentioned this particular method of treating people with two practitioners. Most probably elements of the healing guides were practiced during treatments.

Another researcher, Dave King, alleges that Tatsumi learnt seven basic hand positions from Chûjirô Hayashi before 1931.[75] These were formulated to cover specific acupuncture points on the body.

Hawayo Takata was taught where and how to place her hands on the body during her training with Chûjirô Hayashi in Japan. After a one-year internship she returned to America where she worked intuitively with clients from the late 1930s into the 1970s. She did not appear to use one particular hand position method. After her death, a number of her students came together to create an organization that taught a strict set of 12 hand positions which began at the head. Other students of Hawayo Takata argued that she had taught them to start at the abdomen. Both of these systems, plus totally intuitive systems, are taught in the West.

Researchers today place the beginning of the importance of hand positions with Chûjirô Hayashi. This could mean that what is practiced as Reiki in the West has its origins in Chûjirô Hayashi's system rather than that of Mikao Usui.

The origins of Self-treatment

Parallel to the development of hand positions as a means to heal others, the concept of self-treatment naturally developed. This is where students place their hands on their own bodies in a systemized fashion.

Self-treatment by placing hands on one's own body was not taught directly by Mikao Usui. The recitation of *waka*[76] and the five precepts along with mantras and meditation techniques were the earliest forms of self-development taught to students.

---

[75] Information supplied to the authors by Dave King's website: www.usui-do.org.
[76] Poetry written by the Meiji Emperor and included by Mikao Usui in his teachings.

Self-treatment with hand positions is not mentioned in any original texts, such as the two healing guides referred to previously. It is natural though to place the hands on an area of the body where there is a corresponding problem. There was never any formalized teaching of this until the system of Reiki was taught in the West. Hawayo Takata emphasized that first we must become whole by practicing on ourselves and then we can move on and help others.

Healing Touch in Japan

Using hands to heal is not considered extraordinary in Japan. It was a very popular technique in Japan at the beginning of the twentieth century and it has always been popular through the Japanese deity *Binzuru*. *Binzuru* is known as the 'master of remedies' and is the Buddha of healing. It is believed that he promised to find remedies for human kind for all disease. His abilities are recognized in Japan and many festivals are held yearly in his honour.

In his hands he holds a medicine jar made of precious stone emerald. By being bathed in this Emerald Radiance all illness can be cured. But it is his touch that offers benefits to all who come to him.

From a culture that is grounded in such a strong connection with touch and healing it is easy to imagine the ease with which a healing system using hand positions has evolved.

In Nara, an unusual statue stands just outside the great doors of one of the world's largest wooden structures. This is the Todai ji Temple and it is *Binzuru*, made of wood that has split with age, who is seated there. He wears a cotton cloth cap and shawl with one palm facing towards his followers and the other holding his wooden bowl. Visitors to the temple rub the region of Binzuru's body that corresponds to their own illness or pain. Binzuru consequently relieves them of their problem whether it is physical, mental, emotional or spiritual.

Meditations, Mantras And Symbols

> They (symbols) do not have to fit to any intellectual pattern
> they are to stand alone for all,
> whether *Shintô*, Buddhist, Christian, unbeliever etc.
>
> (Quote by Suzuki san.)[77]

Devices for Enlightenment

Meditations, mantras and symbols appear to have been gradually introduced into Mikao Usui's initial teachings. Much of the information provided here is from the notes and teachings of Mikao Usui that are in the possession of Suzuki san and her fellow students. Meditations, mantras and symbols all work on the same principle. Each method is a different approach yet the end result is the same – eventual enlightenment.

The earliest history begins in 1915 where the mantras and meditations were the first of the three to be taught. The purpose of these teachings was solely to develop spiritual growth. Only later in Mikao Usui's life, around 1923 (once he began working with lay people who were not involved in spiritual practices), were symbols introduced. These symbols were extra tools that made it easier for students to practice Mikao Usui's spiritual teachings.

The Usui Reiki Ryôhô Gakkai and Chûjirô Hayashi do not seem aware of these early teachings. They are known to have worked with the mantras and the symbols as taught by Mikao Usui from 1923 onwards. The mantras and symbols were not included in the *Reiki Ryôhô Hikkei*[78] but were copied by students from their teachers.

According to the student's ability either a meditation, a mantra or a symbol and mantra would be given. These are all different paths leading toward the same destination. The paths are chosen according to the student's abilities.

Another link between these devices is that the energy evoked by some meditations, mantras ,and mantras and symbols is of the same quality. The system offers diverse approaches for different people.

The Use of Meditations

Students received a meditation for their own personal practice. On a regular basis the teacher, Mikao Usui, would discuss their progress

[77] Information supplied to the authors by Andrew Bowling's website: www.usuir eiki.fsnet.co.uk.
[78] Information taken from the *Reiki Ryôhô Hikkei (Spritual Energy Healing Method Manual)*, a manual that is given to Usui Reiki Ryôhô Gakkai members in Japan. For more information about the *Reiki Ryôhô Hikkei* see page 106.

and eventually teach them a new follow-up meditation. This device is not unlike teaching Zen through the use of koans. Here the answer is not reached by logic but rather through an experience, a realization. Depending on the student's ability it may take from a couple of months to a number of years before receiving the new meditation. These meditations are not the same as the known techniques practiced by the Usui Reiki Ryôhô Gakkai.

The Use of Mantras

In Japan the word for mantra is either *kotodama*[79] or *jumon*[80]. The terms *kotodama* and *jumon* accentuate a slightly different aspect of working with sound. For ease of understanding we will use the word mantra to cover all aspects of *kotodama* and *jumon*.

According to Suzuki san's teachings, the mantras (rather than symbols) were the first to be introduced to Mikao Usui's teachings. The mantras taught at this time were pronounced differently as to how they are used in the West today.

Eventually symbols in conjunction with mantras were added for those students who were not sensitive enough to the energy (generally non-Buddhist and non-martial arts practitioners).

Morihei Ueshiba, founder of aikidô and said to be an acquaintance of Mikao Usui, was another martial arts practitioner who worked from a spiritual viewpoint. He too used the chanting of vowel sounds in his spiritual teachings. He was involved with the Oomoto sect who had formulated a number of effective meditation techniques and powerful chants based on *kotodama* theory.[81]

Mantras invoke a specific vibration through sound. Therefore it is most effective when spoken out loud. Mantras must be uttered correctly as a slight alteration creates a different vibration thus producing a different manifestation.[82]

---

[79] *Kotodama* means words carrying spirit. Hiroshi Doi, teacher of Gendai Reiki Hô and member of the Usui Reiki Ryôhô Gakkai, uses the word *kotodama* in place of the word mantra.

[80] *Jumon* is a sound that invokes a specific energetic vibration.

[81] *Three Budô Masters*, John Stevens, Kodansha International, 1995.

[82] Authors' discussion with Hyakuten Inamoto about mantras. Hyakuten Inamoto is a teacher of Komyo Reiki Kai in Kyôto, Japan.

Kotodama and *jumon* were ancient *Shintô* practices that used vibrations to interact with the natural environment. To understand sound's importance it is necessary to experience and learn about vibration. Imagine that you are interested in studying a tree. You could approach it in a number of ways. First you could read a book about it written by someone else (most probably a non-tree), then you could cut a tree down and study it yourself, or lastly you could ask the tree – commune with the tree – go to its vibration and listen.

Primordial sounds are the vibrations of nature that structure the universe. They are the root sounds of every language. We can hear these sounds in the songs of birds, the rushing of streams, the crashing of waves and in the whispering breezes in the leaves of a tree … listening to primordial sounds restores our sense of connection to the whole and enlivens our inner healing energy.

(Excerpt from *The Wisdom of Healing* by David Simon.)

The Use of Symbols

In Japan each symbol is known as a number. For example: Symbol 1, Symbol 2, Symbol 3 and Symbol 4. In the West they are called by the name of the mantra, which is incorrect as the mantra is a separate device.

The West focuses mainly on the symbols rather than the mantras and sees them as very important to the practice of the Western system of Reiki. Over the last 20 years, more and more people have invented new symbols and created new Reiki systems.

Hiroshi Doi[83] states, 'Searching for more additional symbols or regarding symbols as a holy thing is meaningless.'[84]

The symbols have no power of their own – they act merely as a focus for our intent. Until now, the mantras and symbols were not taught in the West as tools to help us focus. The motivation behind creating more symbols and mantras is often to make Reiki 'more powerful'.

[83] Hiroshi Doi is a member of the Usui Reiki Ryôhô Gakkai.
[84] *Modern Reiki Method for Healing*, Hiroshi Doi, Fraser Journal Publishing, 2000, p. 194.

This manner of thinking exists because the original understandings behind these devices has not yet been explored or understood.

According to Hiroshi Doi, the symbols are the training wheels of a bicycle – and once the bike can be ridden the training wheels are taken away. This is the same with the symbols and mantras, but it is necessary to be very careful and not to throw them away too soon. The vibrations must be fully understood before moving on – this may take years and years of practice.

When drawing symbols a few aspects need to be kept in mind by the practitioner. Knowledge of what the action is affects the quality of the outcome. The strength of this outcome is determined by the student's inner connection to the symbol. Ignorance allows for mistakes and a poor bonding with the symbol.

The Use of Mantras and Symbols

There are no traditional Reiki mantras written in *The Reiki Sourcebook* – pseudonyms are used in their place. These are CKR, SHK, HSZSN and DKM.

Symbols have also not been printed on the pages of this book. The rationale behind this is one of respect for Mikao Usui's teachings. Some maintain that the mantras and symbols are secret.

As far as the symbols and Mikao Usui's teachings are concerned – the more they are practiced, the easier it becomes to sense the energy and the sooner the student will find that symbols are irrelevant.

> Progress comes
> To those who
> Train and train;
> Reliance on secret techniques
> Will get you nowhere

> (Quote by Morihei Ueshiba from
> *The Art of Peace* by John Stevens.)

Four traditional mantras and symbols have recently crossed to the West. These are taken from Tatsumi's hand-drawn copies of Chûjirô Hayashi's symbols.[85] This is the closest to the original

---

[85] Chûjirô Hayashi's student Tatsumi gave these hand-drawn copies to Dave King.

symbols that the West has come. In Japan today it is said that the Usui Reiki Ryôhô Gakkai uses slightly different symbols, as does Chûjirô Hayashi's student Chiyoko Yamaguchi[86] and her student, Hyakuten Inamoto. The mantra and the symbol are written independently of one another. In traditional Japanese branches the symbol is not called by the mantra's name as is done in the West.[87]

Of the 12 living students of Mikao Usui only one was taught the mantras and symbols. This student was a farmer while the other members were monks and a nun.

Each mantra and symbol can be practiced independently of other mantras and symbols – CKR and Symbol 1 are not needed to activate the other mantras and symbols as is often taught in the West.

The Mantras and Symbols in Detail

In this section the mantras and symbols are dissected in detail. There are four groupings with one mantra and symbol in each. This has been set up for ease of understanding – the mantra and the symbol, though different devices, work toward the same goals.

The characteristics of the mantras and symbols that are listed for each mantra and symbol are the energetic vibrations that these devices evoke.

When using mantras in conjunction with symbols they must be chanted three times. Many have wondered if 'repeat three times' is a Western addition to the practice of mantras. This does not seem to be the case. In the Usui Reiki Ryôhô Gakkai the five precepts are also chanted three times. They use the Japanese name *gokai sansho* for this practice, which is a Buddhist term meaning to chant the precepts three times. Three is considered to be a divine number.

To draw a symbol there are various approaches that can be taken. Visualize drawing the symbol in the mind's eye, physically with the palm of the hand or with your fingers.

---

[86] Information supplied to the authors by Hyakuten Inamoto.
[87] Taught in these branches: Usui Reiki Ryôhô Gakkai, Usui Reiki Ryôhô, Komyo Reiki, Jikiden Reiki, Method to Achieve Personal Perfection.

Many myths have been created around the mantras and symbols in the West, perhaps because the knowledge behind their origins was unknown. It is unsubstantiated that they originate from Tibet, Atlantis, Egypt or any other country or specific culture.

All of the four symbols are recognizable in Japan. Symbol 1 (or part thereof) is often found inscribed on temple walls. Symbol 2 is related to a seed syllable[88] and can be seen in temples across Japan. Symbols 3 and 4 are Japanese *kanji* and when read in Japanese are the actual names of the mantras used in the West. Though all four mantras are translatable, their technical meanings are less relevant than the vibrations that are invoked with their use. Mantras are simply mental vibrations and they should not carry meaning. Meaning ties us down to everyday associations. By following the vibration of the sound we can cut through these mundane thoughts and reach a space of silence.

Symbols 1 and 2 are clearly 'real' symbols while symbols 3 and 4 are merely Japanese *kanji* that have inaccurately been termed 'symbols'. Plainly these two sets of symbols have separate intentions. The first two symbols invoke an energy (earth and heaven or yin and yang) while the last two 'symbols' create a specific state of mind.

Only after becoming earth energy and heavenly energy can Oneness be experienced.

The Usui Reiki Ryôhô Gakkai shows the mantras and symbols to members but does not actively practice them.[89] The mantra DKM is a Japanese phrase that is a goal for the members to aim towards (and the symbol is simply the *kanji* of the phrase). Chiyoko Yamaguchi also does not use this mantra or symbol.[90]

These mantras and symbols are slightly different to what is taught in the West. This is not surprising, as it is known that in the West The Reiki Alliance standardized all symbols and mantras in 1983. There have also been many variations on these 'standardized' mantras and symbols since then. Chûjirô Hayashi is also known to have

---

[88] Seed symbols are letterforms drawn in a stylized manner of calligraphy to be used for meditation purposes.

[89] Stated by Hiroshi Doi, URRI, 1999.

[90] Chiyoko Yamaguchi did not complete *shinpiden* (Teacher level) fully or formally. She was taught the attunement to help a family member who was hosting a course run by Chûjirô Hayashi.

used slightly different mantras and symbols to that used by the Usui Reiki Ryôhô Gakkai and the West.[91] In Method to Achieve Personal Perfection elements of the mantra are chanted depending on the students' abilities.

It is essentially not necessary to know the literal translation of a mantra. Chanting is about the practice and the vibration it evokes, not the meaning behind the word itself. For interest's sake, *The Reiki Sourcebook* has included the literal translations for each of the mantras.

Some Japanese branches of Reiki today teach that the mantras and symbols are connected to deities.[92] These connections may differ depending on the branch of Reiki using them.

---

[91] Authors' discussion with Hyakuten Inamoto about symbols and mantras.

[92] Deities are gods (in this context – Japanese deities) and connections to them are used in Gendai Reiki Hô, Usui Reiki Ryôhô Gakkai and other traditional Japanese schools.

CKR and Symbol 1

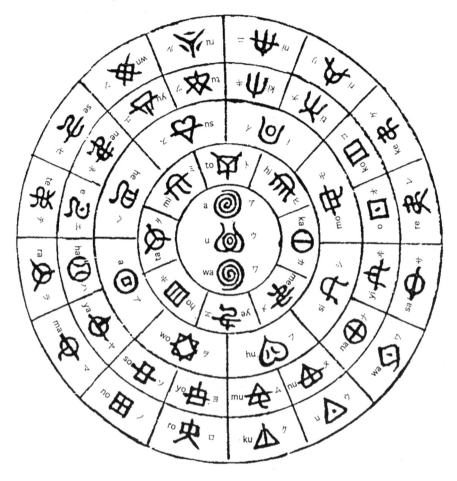

The Futomani Divination Chart stems from the *Hotsuma Tsutae*[93] –
It holds the ancient letters of the traditional Japanese god, Amemioya.

'a' represents Heaven
'u' represents Beginning
'wa' represents Earth

The god, Amemioya, created heaven and the earth by blowing into the chaos of the universe. *In* and *yo* (yin and yang) were formed and light and clear substances became Heaven 'a', and heavy, turbid substances became Earth 'wa'.

Western characteristic: Power
Japanese characteristic: Focus[94]

The energy invoked with this mantra and symbol:
Earth energy[95] – which is heavy, powerful and grounding. The first two mantras and symbols represent earth and heaven. This is a very Shintô concept. Man is said to be the connection between these two energies. The *hara* is stimulated enabling the student to strengthen the connection to Original Energy.[96]

Using the mantra in conjunction with the symbol:
Chant the mantra three times while the symbol is being drawn. It is not necessary to use this mantra and symbol to activate the other mantras and symbols.

Origin of the mantra and symbol:
It has been asserted that CKR and Symbol 1 have a Taoist origin[97] but no verification has, of yet, been presented. An element of Symbol 1 has similarities to a symbol that is used in many global cultures. This element is commonly utilized as an expression for movement

[93] Its first parts, 'Book of Heaven' and 'Book of Earth', were recorded and edited around 660 BC (according to the Nihonshoki calender) by Kushimikatama-Wanihiko. His descendant, Ootataneko, recorded the third part, 'Book of Man', which contains the stories after Emperor Jinmu (660 BC), and offered the complete *Hotsuma Tsutae* to Emperor Keiko (the twelfth emperor) in 126 AD. The origin of the *Hotsuma Tsutae* is controversial. It is guessed to be very old while some researchers challenge the dates written above. Seiji Takabatake provided the Futomani Divination Chart from the Japan Translation Center Ltd, Tôkyô.

[94] Taught in these branches as having this characteristic: Usui Reiki Ryôhô, Method to Achieve Personal Perfection, and other Japanese branches.

[95] Taught as earth energy in Usui dô, Gendai Reiki Hô, Usui Reiki Ryôhô, Method to Achieve Personal Perfection and other Japanese branches.

[96] Original Energy is the energy that you receive from your parents when you are conceived and most importantly it is the energetic connection between you and the universal lifeforce.

of energy. The first symbol, which is found inscribed on Temple Walls, is usually written as a symbol of the earth element in Tendai cosmology with its origins probably in *Hotsuma* symbology. The *Hotsuma Tsutae*, a controversial historical text, is not alone in using a derivation of Symbol 1. Here the letter *'wa'* is translated as an early Japanese letter for *'earth'* and has a physical similarity to an element of Symbol 1. Copies of *Hotsuma Tsutae* have been stored in *iwamuro* (cave storage) in a Tendai temple at *enryaku ji*[98] *(hiei zan, Kyôto)*. These copies were given to *Saichô* (767–822), the founding priest of *enryaku ji*. Tendai priests were also known to give lectures on the *Hotsuma Tsutae*. If there were any link here it would be that Mikao Usui was a practicing Tendai Buddhist said to have trained on *enryaku ji*.

Translation of the mantra:
There are different alternatives when translating the mantra CKR depending on the *kanji* used. Some translations of the mantra CKR from a Japanese Reiki practitioner is:

- Imperial order or command
- Spirit that directly comes from the supreme existence
- Supreme spiritual emptiness (void)

Deity connection:
The deity most often linked to the CKR and Symbol 1 is Daiseishi Bosatsu.

The name means 'He Who Proceeds With Great Vigour'. This is the Buddha who, with great vigour, offers wisdom to awaken the Buddha nature and Buddha wisdom that are in everyone helping them proceed to enlightenment.

---

[97] George Mullen claims to have come across a description of a set of symbols in China identical to those Yûji Onuki had taught him in 1971. Yûji Onuki's Reiki lineage is through Toshihiro Eguchi (a famous Japanese healer) and friend of Mikao Usui. The Usui Reiki Ryôhô Gakkai spokesman, Hiroshi Doi, maintains that Toshihiro Eguchi never studied to become a Reiki teacher and only completed the first levels of Reiki. If this is true then Yûji Onuki did not pass on a lineage from Mikao Usui's teachings rather a lineage from Toshihiro Eguchi's teachings.

[98] Main Japanese Tendai Complex.

SHK and Symbol 2

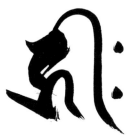

The *kiriku* symbol drawn by a monk at *hiei zan,* Japan

Western characteristic: Mental/Emotional
Japanese characteristic: Harmony

The energy invoked with this mantra and symbol:
Heavenly energy – which is light. The first two mantras and symbols represent earth and heaven. This is a very Shintô concept. Man is said to be the connection between these two energies. It helps to increase one's intuition and stimulate the upper *hara* center, in turn creating more psychic ability and a stronger connection to spirit.

Using the mantra in conjunction with the symbol:
Chant the mantra three times while the symbol is drawn.

Origin of the mantra and symbol:
Symbol 2 originated from the sacred *siddham* script and physically appears to be based on a seed syllable called *kiriku* (also known as *hrih* in Sanskrit). *Kiriku* calls upon the energy of Amida Nyorai. Amida Nyorai is the main deity in Pure Land Buddhism. Tendai utilizes Pure Land Buddhist principles and Mikao Usui was a Tendai lay priest[99] therefore it would be within reason to see a connection between the two.
   A seed syllable is a letterform used solely for meditation and is a part of esoteric Buddhism practiced in China and Japan. Calligraphy

[99] Information supplied to the authors by Chris Marsh. Mikao Usui was also buried in a Pure Land Buddhist graveyard.

in the *siddham* script is a living art. To use for the purpose of meditation, the character is drawn large in either formal or soft style on a scroll and hung on a wall.

Translation of the mantra:
Translations of the mantra SHK from a Japanese translator is:
- One's disposition
- Natural tendency
- Mental habit

Deity connection:
The deity most often linked to SHK and Symbol 2 is Amida Nyorai. The Sanskrit for Amida is 'Infinite Light'. Amida's compassion is therefore also infinite. In Pure Land schools of Buddhism, Amida Nyorai is the main deity.[100] Spiritual peace of mind lies in being able to attain salvation by relying on his powers.

HSZSN and Symbol 3

> A monk asked Ummon, 'What is the teaching of the Buddha's lifetime?'
> Ummon said, 'Preaching facing Oneness.'
>
> Oneness is absolute truth.
> To face oneness means to face everything –
> yourself, the world, every being, and everything –
> in its absolute truth.

(Koans – The Lessons of Zen)

Western characteristic: Sending energy across a distance
Japanese characteristic: Connection

The energy invoked with this mantra and symbol:
A state of mind is created with this mantra and *kanji*. This creates Oneness for all things. Therefore it is not about sending distant

---

[100] Mikao Usui's Memorial Stone is in a Pure Land Buddhist temple. Pure Land Buddhism was propagated in Japan by the Tendai monk Honen in the year 1175.

healing but about becoming One with the recipient to allow healing to take place. The student is reminded that this connection already exists.

Oneness comes repeatedly to the fore with any research completed about Mikao Usui's teachings. It is an undeniably Japanese perspective that has strong roots in Buddhism and martial arts – two main aspects of Mikao Usui's life.

Using the mantra in conjunction with the symbol:
Chant the mantra three times while the *kanji* is drawn.

Origin of the mantra and symbol:
This 'symbol' is made up of five separate *kanji* permitting it to be read as a sentence in either Japanese or Chinese. Clearly this could not be an Altlantian, Tibetan or Egyptian symbol as *kanji* is not in the make-up of these languages (where these languages are known). The *kanji* of Symbol 3 is the written form of the mantra HSZSN. If students wish to know if they have the correct 'symbol' simply have HSZSN (the complete mantra – not this pseudonym) written into Japanese *kanji*.

Translation of the mantra:
Translating *kanji* is unique. Each singular *kanji* can be translated to have many varied meanings. Depending on the translator there will be different versions of HSZSN. Here are some examples:

- My original nature is a correct thought[101]
- I am correct consciousness[102]
- Right consciousness is the origin of everything[103]

By returning to one's Original Nature a state of correct consciousness is achieved and it is in this state that Oneness is attained. True nature is Oneness.

Deity connection:
The deity most often linked to the HSZSN and Symbol 3 is Kannon.

[101] Authors' personal translation.
[102] Authors' personal translation.
[103] Hiroshi Doi's translation.

No other Buddha is worshipped by as many people as Kannon. This is the 'Bodhisattva Who Perceives the Sounds of the World'. Kannon made a vow to hear the voice of the people and the sounds of the conditions of the world. Salvation was immediately granted to the suffering and the afflicted as well as dispelling the evil and calamities that surround them.

DKM and Symbol 4

> To unify mind and body and become one with the universe is the ultimate purpose of my study
>
> (Motto of Koichi Tohei.)

Western characteristic: Embodiment of Mastership
Japanese characteristic: Empowerment

The energy invoked with this mantra and symbol:
A state of mind is created with this mantra and *kanji*.

Using the mantra in conjunction with the symbol:
Chant the mantra three times while the *kanji* is drawn.

Origin of the mantra and symbol:
This 'symbol' is made up of three separate *kanji* permitting it to be read as a sentence in either Japanese or Chinese. The *kanji* of symbol 4 is the written form of the mantra DKM. If students wish to know if they have the correct 'symbol' simply have DKM (the complete mantra – not this pseudonym) written into Japanese *kanji*.

DKM is used in a text of the Mikkyô tradition of Tendai called *ko myo ku*. This is practiced in *ju hachi dô*, a traditional Mikkyô style that is common to all esoteric ritual patterns. In the *ko myo ku* one merges with the 'Light Wisdom' of the Original Buddha Nature (Dainichi Nyorai). This manifests as the pure light of one's radiant self; a natural energetic force. Reaching this purity in one's life ties in with using light as a healing force and working towards enlightenment.

Translation of the mantra:
Translating *kanji* is unique. Each singular *kanji* can be translated to
have many varied meanings. Here are some translations of DKM:

- Great enlightenment[104]
- Zen expression for one's own true nature or Buddha-nature
  of which one becomes cognizant in the experience of
  enlightenment.[105]
- Great Bright Light[106] (void)

Deity connection:
The deity most often linked to the DKM and Symbol 4 is Dainichi
Nyorai. This is the Great Shining Buddha because this Buddha is
the life force of the Buddhas that illuminates everything. Dainichi
Nyorai dispels the darkness of the world by casting light everywhere,
giving life to and nurturing all living things.

Reiju and Attunements

reiju – (lit. Japanese) spiritual offering
attunement – an initiation ritual for students of the system of
    Reiki

What is a *Reiju* or an Attunement?

Reiju is the Japanese term for what was first called an initiation in
the West and is currently known as an attunement. There are differences in the actual rituals behind this practice depending on who
performed them and when.

Reiju is a ritual initially used and taught by Mikao Usui and
appears to have a twofold action:

- A sense of reconnection to one's true self.
- A clearing of the meridians allowing the student to conduct
  more energy through the body.

[104] Translated by Hyakuten Inamoto.
[105] Encyclopedia of Eastern Philosophy and Religion.
[106] Japanese translator.

Ritual

Ritual is in use by every living being throughout our planet. Often there is no awareness of this or the effect it creates. By working consciously with ritual an even stronger effect can be achieved.

The purpose of ritual can be seen from a number of different levels:

- The mind's fundamental method of learning is through symbolism. Ritual uses symbolism. The mind responds quickly to this as communication is taking place in its own language. An example is where the baby falls asleep quickly when rocked. In fact the baby will fall asleep with or without the rocking but it is the ritual that brings about the state of mind faster.
- When ritual is based on movement then that movement is used as a focusing point. Eventually the movement may be left out when the intent becomes clear enough to focus on its own. Learning the movement of ritual without the intent is ineffective. Intent needs to be focused and clear and this grows with the repetition of ritual.
- Ritual provides a structured approach to experiential learning. This can be seen as a form of protection against drifting off into a fantasy world. It keeps practitioners on track so that the learning that others may have begun (perhaps centuries earlier) is continued.
- By gaining an understanding of the meaning behind the physical movement or ritual it can expand knowledge of the method as a whole. It is not often that a challenge to complete something so structured and rigid is taken on. On true understanding of this structural conformity the exact nature can be hit upon.

Origins of the *Reiju*

Reiju appears to originate from Tendai Buddhism. This is not surprising as Mikao Usui was a Tendai practitioner throughout his life. Two separate respected Tendai teachers have related that the *reiju* mirrors a

Tendai ritual called *go shimbô* also known as Dharma for Protecting the Body. *Go shimbô* is a purification process and is one of the first Mikkyô rituals that one completes. These esoteric teachings are passed from teacher to student and are not available for the general public.

Hiroshi Doi writes, 'As a result of extensive study and experiments, he [Mikao Usui] successfully developed techniques for passing on Reiki hô (*Reiju*) and for heightening spirituality (**hatsurei hô*). In these techniques, some of the techniques in kôshin dô and Mikkyô are incorporated.'[107]

Another Japanese Tendai teacher explained that over the years there have been many small healing schools and practices that in some way are offshoots of the Mikkyô tradition, and that they all claim connection to Tendai for their orthodoxy.

Purpose of *Reiju*

Mikao Usui created the *reiju* to give people tools to reconnect to their original nature and heal themselves. *Reiju* was just the first step. The recipients were also asked to practice with the mind and the body using the five precepts and *waka* and the physical techniques respectively. Those that repeatedly practiced these elements and received ongoing *reiju* naturally became students of Mikao Usui.

The *reiju* ritual that Mikao Usui practiced did not use symbols or mantras.

The same *reiju* is repeated at each meeting of the student and teacher. This confirms the understanding that students take in as much energy as they can at each *reiju*. By receiving repeated *reiju* the students enhance their own energy levels. The teacher is merely a channel for the energy to move through. Though this is true – the more the teacher energetically evolves, the higher the vibration level is and the more energy that is channeled. This also supports the notion that the teacher does not have any special 'power' over the students – personal development is solely up to the student and the amount of work that the student completes. Traditionally the study of Mikao Usui's teachings in Japan is not taken lightly and is a commitment that one might carry throughout one's life. The practitioner must be fully aware of

---

[107] *Modern Reiki Method for Healing*, Hiroshi Doi, Fraser Journal Publishing, 2000.

what he/she is doing and why, before learning the *reiju*. Chris Marsh said that the *reiju* is performed in a state of mindfullness, with compassion, unconditionally without attachment to any given outcome. If the giver is not in the right place spiritually and emotionally they should not be giving *reiju* at all.

Types of *Reiju*

Below are three major directions that have evolved from Mikao Usui's teachings within Japan.

The 12 Living Students of Mikao Usui

There are said to be 12 students of Mikao Usui still alive. Suzuki san is the only one who has taught Mikao Usui's teachings to a Westerner. Chris Marsh (martial arts practitioner and professional musician) is her student and he is passing on the information, with her consent, that she has shown and spoken to him about. When Chris Marsh met all 12 students he received *reiju* from each individual.

Usui Reiki Ryôhô Gakkai

The Usui Reiki Ryôhô Gakkai performs *reiju* at each gathering of members. This is not to say that this society uses the exact attunement that Mikao Usui developed. Within the society it is also likely that changes have been made throughout the last century.

Hiroshi Doi claims that the *reiju* is the same for each level – there are no differences as it is the student's ability to draw on more energy that creates the differences not the *reiju* itself. No symbols or mantras are used in the *reiju* and it is definitely not based on the Indian chakra system.

At the URRI[108] workshop 1999 Hiroshi Doi taught a *reiju* that he said was re-created from that used by Kimiko Koyama, sixth President of the Usui Reiki Ryôhô Gakkai. There are also similarities between this 'created' *reiju* and the *reiju* used by Suzuki san.

[108] Usui Reiki Ryôhô International is an organization that promotes traditional Japanese Reiki teachers and their teachings through workshops that are held annually in different countries throughout the world.

At the URRI workshop 2002 Hiroshi Doi taught what he called the *'Original Usui Reiju Used in Gakkai'*. It is a different *reiju* to his earlier presentation in 1999.

Whichever *reiju* the Usui Reiki Ryôhô Gakkai practice it is likely to be closer to the original than that used in the West as it has been kept within the one community.

Chûjirô Hayashi

Chûjirô Hayashi was a student of Mikao Usui and was also a member of the Usui Reiki Ryôhô Gakkai. He broke away from it in 1931 to create his own clinic.

Hawayo Takata studied with Chûjirô Hayashi from 1936 to 1938 and thereafter took the teachings to the West.

In the West what is called an attunement today might be one of a multitude of different attunement versions. There are in fact so many that are being taught that no one is really sure what the 'original' is. Most are re-creations of re-creations of re-creations ... Some practitioners have added more symbols to the attunements, others extend the process to include extra movements and unending repetition, link individual attunements to chakras or include the playing of singing bowls etc ...

This uncertainty promotes a disregard for this mystical process leaving it open for more distortions.

Albeit that there are so many versions of attunements[109] there are also general similarities in the Western attunement:

- The use of mantras and symbols
- Each level has a slightly altered attunement

These elements denote a distinctly different ritual to the *reiju* taught by Mikao Usui.

This tells us one thing: the attunements have all came from one source – Chûjirô Hayashi via his student Hawayo Takata.

To further back this up there are the similarities of attunements from two more students of Chûjirô Hayashi. One is Tatsumi who taught a simpler, non-elaborate attunement. The other is Chiyoko

---

[109] It is possible to buy manuals on the Internet with over 20 different attunement processes in them.

Yamaguchi who, until the age of 82 was teaching in Kyôto. Chiyoko Yamaguchi's attunement is simpler still with only 2 hand positions. Both Tatsumi and Chiyoko Yamaguchi[110] use symbols and mantras and alter the attunement for each level. Therefore, the attunement process can be traced back to Chûjirô Hayashi. Though Chiyoko Yamaguchi does not use Symbol 4 in her attunement.

It is unknown whether Mikao Usui taught Chûjirô Hayashi this ritual or if he created it himself. It is known that Japanese practitioners today say that the West practices Hayashi's Reiki not Usui's teachings. It may be the case that Chûjirô Hayashi took the *reiju* and adapted it to fit in with his idea of teaching over a short period of time. This is unlike the Usui Reiki Ryôhô Gakkai who repeat *reiju* at each meeting.

Chûjirô Hayashi may have believed that he made the *reiju* more 'powerful' by including the symbols and mantras into the process. This, therefore, allowed students to receive their certificates at the end of the 5-day training without the obligation of any ongoing meetings, tutoring or repeated performing of *reiju*.

This particular arrangement is very much a forerunner to the Western style of teaching where there is no continuity of study with the teacher. It is also representative of the concept that symbols add more 'power' to one's Reiki practice. Traditionally, mantras and symbols are not considered to be 'powerful' but simply to aid in the understanding of energy. This Western misconception may very well have begun in the practice of Chûjirô Hayashi.

There have been suggestions that Chûjirô Hayashi was actually unaware of the exact workings of the *reiju* and therefore created his own ritual and that is what is called an attunement today. The basis for this statement is that he only studied with Mikao Usui for the limited period of 10 months. According to Chris Marsh, there is a record stating that Chûjirô Hayashi started *shinpiden* in 1925. As Mikao Usui died not long after this there is the suggestion that he may not have finished this training and therefore may not have learnt the *reiju*. Toshitaka Mochizuki states in his book, *Iyashi No Te*

[110] Chiyoko Yamaguchi does not teach DKM and Symbol 4 or use them in the attunement – this might be because she was taught by a relative and never formally learnt *shinpiden* or because Chûjirô Hayashi altered his teaching of the mantras and symbols and attunements according to who his students were.

(Healing Hands), in 1995, that Chûjirô Hayashi was one of 19 teachers appointed by Mikao Usui before he died.

Saihôji Temple

Of late the fellow disciples consulted with each other about building the stone memorial in a graveyard at Saihôji Temple in Toyotama gun so as to honor his merits and to make them immortalized

(Excerpt from Mikao Usui's Memorial Stone, translated by Hyakuten Inamoto.)

Mikao Usui's memorial is at the Pure Land Buddhist Saihôji Temple in Tôkyô. The exact address is Toyotama district, 1-4-56 Umesato, Suginami Ku, Tôkyô.

Here the memorial stone can be seen that was engraved and erected by his students in February 1927, one year after his death. The ashes for the Usui family are also placed here.[111]

This is a site that all students of Mikao Usui's teachings would do well to visit. The peace and serenity of the Saihôji Temple is a wonderful reminder of the origins of these teachings. The connection to their past is here to be experienced, steeped in Japanese culture.

Most funeral ceremonies held in Japan are Buddhist. The body is first cremated with the relatives picking the bones out of the ashes with chopsticks and passing them from person to person.

A meal may be offered to the guests at the crematorium. The actual funeral then takes place. Guests offer money to the relatives and receive a small gift in return. A final meal is taken.

The urn filled with ashes is placed on an altar at the family's house for 35 days. Incense sticks are burned around the clock and, during this period, visitors drop by to burn a stick of incense and extend their sympathy to the family.

Finally, after the 35 days, the urn is buried at a Buddhist gravesite. There are many occasions throughout the year when family members visit their ancestors' gravesites.

[111] Dave King alleges that only some of Mikao Usui's ashes are at this site and the rest are in a secret shrine in Tôkyô. The Japanese practitioners the authors spoke to were unaware of the existence of another shrine.

Directions to the Gravesite

To find Mikao Usui's gravesite take the metro to the shin koenji station. Leave the station through the south exit. If you're unsure which is north or south then it is best to take note which direction you are coming from. If you are arriving from the Tôkyô central direction then exit from the left side of the train.

At the south exit turn to the right and follow the sidewalk. At the first main road cross over the street to your right. Here there is a small side street with the numbers 1-4-56 written on the signpost.

Walk down this street until you arrive at its end. To your right is the shingled roof of the entrance gate to the Saihôji Temple.

Walk under the gate and straight ahead of you is the main temple. To your right is the central path of the memorial grounds. Begin to walk along this central path and immediately to your right you will find an alcove where you can purify yourself with the aid of a wooden ladle and water from the temple well.

This method of purification is offered to all who visit the Saihôji Temple (and is a general rule of etiquette in temples throughout Japan). The ladle is provided to scoop up the water to wash the visitors' hands and mouth. Do remember that it is impolite to drink this water. The correct custom is to scoop water holding the ladle in your right hand and wash your left hand. Take the ladle in your left hand and now wash the right hand. Return the ladle to your right hand and place some water in your left hand using it to rinse your mouth out. Shake the ladle sideways. The little remaining water will remove any dirt that may have become attached to your hands from the handle.

Wooden pails line the walls of the alcove and visitors pump them full of water from the temple well.

Carry the pail of water and ladle with you as you return to walking down the central path. This graveyard is cool and green – dotted with large trees. People wander along its cobbled pathways visiting those who are no longer with them in their daily lives.

When you pass a red wall turn to the left. Follow this path, and then take the second path to the left. You are almost there. Look up and you can see the large memorial stone dedicated to the life and works of Mikao Usui peering through the pine trees. It is the second site on your right.

Follow the short path into the gravesite. It is about 10 by 10 feet (3½ × 3½ metres) in size. To your right a red berry tree stands next to a stone lantern or *tôrô*. *Tôrô* were first brought to Japan from China in the sixth century along with the introduction of Buddhism. Though they come in all shapes and sizes their one common factor is the hollow upper tier that is used for illumination purposes where a candle or oil lamp can be placed.

There is also a great granite-like stone on the ground with a fist sized indentation in its center that gathers the daily dew dripped from overhanging pine trees.

In front of you is the altar and gravesite marker. Here students come to demonstrate their respect to the man who has reminded them of their connection to the source. Purify the altar with the water ladled from your pail. Light your incense and place flowers in both of the vases.

Below, and in front of, this altar, the Usui family Chiba crest or *mon* can be seen elegantly carved out of stone. The Chiba crest is a circle with a dot at the top. The circle represents the universe, and the dot or Japanese star represents the North Star. The North Star never moves while the universe circumambulates it. These crests are handed down from generation to generation and originated in the eleventh century when soldiers affixed them to the banners that they carried into battle. There are around 200 basic crests in Japan today with about 4000 individual variations. The most famous crest is the 16-petalled chrysanthemum inherited by the Imperial family.

At the back of the altar is a rectangular pole about 6 feet high. On the front side it states that this marker is the gravestone for the entire Usui family. This marker was erected one month after the memorial stone had been placed at the site by students from the Usui Reiki Ryôhô Gakkai.

The left side of the marker has written the posthumous names of both Mikao Usui and his wife, Sadako. Mikao Usui's name, given after his death, is *Reizan-in Shuyo Tenshin Koji* 靈山院秀誉天心居士.

The back of the marker explains when the marker was erected and by whom. This was exactly one year after Mikao Usui's death on 9 March 1927. It was their son, Fuji, who erected the marker. On the left side of the marker is the inscription recording the date of the death of their daughter, Toshiko Usui. Between the *tôrô* and the gravesite marker is a small square tablet raised off the ground. This is the gravesite marker for their son, Fuji Usui.

Turn to your left and there the great monolithic memorial stone stands. Composed by Masayuki Okada with brush strokes written by Jûzaburô Ushida[112] in 1927.

This memorial relates the story of Mikao Usui's life – his trials and accomplishments. It also recounts his basic teachings of the five precepts, and reminds all that the purpose of his teachings was not just to heal illnesses but also to combine a right mind and a healthy body. This in turn creates enjoyment and happiness in life.[113]

Mikao Usui
9 March 1926

Sadako Usui
17 October 1946

Toshiko Usui
23 September 1935 (22 years old)

Fuji Usui
10 July 1946 (39 years old)

Reiki Ryôhô Hikkei

Our Reiki Ryôhô is something absolutely original and cannot be compared with any other (spiritual) path in the world.

(Excerpt from the *Reiki Ryôhô Hikkei* as translated in Frank Arjava Petter's book,
Reiki – The Legacy of Dr Usui.)

[112] Jûzaburô Ushida was the second President of the Usui Reiki Ryôhô Gakkai.
[113] There is a full translation of the Mikao Usui Memorial Stone, translated by Hyakuten Inamoto, on page 339.

What is the *Reiki Ryôhô Hikkei*?

Frank Arjava Petter first wrote about the manual he came across in Japan in his book *Reiki, The Legacy of Dr. Usui* in 1998. This was yet another eye opener for Reiki practitioners in the West. First there had been the discovery of the wonderfully informative memorial stone and now there were actual written notes. The surprise was great, namely, because Hawayo Takata had said that the system of Reiki was an oral tradition and allowed no note taking in her classes.[114]

The *Reiki Ryôhô Hikkei (Spiritual Energy Healing Method Manual)* is a 68-page document divided up into four sections that is handed out to *shoden* (Level 1) members.[115] It is comprised of an introduction or explanation by Mikao Usui with the five precepts; a question and answer section with Mikao Usui; the *Ryôhô Shishin*, or *Healing Method's Guideline*, with specific hand positions; and the *gyosei* (*waka*, poetry, of the Meiji Emperor).

Origins of the *Reiki Ryôhô Hikkei*

Kimiko Koyama[116] published this teaching manual for the fiftieth anniversary of the Usui Reiki Ryôhô Gakkai. It is still handed out to members today and is also available on the 'black market' in Japan at an expensive price.[117]

Recently some practitioners have alleged that the *Reiki Ryôhô Hikkei* may not have come from Mikao Usui at all. Elements of the manual are certain to have been derived from Mikao Usui as another manual from around the 1920s has also turned up.[118] The term manual is used loosely here. It is in fact a number of handouts comprised of the *gokai* or five precepts, meditations and over 100 *gyosei* (*waka*, poetry, from

[114] Though this is said to be the case a number of her students did receive a manual called the *Ryôhô Shishin* written by Chûjirô Hayashi. It appears to be almost identical to the healing guide in the *Reiki Ryôhô Hikkei*.

[115] Frank Arjava Petter included only three sections in the book *Reiki – the Legacy of Dr Usui* and placed the fourth section, the *Ryôhô Shishin*, in a later book called *The Original Reiki Handbook of Dr Mikao Usui*.

[116] Kimiko Koyama was the sixth President of the Usui Reiki Ryôhô Gakkai.

[117] The *Reiki Ryôhô Hikkei* is available at this website: http://member.nifty.ne.jp/okojo/hikkei.htm.

[118] Information supplied to the authors by Andrew Bowling's website: www.usuireiki.fsnet.co.uk.

the Meiji Emperor). There are no specific hand positions included in this manual. The meditations in this manual were not printed in the later *Reiki Ryôhô Hikkei* either. From this it can be seen what changes may have occurred within Mikao Usui's teachings. Most obviously the earlier teachings were focused on self-development and the latter teachings on healing others. The meditations are definitely to aid the student's own ability while the healing guide directs the practitioner when working on clients. No one is certain at what point these latter teachings took place and whether it was during Mikao Usui's lifetime or not. In many ways it is irrelevant whether the manual was formed during Mikao Usui's lifetime or not. It is understood that it is a representation of Mikao Usui's teachings in the late 1920s and 1930s.

Reiki Ryôhô Hikkei Summarized

Below is a brief summary of what is included in the Usui Reiki Ryôhô Gakkai manual called the *Reiki Ryôhô Hikkei*.

Part I – *Usui Reiki Ryôhô Kyôgi* or *Usui Spiritual Energy Healing Method Doctrine*
This is an explanation by Mikao Usui as to why he taught publicly.

He maintains that the happiness of humanity is based on two elements: working together and the desire for social progress. This cannot happen if any one individual attempts to possess Reiki.

This method is original and cannot be compared with any other spiritual path and therefore it should be available for all.

Through this spiritual method people will become happy and healthy and that is something that is clearly needed today (there was a great deal of military action at the turn of the twentieth century in Japan).

Part II – Explanation of Instruction for the Public
The origins of this section may lie in the system where students wrote their questions for Mikao Usui in their 'manuals' and consequently also wrote the answers once they were provided. In those days there were no photocopiers to quickly print off information for students and everything was hand written. Below is a condensed version of Mikao Usui's responses:

- Mind and body are one. Once the spirit is healed, humanity will find its true path resulting in a healthy body.
- The method is a spiritual secret of freeing the body and mind.
- It is a spiritual and a physical method. Physical in that energy and light radiate from the mouth, the eyes and the hands of the practitioner. This can heal chronic and acute illnesses.
- It is unnecessary to believe in it. Though, even after the first treatment the benefits are noticed and therefore it is only natural to come to believe in it.
- It not only works on physical illness but also bad habits and psychological imbalances. By practicing, students become aligned with God energy, which in turn gives a desire to help fellow human beings.
- Mikao Usui was not initiated into the method by anyone. During fasting he sensed an intense energy and thereafter realized he had been given the spiritual art of healing. He cannot explain how it works scientifically.
- The method does not use medication.
- It is a spiritual method not a scientific one. The part of the body that has the problem just needs to be touched, that's all.
- Allopathic medicine does not treat the spiritual aspect of human beings.
- In 1922, the Japanese Government's position as far as Reiki was concerned was that this method had nothing to do with the medical faculty as it then stood.
- Anyone can learn it; men, women, old and young. Mikao Usui had at the time of writing taught over one thousand students and not one had been unable to practice it. It is simple to learn yet effective to perform.
- First, healing one's self must take place before healing others.
- *Okuden*, the second level, consists of techniques such as tapping, stroking, pressing and distant healing. First enthusiasm for the method must be learnt with much personal practice.

Part III – *Ryôhô Shishin* or *Healing Method's Guideline*
This guide is split into 11 chapters as listed below:
1. Basic Treatment of Specific Body Parts
2. Nerve Disorders
3. Respiratory Disorders
4. Digestive Disorders
5. Circulatory and Cardiovascular Disorders
6. Metabolic Imbalances and Blood Disorders
7. Urogenital Disorders
8. Surgical and Dermatological Disorders
9. Pediatric Disorders
10. Gynecological Disorders
11. Contagious Diseases

Part IV – *125 Gyosei* (*waka*, poetry written by the Meiji Emperor)

Akino yono tuskiwa mukashini kawaranedo
yoni nakihito no ooku narinuru (Tsuki)

> While a moon on an autumnal night remains just
> the same as ever,
> in this world the number of the deceased
> has become larger. (Moon)

Asamidori sumiwataritaru ohzorano
hiroki onoga kokoro to mogana (Ten)

> As a great sky in clear light green
> I wish my heart would be as vast. (Sky)

Atsushitomo iware zarikeri niekaeru
mizutani tateru shizu wo omoheba (Orinifurete)

> Thinking of lowly people standing in a boiling hot
> paddy field
> I hesitate to utter "it's hot". (Upon occasion)

Amata tabi shigurete someshi momijiba wo
tada hitokaze no chirashi kerukana (Rakuyou-fu)

> Maple leaves tinted by frequent showers
> in late autumn
> just a whiff of wind scattered. (Fallen Leaves-Wind)

Shiori

Along with this manual, Usui Reiki Ryôhô Gakkai members also receive the *shiori*. This is a booklet exclusively for members and was written by Hôichi Wanami[119] and Kimiko Koyama. It contains:[120]

- The purpose, history and administrative system of the Usui Reiki Ryôhô Gakkai and includes the names of 11 of the 21 shinpiden students taught by Mikao Usui.
- How to strengthen Reiki and includes techniques such as *byôsen reikan hô*, *gedoku hô*, *kôketsu hô*, and *nentatsu hô*.
- A teaching from Mikao Usui.
- A guide to treatment.
- Characteristics of Reiki Ryôhô (Spiritual Energy Healing Method).
- Remarks by medical doctors.
- Explanation of the *Ryôhô Shishin (Healing Method's Guideline)*.

---

[119] Hôichi Wanami was the fifth President of the Usui Reiki Ryôhô Gakkai.

[120] Information supplied to the authors by Hyakuten Inamoto.

6   Reiki in Japan

Post Mikao Usui

The Private Teachings

Mikao Usui died in 1926 leaving his legacy, his teachings, to the world. He once said that he wished to 'release this method to the public for everyone's benefit'.[1] His intention has been realized with practitioners in every country of the world today. Yet, in Japan itself, there has been a reticence to bring his teachings into the public eye by many traditional Japanese practitioners.

There were only a handful of books written by Mikao Usui's students in the first half of the last century. Some of these were:

- *Te No Hira Ryôji Nyûmon (Introduction to healing with the palms)*, Toshihiro Eguchi and Kohshi Mitsui, 1930
- *Reiki To Jinjutsu – Tomita Ryû Teate Ryôhô (Reiki and Humanitarian Work – Tomita Ryû Hands Healing)*, Kaiji Tomita, 1933
- *Te No Hira Ryôji Wo Kataru (A story of healing with the palms)*, Toshihiro Eguchi, 1954

Looking at the system of Reiki in the West it can be difficult to see where it connects to what was once practiced in Japan in the early 1900s. So many alterations and additions by so many individuals

[1] Information supplied by the *Reiki Ryôhô Hikkei*.

have created a method that Mikao Usui would not recognize as his teachings. Aura cleansings, dragon breaths and the chakra system were not a part of his vocabulary. These changes may also not have been welcomed by traditional Japanese practitioners. Fundamental Japanese culture is based on respect. Within that there is a deep respect for the *kokoro* or the true nature of Mikao Usui's teachings. Traditional Japanese practitioners are respectful and protective of them. For this reason it has been difficult to trace the teachings in Japan. Once they moved to the West they spread like a wild fire that could not be contained (especially after Hawayo Takata's death in 1980). The system of Reiki as it is practiced in the West is perceived to have lost touch with its *kokoro*. For example, in America one teacher has 'Reiki Master' on the number plates of his car. This type of foreign approach has validated and strengthened many traditional Japanese practitioners belief's that Mikao Usui's teachings should be practiced quietly, without advertising and within the parameters of the culture.

> Focus on your feet rather than getting on a horse
> Focus on your ki rather than your feet
> Focus on kokoro rather than your ki
>
> (Excerpt from Funakoshi Gichin in 'Tanpenshu'
> by Patrick and Yuriko McCarthy.)

When the American born Hawayo Takata wanted to learn Chûjirô Hayashi's teachings in Japan in 1935–36 she was told that she could not become a practitioner because she was a foreigner. After proving her sincerity and commitment to his teachings she was made an exception to the rule. An article written by a student of Chûjirô Hayashi in Japan in 1928[2] (just two years after Mikao Usui's death) said that Usui Reiki Ryôhô Gakkai members do not like to advertise or to make their teachings public. It seems their attitude has not changed up until today.

---

[2] 'A Treatment to Heal Diseases, Hand Healing', Shûô Matsui in the magazine *Sunday Mainichi*, 4 March 1928, translated by Amy, to be viewed at www.reiki.net.au.

Traditional Teachers

Exactly who these traditional Japanese practitioners are today is somewhat unclear because of their lack of interest in standing in the public arena. Throughout the last decade interest in traditional Japanese practitioners has been growing. Prior to this there was little curiosity due to a claim in America that Hawayo Takata was the only Reiki Master in the world.[3]

The names of 11 of 21[4] teacher students of Mikao Usui have been recorded in a booklet used by the Usui Reiki Ryôhô Gakkai called the *shiori*.[5] From those 21 stem a small number of traditional Japanese practitioners claiming to teach what he taught without Western influence. There have been many other Japanese offshoots of Mikao Usui's teachings but they are no longer directly linked to him.

The most well known group, though reclusive, stemming directly from Mikao Usui is the Usui Reiki Ryôhô Gakkai. The Usui Reiki Ryôhô Gakkai was comprised of naval men as its senior members plus Mikao Usui himself (according to the Usui Reiki Ryôhô Gakkai). Thanks to one of its recent members, Hiroshi Doi, there has been a better understanding in the West of how that society practices and what this might mean for the system of Reiki in the West. Interestingly, in the 1930s it was one of the Usui Reiki Ryôhô Gakkai, Chûjirô Hayashi, who crossed out of Japan and into the West with the American student, Hawayo Takata. This was the first step into the West for these teachings.

A couple of Chûjirô Hayashi's students are still alive, though elderly. Chiyoko Yamaguchi[6] is in her 80s and was taught Levels 1 and 2 by Chûjirô Hayashi. Many of her family members were practitioners and from one of them she was taught to perform the attunement. Chiyoko Yamaguchi assists her son, Tadao, teaching a style that they now call Jikiden Reiki. Also alive are some of their family members who are practitioners but are not teachers in the system.

---

[3] Advertising Poster for a workshop by Hawayo Takata states: The Only Teacher of the Usui System of Reiki in the World Today, 27-31 July 1975.

[4] Hiroshi Doi states that there were 21 teacher students of Mikao Usui while Toshitaka Mochizuki suggests 19 in his book, *Iyashi No Te*.

[5] For more information about what is included in the *shiori* see page 11.

[6] Chiyoko Yamaguchi died at the age of 82 in August, 2003.

Students of Mikao Usui are alleged to still be alive today. At present there is little known about them directly but their information is being passed on to the West through a small number of practitioners. Suzuki san, born in 1895, is one of this group of 12 students of Mikao Usui who are still alive today. She has only just begun to pass on notes and teachings to the general public via a student.

Another nun, Mariko Obaasan, also known as Tenon in, was born in late 1897, and is from a group of five nuns who may have studied with Mikao Usui. One of these five nuns, Yuri in, who was born in 1896, is said to have died in 1997. There are said to be more traditional teachers in Japan. Masaharu Ueno (a President of Cosmo Bright) and Mr Okajima (manager of Modern Reiki Healing Center in Osaka) both claim to have received *reiju* early on in their lives.[7]

Popularity of Hands-on Healing

According to Toshitaka Mochizuki's book, *Iyashi No Te (Healing Hands)*, tens of millions of people have been affected by Mikao Usui's teachings over the past 100 years.

Some of the better-known hands on healers who trained with Mikao Usui in Japan were Toshihiro Eguchi and Kaiji Tomita.

Toshihiro Eguchi was a friend of Mikao Usui and may have studied with him in 1921, returning in 1923 to present his own healing concepts.[8] It is also said that he studied from 1925 to 1927, first with Mikao Usui and after his death, with his school.[9] In 1928, he left the Usui Reiki Ryôhô Gakkai and with his experience as a schoolteacher established his own *Tenohira Ryoji Kenkyû Kai* (Hand Healing Research Center). It's believed he ran a healing community called Ittoen for a number of years. Reiki practitioners are currently conducting research into this subject, as it appears he may have had a greater influence on the Western system of Reiki than was previously believed.[10] It is unknown whether he actually studied through to the teacher level with Mikao Usui. Hiroshi Doi has stated that he did

[7] *Modern Reiki Method for Healing*, Hiroshi Doi, Fraser Journal Publishing, 2000.
[8] Information supplied to the authors by Dave King's website: www.usui-do.org.
[9] *Modern Reiki Method for Healing*, Hiroshi Doi, Fraser Journal Publishing, 2000.
[10] Information supplied to the authors by Chris Marsh.

not study to this level. Toshihiro Eguchi introduced hundreds of thousands of students to his style of hands-on healing. In Japan, a number of his students such as Yasukiyo Eguchi, Kohshi Mitsui and Goro Miyazaki are also well known.[11] Goro Miyazaki taught Mieko Mitsui who taught The Radiance Technique in New York and Japan – a Western form of Reiki founded by Barbara Weber Ray.

Kaiji Tomita studied Mikao Usui's teachings around 1925 and founded *Tomita Teate Ryôhô* (Tomita Hands-on Healing Method). Kaiji Tomita taught Reiki in four levels – *shoden, chuden, okuden* and *kaiden*. Each level required five days (two hours for each day) to be completed. The last level, *kaiden*, required 15 days. Kaiji Tomita wrote a book in 1933 called *Reiki To Jinjutsu – Tomita Ryû Teate Ryôhô* (*Reiki and Humanitarian Work – Tomita Ryû Hands Healing*). It describes around 20 case histories, a major technique that he uses to generate energy called **hatsurei hô* and a five-day plan to work on yourself. It is a technical book with many hand positions for specific illnesses listed. He had more than 200,000 students and his most famous student was Asuke Jiro who wrote, *Therapy with Hands*.[12]

Toshitaka Mochizuki actually claims that Mikao Usui was the nucleus from which many other forms of spiritual healing took place in the early 1900s in Japan. Some of these other spiritual healing groups working at the time were:[13]

Tairedô by Morihei Tanaka
Jintai Rajiumu Gakkai (Human Radium Society) by Dobetsu Matsumoto
Shinnôkyô Honin by Taiman Nishimura
Toyo Jindo Kyokai by Shunnichi Ema
Teikoku Shinrei Kenkyû Kai (Imperial Society of the Spirit) by Kinji Kuwata
Dainihon Tenmei Gakuin (Japanese Tenmei Institute) by Kumagoku Hamaguchi
Shurei Tanshinkai by Saiko Fujita
Seido Gakkai by Reizen Ôyama
Reiki Kangen Ryôin by Koyo Watanabe

[11] *Iyashi No Te*, Toshitaka Mochizuki, Tama Shuppan, 1995.
[12] *Modern Reiki Method for Healing*, Hiroshi Doi, Fraser Journal Publishing, 2000.
[13] *Iyashi No Te*, Toshitaka Mochizuki, Tama Shuppan, 1995.

Nipon Shinrei Gakkai (Japanese Society of the Spirit) by Tôko Watanabe
Shinshin Kaizen Kôshû Kai (Psychophysical Improvement Academy) by Reizen Yoshiwaza
Reidô Shûyô Kai by Shûsen Oguri
Shizen Reinô Kenkyû Kai (Institute of Investigation of the Natural Mystical Capacity) by Reikô Takeda
Shizenryô Nôryokuhô Denshû Kai (Institute of the Capacity of Natural Therapies) by Reijin Oze
Seiki Ryôhô Kenkyû jo (Institute of Treatment of Spirit) by Jôzô Ishi
Katsurei Kai by Yoshikatsu Matsuda
Dainihon Reigaku Kenkyû Kai (Japanese Institute of Studies of the Spirit) by Reikô Saito
Yôki Jutsuryôin by Yoshitaro Ueda
Reinôin by Reisei Katayama

Many of the founders of these hands-on healing schools changed their first names to indicate the field that they worked in. For example the names Reizen, Reikô, Reijin and Reisei all allude to working with spiritual energy.

At the turn of the twentieth century there were also a number of spiritual movements in Japan that influenced each other. Some of these were the Seiki therapy, Fuji System, Ishii system and the Master Masaharu Taniguchi's Seicho No Ie (The Home of Infinite Life, Wisdom and Abundance).[14]

Usui Reiki Ryôhô Gakkai[15]

… the Society's goal was 'keeping good health and enhancement of body and spirit. Peace prosperity and happiness in family, society, country and world'.

(Excerpt from *Modern Reiki Method for Healing* by Hiroshi Doi.)

---

[14] *Iyashi No Te*, Toshitaka Mochizuki, Tama Shuppan, 1995.

Usui Reiki Ryôhô Gakkai Members

The memorial to Mikao Usui, which was erected in 1927, writes that students remained in Tôkyô and carried on practicing and teaching after his death. Their group was called the Usui Reiki Ryôhô Gakkai or Society of the Usui Spiritual Energy Healing Method. This society they claim began with Mikao Usui as President in April 1922[16] followed, after his death, by Jûzaburô Ushida.[17] Today this society has its seventh President.

Some researchers believe that Mikao Usui was not the first president of the Usui Reiki Ryôhô Gakkai and that it was in fact founded after his death.[18] It is understood that Mikao Usui formalized his teachings after his meditation on *kurama yama* in March 1922 but whether this was the inauguration of the Usui Reiki Ryôhô Gakkai or simply the creation of his official seat of learning is as yet unknown.

The early members of the Usui Reiki Ryôhô Gakkai appear to mainly be naval officers. The military was quite powerful at this period in Japanese history. First there was World War I and then there was a build up toward the military conflict with China in Manchuria. Japan was expanding its borders and a large sum of the male Japanese population was involved. The military held influential positions in the society. It has been suggested that Mikao Usui was pressurized into teaching many of the naval men. This may be a reason for the more practical and basic elements of his teachings that evolved – such as the hand positions.[19]

Here is a list of Presidents and their details from Mikao Usui to modern day:[20]

---

[15] Much of the information gathered in this chapter about the Usui Reiki Ryôhô Gakkai has been passed down from Hiroshi Doi to his translator and students. Frank Arjava Petter and Dave King have also shed light on traditional teachings in Japan.

[16] *Modern Reiki Method for Healing*, Hiroshi Doi, Fraser Journal Publishing, 2000.

[17] Jûzaburô Ushida wrote the brushstrokes for the text for Mikao Usui's Memorial Stone.

[18] Information supplied to the authors by Andrew Bowling's website: www.usuireiki.fsnet.co.uk.

[19] Information supplied to the authors by Andrew Bowling's website: www.usuireiki.fsnet.co.uk.

[20] *Iyashi No Te*, Toshitaka Mochizuki, Tama Shuppan, 1995.

1. Mikao Usui (1865–1926)
2. Jûzaburô Ushida (Rear Admiral 1865–1935)
3. Kanichi Taketomi (Rear Admiral 1878–1960)
4. Yoshiharu Watanabe (Schoolteacher ? –1960)
5. Hôichi Wanami (Vice Admiral 1883–1975)
6. Kimiko Koyama (1906–99)
7. Masaki Kondô (University Professor)

An ex-Naval surgeon called Chûjirô Hayashi joined the Usui Reiki Ryôhô Gakkai in May 1925. He broke away in 1931 further developing his own branch called the *Hayashi Reiki Kenkyû Kai*.

In November 1925 Jûzaburô Ushida and Kanichi Taketomi, both naval men, became members of Mikao Usui's seat of learning.[21]

Fumio Ogawa joined the Usui Reiki Ryôhô Gakkai in 1942 and completed six levels in 14 months. His certificates were displayed in a Japanese magazine called *Twilight Zone* in 1986.[22]

Hiroshi Doi said that during World War II the Usui Reiki Ryôhô Gakkai moved quite often because of aerial bombing. It has also been suggested that the Usui Reiki Ryôhô Gakkai needed to be careful in case it became associated with the underground Peace movement. During World War II, naval members could no longer participate in meetings but the Usui Reiki Ryôhô Gakkai did have members who were not naval men and has continued through to modern times.

Usui Reiki Ryôhô Gakkai Teachings

There are three major levels in the Usui Reiki Ryôhô Gakkai. These are *shoden*, *okuden* and *shinpiden*, the teacher level.[23] Within these levels there are six levels of proficiency. The lowest being 6 and the highest being 1. Mikao Usui rated himself as a 2 with the knowledge that there was always more to be achieved. *Shoden* includes the first four levels of proficiency. At each stage new techniques are learnt, with the member progressing to the next level of proficiency on satisfactorily accomplishing the technique.

[21] Information supplied to the authors by Dave King's website: www.usui-do.org.
[22] Information supplied to the authors by Rick Rivard's website: www.threshold.ca/reiki.
[23] For more information about the traditional Japanese levels see page 131.

The society's meetings, or *kenkyû kai*, are held three times a month. Once new members receive the regular *reiju* they begin at the sixth level of proficiency. The *reiju* does not change with each level – it remains the same. No mantras or symbols are used in the Usui Reiki Ryôhô Gakkai's *reiju* either. In fact the society does not use mantras and symbols but is aware of them.[24] The mantras and symbols are different to how they are taught in the West.

At each meeting *gyosei* (*waka*, poetry, written by the Meiji Emperor) is read aloud by all members and **hatsurei hô* is practiced. Members receive *reiju* from the *shihan* or senior teacher. At the end, the *gokai* (five precepts) are repeated three times by all present.[25] After the *shûyô kai* there is the *jisshû kai*, the practical gathering, where some techniques are practiced.

Each member is supplied with the *Reiki Ryôhô Hikkei*,[26] which contains the five Reiki precepts, an interview with Mikao Usui, a guide to healing using specific hand positions and *gyosei*. Booklets, *shiori*, are also provided and these are exclusively for Usui Reiki Ryôhô Gakkai members. They were written by Hôichi Wanami and Kimiko Koyama and contain information including original teachings and techniques such as **byôsen reikan hô*, **gedoku hô*, **kôketsu hô*, and **nentatsu hô*.[27]

Usui Reiki Ryôhô Gakkai Protocol

The Usui Reiki Ryôhô Gakkai does not accept foreigners as members and is a very private society. Members are not even meant to tell people that they belong to it.[28] Many requests have been made to the society from Westerners intrigued to know how it works and what its history is but few have met with its members. A Reiki Master calling on Phyllis Lei Furumoto's behalf contacted Hiroshi Doi on 14 De-

---

[24] Information supplied to the authors by Hyakuten Inamoto.
[25] *Modern Reiki Method for Healing*, Hiroshi Doi, Fraser Journal Publishing, 2000.
[26] Information taken from the *Reiki Ryôhô Hikkei* (*Spriutal Energy Healing Method Manual*), a manual that is given to Usui Reiki Ryôhô Gakkai members in Japan. For more information about the *Reiki Ryôhô Hikkei* see page 106.
[27] Information supplied to the authors by Hyakuten Inamoto.
[28] Information supplied to the authors by Hyakuten Inamoto.

cember 1996. Hawayo Takata's granddaughter was to travel to Japan and wanted to meet with the President, Kimiko Koyama, who was 91 at the time. This would have been an historic visit of West meets East but one of Phyllis Lei Furumoto's teacher students made claims that insulted Kimiko Koyama and the meeting was cancelled.[29]

The Usui Reiki Ryôhô Gakkai may be joined by invitation only. At this point the person becomes an honorary member until full membership is offered. The society today charges US$90 on the initial entry to the society and then US$15 at each meeting.[30] There were once 80 divisions of the Usui Reiki Ryôhô Gakkai throughout Japan but today there are only five. All the teaching takes place in Tôkyô itself. There are 11 *shinpiden* in the Usui Reiki Ryôhô Gakkai and that includes the five *shihan* or Masters. The majority of members are long standing and there are only about 500 throughout the whole of Japan.

The society's function today is generally described as a support group for its members. The members are supported on a more personal level than would occur in a school. Hiroshi Doi's first impression was his amazement at how different it was from the Western style Reiki of Mieko Mitsui and yet it still came from the same root.

Chûjirô Hayashi (1880–1940)

Family and Career

Chûjirô Hayashi was born on 15 September, 1880 in Tokyo. He was a Sôtô Zen practitioner who naturally included Shintô practices, as is common in Japan, into his religious routine.[31] He was not a Christian. He was also married with two children. His son, Tadayoshi, was born in 1903 and his daughter, Kiyoe, was born in 1910. In 1902, Chûjirô Hayashi was on harbour patrol during the Russo-Japanese War. In 1918 he became commander of the defence station of Port Owinato.[32]

---

[29] *Modern Reiki Method for Healing*, Hiroshi Doi, Fraser Journal Publishing, 2000.
[30] Information supplied to the authors by Rick Rivard's website: www.threshold.ca/reiki.
[31] Information supplied to the authors by Hyakuten Inamoto.
[32] *Die Reiki-Techniken des Dr. Hayashi*, Petter, Yamaguchi, Hayashi, Windpferd, 2003.

Meeting Mikao Usui

In May 1925, he became a student of Mikao Usui's seat of learning in Tôkyô.[33] He was a retired naval officer (still in the reserves) and surgeon and was about 45 years old when he met Mikao Usui.[34] He had but 10 months to learn the complete teachings before Mikao Usui died of a stroke.

A number of other naval officers joined the same school not long after Chûjirô Hayashi. Once Mikao Usui died they continued on with his work using the title Usui Reiki Ryôhô Gakkai. Chûjirô Hayashi remained as a member until 1931 when he began developing his own clinic and school called the *Hayashi Reiki Kenkyû Kai* or Hayashi Spiritual Energy Research Society. He is said to have left the Usui Reiki Ryôhô Gakkai due to differences with the then President Jûzaburô Ushida.

Chûjirô Hayashi's Clinic

Unique to the system at this time his clinic was known to have a treatment room where eight clients could be treated. These clients would lie down on futons or low tables and have two practitioners working on them. According to Hawayo Takata one would begin at the abdomen and the other at the head. Chûjirô Hayashi's wife, Chie, was the receptionist and hostess. She continued on with his work after he died.[35]

Chûjirô Hayashi's Teachings

Chûjirô Hayashi was known to have a healing guide called the *Ryôhô Shishin*. It appears to be an almost exact copy of the *Reiki Ryôhô Hikkei*'s own healing guide. Today researchers think that Chûjirô Hayashi may well have written the *Reiki Ryôhô Hikkei*'s *Ryôhô Shishin* at Mikao Usui's request. As he was a doctor with knowledge of anatomy and human disease this is not an illogical assumption.

[33] This seat of learning may well have been called the Usui Reiki Ryôhô Gakkai at this stage.
[34] Transcript of tape of Hawayo Takata telling the story of Dr Hayashi, 1977.
[35] Information supplied to the authors by Chiyoko Yamaguchi.

Another student of Chûjirô Hayashi, Tatsumi, trained in 1927 to become a teacher. Tatsumi did not appreciate the changes that Chûjirô Hayashi had made and finally left in 1931. Tatsumi said he was initially taught in a class with five other students and that he often saw Jûzaburô Ushida and Kanichi Taketomi (Usui Reiki Ryôhô Gakkai members) at the school. Kanichi Taketomi was also an officer in 1918 at Port Owinato with Chûjirô Hayashi. Students volunteered in the clinic practicing for eight hours a week on clients. After three months it was possible for them to move to the second level. Nine months later they might progress to the third level and aid in the running of the clinic. After two years students would achieve *Shinpiden* with the knowledge of how to teach and perform attunements.[36] Students received *reiju* in a dark room while sitting in *seiza*. *Waka*, poetry, was then recited before *reiju* was performed. The 5 precepts were then chanted and **reiki mawashi* would be practiced.[37]

Shûô Matsui became a student of Chûjirô Hayashi in 1928. The first level was completed in five lots of one and a half hour sessions. He wrote that it was very expensive and was surprised that the modest people who ran the clinic would charge money and have a grading system. He said he did not intend to begin the second level but shared many stories of people he had helped, over 100 to be exact. Shûô Matsui also mentions that there are more grades but claims that he was unaware of exactly how many there were.[38]

Hawayo Takata's experience with Chûjirô Hayashi was a little more difficult as she was considered to be a foreigner. First, she received treatments for ill health for six months in 1935. In 1936 she volunteered at the clinic over the period of a year while staying at the Hayashi's home. On 21 February 1938, as Chûjirô Hayashi was leaving Hawaii after having helped her to set up a clinic, he awarded her a Master certificate.

Chiyoko Yamaguchi studied with Chûjirô Hayashi in 1938[39]. Many of her family members were already practitioners by that time. She said that she learnt both *shoden* and *okuden* together over five con-

---

[36] Information supplied by Dave King.

[37] *Die Reiki-Techniken des Dr. Hayashi*, Petter, Yamaguchi, Hayashi, Windpferd, 2003.

[38] 'A Treatment to Heal Diseases, Hand Healing' by Shûô Matsui in the magazine *Sunday Mainichi*, 4 March 1928, translated by Amy to be viewed at www.reiki.net.au.

[39] Chiyoko Yamaguchi died at the age of 82 in August, 2003.

secutive days and this is what she teaches in Jikiden Reiki today.[40] This cost 50 yen which was extremely expensive at this time (the equivalent of thousands of US dollars today).[41]

This leads to the conclusion that Chûjirô Hayashi taught *shoden* independently from *okuden* in 1927 with Tatsumi, 1928 with Shûô Matsui and between 1936 and 1938 with Hawayo Takata. In 1938, Chiyoko Yamaguchi was taught *shoden* and *okuden* together over a five-day period.

Unfortunately, Chiyoko Yamaguchi no longer has her certificates and other notes, as they were lost when she and her late husband fled Manchuria at the end of World War II.[42] She has only recently begun teaching students with her son, Tadao, in a branch they have called Jikiden Reiki. It appears she never learnt to become an official teacher but was taught the attunement from a relative who was hosting a course for Chûjirô Hayashi. The mantras and symbols Chiyoko Yamaguchi uses are slightly different to those taught by Tatsumi as well as to those taught by the Usui Reiki Ryôhô Gakkai. Interestingly, she was also not taught Symbol 4. This may be because she did not officially study to become a teacher.[43] It may also indicate that there was no Symbol 4 used in the attunement process at that time.

What is considered to be the system of Reiki in the West is proposed by traditional Japanese practitioners to be Chûjirô Hayashi's teachings rather than Mikao Usui's.

The attunement process that is performed today, in all its variations, utilizes mantras and symbols. This is not the case in the Usui Reiki Ryôhô Gakkai or other traditional Japanese teachings where these methods of attunement are called *reiju* and are practiced without mantras and symbols. This is a major difference between what Chûjirô Hayashi taught and Mikao Usui's teachings.

Mantras and symbols were only taught to those who had difficulty with sensing the energy. Chûjirô Hayashi may have believed that his students who did not have enough experience with energy work were aided by the inclusion of symbols into the ritual.

[40] Information supplied to the authors by Chiyoko Yamaguchi.
[41] Information supplied to the authors by Hyakuten Inamoto.
[42] Information supplied to the authors by Chiyoko Yamaguchi.
[43] Information supplied to the authors by Hyakuten Inamoto.

Though Chûjirô Hayashi changed the teachings his respect for Mikao Usui remained. Even after leaving the Usui Reiki Ryôhô Gakkai, a scroll of the *gokai* was hung in his clinic. Chiyoko Yamaguchi also displays a copy of these precepts in her treatment room and offers a copy to her teacher students.

Chûjirô Hayashi's Legacy

Chûjirô Hayashi wrote in 1938 that he had trained 13 Reiki Masters.[44]

On 10 May 1940 Hawayo Takata reported that he died ceremoniously of a self-induced stroke in his country house in Atami with his family, colleagues and friends around him. Chiyoko Yamaguchi, a student of Chûjirô Hayashi, emphatically recounts that Chie Hayashi had personally told her that he had killed himself by 'breaking an artery'.[45] Others say that as he was a military man the honourable method of death would certainly have been *seppuku* (the cutting of the *hara* or abdomen). Chûjirô Hayashi informed his wife and Hawayo Takata that his reason for suicide was that he did not wish to be called upon to enter World War II.

Chie Hayashi stayed on at her husband's clinic becoming the second President of the *Hayashi Reiki Kenkyû Kai*.[46] Hawayo Takata told a story that she was, in fact, the successor but felt that she could not remain in Japan and asked Chie Hayashi to manage it for her. After World War II, Hawayo Takata stated that she returned it to Chie Hayashi, as she had no desire to live in Japan.

Modern Japan

Westerner Practitioners in Search of their Roots in Japan

The Usui Reiki Ryôhô Gakkai would happily have continued to exist in peace but this was not likely to be the case.

---

[44] Hawayo Takata's Master certificate.
[45] Information supplied to the authors by Chiyoko Yamaguchi.
[46] Information supplied to the authors by Chiyoko Yamaguchi.

Since Hawayo Takata's death in 1980 many foreigners have attempted to contact traditional Japanese practitioners. These curious Westerners have changed the face of the modern system of Reiki in both Japan and the West. This has occurred through the exchanging of information between the two worlds.

Mieko Mitsui, a Japanese Reiki practitioner living in New York, visited her native country in 1985. She began a revival of Reiki in Japan and taught the first two levels of The Radiance Technique[47] to many Japanese. During one stay she met a member of the Usui Reiki Ryôhô Gakkai, most probably Fumio Ogawa. Mieko Mitsui's interest was sparked and she began researching the roots of the system in Japan. There was an article in a Japanese magazine called *Twilight Zone* that had a photo of Fumio Ogawa reading from a book about Reiki.[48] In the same article there was a photo of Mieko Mitsui demonstrating Reiki.

In 1991, Frank Arjava Petter moved to Japan with his Japanese wife, Chetna, to live. Briefly returning to Germany, his homeland, he studied all three levels of the system of Reiki. He claims that before long he became the first teacher to teach all three levels openly in Japan.

From 1993, Frank Arjava Petter and Chetna began researching the system of Reiki's traditional roots. A female member of Mikao Usui's family had left a clause in a will saying that Mikao Usui's name must never be mentioned in her house. Her relative informed Frank Arjava Petter that a number of people had been in contact to find out about Mikao Usui but she preferred to be left alone because of family reasons.[49] One of these people was undoubtedly Mieko Mitsui who had received a similar reception a number of years earlier.[50] Their research also brought them to a current member of the Usui Reiki Ryôhô Gakkai in Japan. She declared that she didn't want anything to do with a system of Reiki that came from outside of Japan. However, she did offer a small amount of information that led them to Mikao Usui's memorial stone in Tôkyô.

---

[47] For more information about Reiki branches see page 171.
[48] Fumio Ogawa was reading a book by Barbara Weber Ray, founder of The Radiance Technique.
[49] *Reiki Fire*, Frank Arjava Petter, Lotus Press, Twin Lakes, 1998.
[50] 1986 article 'Mysterious Report 28' from *The Twilight Zone* by Shiomi Takai – translated by Shiya Fleming for Rick Rivard's website: www.threshold.ca/reiki.

The discovery of Mikao Usui's memorial stone has been a milestone in the history of modern Reiki for hundreds of thousands of practitioners around the world. It is now possible to connect to a tangible history. Funnily enough it appears that Hawayo Takata had told many of her students about the memorial stone but there had never been great interest in it. Fran Brown's book, *Living Reiki – Takata's Teachings*, writes briefly about Mikao Usui's memorial stone and her book was published in 1992 – a number of years before Frank Arjava Petter heard of it and consequently published his first book.

Frank Arjava Petter also gradually made contact with other Japanese people associated with Mikao Usui's traditional teachings in Japan. Among these was Fumio Ogawa who is given a special mention of thanks in Frank Arjava Petter's third book for openheartedly sharing information with him. His stepfather, Kôzô Ogawa, ran a center in Shizuoka for Mikao Usui during his lifetime. Kôzô Ogawa had trained the mother of another contact called Tsutomu Oishi. In 1997, Tsutomu Oishi provided Frank Arjava Petter with a photo of Mikao Usui with the five precepts in the left-hand corner. He also gave a copy of the *Reiki Ryôhô Hikkei* (Frank Arjava Petter translated the *Reiki Ryôhô Hikkei* in two of his first three books).[51]

Dave King first met a student of Toshihiro Eguchi[52] called Yûji Onuki, in Morocco in the 1970s. Both Dave and his friend Melissa studied with him not knowing that what he may have been teaching was a variant on the system of Reiki. In 1995, Dave King met Tatsumi, a teacher student of Chûjirô Hayashi, in an out of the way Japanese village. Tatsumi had become a student of Chûjirô Hayashi's in 1927. Due to the changes in the system that were taking place Tatsumi left Chûjirô Hayashi's clinic in 1931. Though Tatsumi had never taught these teachings he still had the paperwork. These included handwritten notes from Chûjirô Hayashi's teachings and copies of the four traditional symbols. Dave King made copies of Tatsumi's notes and symbols. He was also taught Tatsumi's attunement, which he passed on to Rick Rivard who then taught it to students at the URRI in Vancouver, 1999. This attunement has become popular amongst

---

[51] Information supplied to the authors by Frank Arjava Petter.
[52] Toshihiro Eguchi was a student of Mikao Usui and a well-known healer in his own right. Hiroshi Doi states that he did not attain the teacher level of Mikao Usui's teachings.

practitioners wishing to practice in a more traditional Japanese manner. Today, Dave King denies having passed on the full information relating to the attunement (or transformation as he calls it).[53]

In his most recent research Dave King states that he is in contact with a Tendai nun called Mariko Obaasan who was a student of Mikao Usui.

Another Tendai nun, Suzuki san, is believed to exist and she, too, is teaching some Westerners. Though the two nuns are not said to be the same person – coincidentally they are both over 100 and are Tendai practitioners who have studied with Mikao Usui.

Suzuki san is a member of a group of 12 practitioners who are aged between 98 and 112. She is a cousin of Mikao Usui on his wife's side. The information is intriguing. A student of Suzuki san, Chris Marsh, is writing a book about this group of 12 and their teachings. Hopefully this will completely verify the teachings and add clarity to the understanding of Mikao Usui's life and teachings.

The modern system of Reiki has become increasingly popular in Japan. The majority of it is influenced by either Mieko Mitsui's Radiance Technique or Frank Arjava Petter's Independent style of Reiki – both Western based.

Japanese Practitioners Contact the West

Andrew Bowling was inquisitive about the system of Reiki in Japan. One day he noticed an e-mail address from Japan on a Reiki forum list on the Internet. Curious, he contacted the Japanese practitioner. This practitioner connected him with someone who had a fascinating story. His name was Hiroshi Doi and he was a member of the Usui Reiki Ryôhô Gakkai, a traditional society. He said that the Usui Reiki Ryôhô Gakkai was created by Mikao Usui and was in no way affiliated with the system of Reiki that was taught in the West. Gradually, he began to share information about the history of the teachings in Japan and the place of the Usui Reiki Ryôhô Gakkai within that. Andrew Bowling then teamed up with Rick Rivard and Tom Rigler to spread this exciting information throughout the West with Hiroshi Doi's approval.[54]

---

[53] Information supplied to the authors by Dave King.
[54] Information supplied to the authors by the article, 'Andy's Story', www.reiki.net.au.

Hiroshi Doi has influenced both Japan and the West in recent times. He is the initiator of what is known as Usui Reiki Ryôhô. This new branch of Reiki is based on the techniques and concepts of traditional teachings from Mikao Usui and the Usui Reiki Ryôhô Gakkai. The Usui Reiki Ryôhô Gakkai no longer practices all of the techniques taught in this branch. There has also been confusion between what is Usui Reiki Ryôhô Gakkai information and what is from Hiroshi Doi himself. Hiroshi Doi's own interest is in combining what he considers to be the best aspects of both the Western and Japanese systems of Reiki. Today he teaches his own branch of Reiki called Gendai Reiki Hô, which exemplifies this objective.

Hiroshi Doi was interested in all sorts of energy techniques and has studied many facets of it. His own history as he explained includes a number of different energetic lineages.

Interestingly, in 1982, he learnt a method called *teate*, which later turned out to be teachings from the Usui Reiki Ryôhô Gakkai. His teacher, Hiroshi Ohta, had unofficially been taught by Asaka Sasaki. Asaka Sasaki, a Usui Reiki Ryôhô Gakkai teacher from the Hiroshima section, taught unofficially. In post-World War II Japan, the society had temporarily been closed. As a result, Hiroshi Ohta was allowed to teach but not as a certified Usui Reiki Ryôhô Gakkai teacher.

Hiroshi Doi was also one of the first Japanese to study Levels 1 and 2 with Mieko Mitsui. She taught Barbara Weber Ray's Radiance Technique but was only permitted to teach the first two levels. He then went on to study all three levels of a system of Reiki called Neo Reiki (another branch that mixes both Western and Japanese styles together) with Manaso.[55]

His interest heightened by his experiences with the system of Reiki, Hiroshi Doi was fortunate to meet a member of the Usui Reiki Ryôhô Gakkai at a crystal workshop. This was his introduction to the society and he officially joined on 22 October 1993. Here he studied with Kimiko Koyama, the society's sixth President before she died in December 1999. It is the Usui Reiki Ryôhô Gakkai lineage that Hiroshi Doi uses today, with their consent, although he is not officially a teacher in the society. Hiroshi Doi continues broadening his Reiki

---

[55] Manaso learnt from Osho (Bagwan) in India and Alpan. He organizes tours for learning Reiki by swimming with the dolphins.

knowledge and more recently has studied with Chiyoko Yamaguchi in Kyôto.

With the advent of organized projects such as the URRI (Usui Reiki Ryôhô International) there has been a worldwide interest in Mikao Usui's traditional teachings. These projects have been held annually in different countries around the globe and introduce Western practitioners to teachers from Japan.

Some Western teachers have made or attempted to make contact with the Usui Reiki Ryôhô Gakkai apart from those who have contact with Hiroshi Doi. Fran Brown, a student of Hawayo Takata, teaches regularly in Japan and has met with some of their members. Phyllis Furumoto had planned to visit Usui Reiki Ryôhô Gakkai members in Japan but this was supposedly foiled during the initial communication process and nothing happened. Frans and Bronwen Stiene met a Usui Reiki Ryôhô Gakkai member, who preferred to remain unnamed, in 2001.

There is a renewed interest in traditional forms of Reiki within Japan. Research is now being instigated by the Japanese rather than just by probing Westerners.

More traditional Japanese Reiki books are continuing to be published. Hiroshi Doi's book, which was published in Japanese, has been translated into English. Toshitaka Mochizuki, highly influenced by The Radiance Technique teachings, has written a book that includes some interesting historical facts and photos. It has also been translated into English. Tadao Yamaguchi has recently co-written a book with Frank Arjava Petter focusing on Mikao Usui's student, Chûjirô Hayashi. As mentioned earlier, Chris Marsh is writing about Mikao Usui's life and early teachings.

As we move deeper into the new millennium, progress is gradually being made in this connection between the West and Japan.

Japanese Reiki Levels

Japanese words are increasingly being incorporated into the modern-day system of Reiki. This can create confusion. Here is some insight into the names of various Japanese levels attributed to the teachings of Mikao Usui.

At the turn of the twentieth century when Mikao Usui first started teaching he had no need for recognized levels – it was just the teachings and students would be given further teachings after they had progressed on their spiritual path.

Mikao Usui's close association with members of the martial arts world and his own experience within it may have led him to create levels once the teachings became more formalized.[56]

According to Dave King, Mikao Usui started to use these *jûdô* levels in 1923: *rokkyû, gokyû, yonkyû, sankyû, nikyû, ikkyû, shodan, nidan, sandan, yondan, godan, rokudan* and *shichidan*. He states that the first four levels correspond to *shoden* and the next three to four levels correspond to *okuden zenki* and *okuden kôki*. The last five levels he asserts are not taught today.[57]

In 1928, Shûô Matsui, a student of Chûjirô Hayashi, writes about the levels *shoden* and *okuden* and mentions that there were further unknown levels.[58]

Kaiji Tomita, founder of *Tomita Teate Ryôhô*, studied with Mikao Usui around 1925 and created his own *Teate Ryôhô Kai* after Mikao Usui's death. The levels he used were *shoden, chuden, okuden* and *keiden*[59]

The levels on Fumio Ogawa's certificates read *rokkyû, gokyû, yonkyû, sankyû, okuden zenki* and *okuden kôki*. These dated from 1942 to 1943.[60] Here the first four certificates may well account for *shoden*. His stepfather, Kôzô Ogawa – a senior member of the Usui Reiki Ryôhô Gakkai, was his teacher.

The terms *shodan, okudan* and *shinpeten* were written in Hawayo Takata's diary notes (possibly instead of *shoden, okuden* and *shinpiden*).[61] These slight spelling changes represent different

[56] Information from Chris Marsh states that Mikao Usui received *menkyo keidan* in martial arts. Some of the martial arts people he apparently knew were Morihei Ueshiba (founder of aikidô), Jigorô Kanô (founder of jûdô) and Gichin Funokoshi (the father of modern karate).
[57] Information supplied to the authors by Dave King.
[58] 'A Treatment to Heal Diseases, Hand Healing', Shûô Matsui in the magazine *Sunday Mainichi*, 4 March 1928, translated by Amy, to be viewed at www.reiki.net.au.
[59] *Modern Reiki Method for Healing*, Hiroshi Doi, Fraser Journal Publishing, 2000.
[60] Information supplied to the authors by Rick Rivard's website: www.threshold.ca/reiki.
[61] *The Gray Book – Reiki*, Alice Takata Furumoto, 1982.

understandings of the terms in the first two cases. Hawayo Takata did spell some Japanese terms incorrectly in her diary notes (the incorrect spelling of *shinpeten* was crossed out and replaced with the almost correct *shinpeden*) and therefore it might just simply have been a spelling error. *Dan* (rather then *den*) is for levels that are used in Japanese martial arts such as karate, aikidô and jûdô. *Dan*, therefore, means level while *den* means teachings.

Each of the levels used in Mikao Usui's teachings represent that the student is beginning that level rather than having already achieved it.

The levels taught in the Usui Reiki Ryôhô Gakkai today are:

- *Shoden* – (lit. Japanese) first teachings. It can also mean the receiving of the first full transmission.
- *Okuden zenki* – (lit. Japanese) first stage of hidden teachings.
- *Okuden kôki* – (lit. Japanese) second stage of hidden teachings.
- *Shinpiden* – (lit. Japanese) mystery teachings.

These levels have within them different levels of proficiency that need to be accomplished. In total, it is understood that there are six levels of proficiency in the Usui Reiki Ryôhô Gakkai teachings. The teacher measures the progress of the student/member allowing them to move on to the next level when ready.

Certification in Usui Reiki Ryôhô, taught in the West today, generally uses the three levels – *shoden, okuden* (incorporating both *zenki* and *kôki*) and *shinpiden.*

Japanese Traditions

The Japanese are shrouded in a certain mystique as far as most Westerners are concerned. Their rituals are inextricably linked with so much historical and religious tradition that they may seem unfathomable to a foreigner. Westerners can sense the beauty of these traditions and often desire to imitate them. This is the point where possible disconnection from the source may allow the original beauty to fade. Another way of looking at it is that the *ki* is being weakened.

The system of Reiki is a Japanese practice that has a mystique all of its own. As with all things Japanese, certain traditional elements exist within these teachings of Mikao Usui. In the West, there is an uncertainty as to how these Japanese elements should be applied or dealt with. Often they are introduced into a Western Reiki course as a fad rather than something beneficial. Understanding the roots of a Japanese custom will strengthen practitioners' certainty in their practice promising a stronger sense of connection to the source.

A number of basic Japanese energetic and practical terms are discussed here to help clarify their meanings for Western practitioners.

Ki

Ki or Energy was first written about in a Chinese document, *Huang Ti Nei Ching Su Wen*, or The Yellow Emperor's Classic of Internal Medicine (also commonly known as the *Nei Ching*).

The *Nei Ching* is written on the subject of healing. Chinese folklore claims the *Nei Ching* was written during the mythological life of Emperor *Huang ti* (2697 to 2599 BC), but the text is historically dated at approximately 300 BC.

In the *Nei Ching, ki* is described as the Universal Energy that nourishes and sustains all life forms. It flows through the universe and each individual. A non-restricted flow of *ki* in the body allows one to remain healthy, while a diminished flow of *ki* in the body leads one to illness.

The *Nei Ching* describes how *ki* circulates through the body and is directed by invisible channels known as meridians.

Ki is considered an integral element to everyday Japanese life. Many Japanese traditions are based on a strong connection to *ki* apart from the martial arts and religious training. The success of the world-renowned tea ceremony called *sadô*, the ancient game of *go* and the art of calligraphy or *shodô* are all based on the practitioners' ability to channel free-flowing *ki*.

Teachings from the *Nei Ching* traveled from China to Korea and eventually across to Japan in the seventh century along with Buddhist sutras, historical books, medical books, works on astronomy, geography and the occult arts.

Ki was practiced solely for medical purposes until the twelfth century when the *samurai* introduced it into their art.

Hara

The word *hara* literally means stomach, abdomen or belly. Energy is stored in this point of the body from where it expands through out the whole body. Though the abdomen is generally called the *hara* there are, in fact, two more energetic centers in the body. One is the head and the other is the heart. By linking all three areas the practitioner creates unity and balance. Throughout *The Reiki Sourcebook* we refer to these centers as the three *haras*; lower, middle and upper. Most important, however, is to first develop the lower *hara*, as this is the body's central axis point.

A strong *hara* in a practitioner is indicated by a firm and collected stance. The shoulders are low and hanging loose. The legs are slightly apart with the body weight evenly distributed. The *sumô* wrestler is a good example as the body is large and heavy yet somehow quick and nimble. It is not their physical strength that wins their fights. The lower *hara* is like a building block. It is from this point that strength is developed. It is the base of the pyramid and it needs to be strong and stable.

In the West people are too afraid of being large and of carrying a protruding belly. The belly is culturally rejected and therefore the natural instinct for gravity within the body is lost. Instead the shoulders are built up at the gym creating a broad top of the body and a small abdomen. This is the shape of an upside down pyramid – one that is unstable and ready to topple at any time. Sticking out the chest strengthens the connection to the ego. This expresses a disconnection between mind and body with the axis of gravity in an unbalanced point of the body.

Many New Age practitioners focus on energetically building the energy in the head, the purpose being to develop the intuitive and psychic abilities of the practitioner. By working solely on this area of the body it is easy for the practitioner to become, once again, top heavy and unbalanced. Though there are a great many psychics practicing today who are genuinely helping others heal and grow, it is often interesting to see that their own lives are confused and unbalanced. This is an excellent example of the instability created by not first building the lower *hara*.

Re-establishing this connection with the Original Energy[62] through the *hara* will ensure good health and recovery from illness. There is always access to a reliable source of strength whenever needed.

An inner attitude results from focusing on the *hara*. From this central point there is an ability to cope with everyday tasks and sudden emergencies with an ease of understanding. This allows appropriate action to be taken in a balanced and unprejudiced manner.

Gasshô

Literally *gasshô* means 'to place the two palms together'. It actually has several interpretations at different levels.

Initially it is a sign of reverence. It also says, 'I revere the Buddha nature in you' – a non-judgmental manner of showing respect for all beings.

> This Bodhisattva constantly bowed with palms together in the act known as gasshô before anyone he encountered, for he recognized the potential for enlightenment in all beings.
>
> (Excerpt from *River of Fire – River of Water* by Taitetsu Unno.)

The *gasshô* brings all opposites together. It creates unity within the body by bringing the left- and right-hand side together. All opposites become one.

It is possible to see how focused an individual is by their *gasshô*. If their concentration is poor their *gasshô* will be loose and sloppy. A firm *gasshô* indicates a quiet and focused mind. This action creates the integration of mind and body as one.

There are many varieties of *gasshô*. When performing *gasshô* the eyes must be kept on the tips of the middle fingers. One style has been included to direct practitioners in a correct application of the *gasshô*.

---

[62] Original Energy is the energy that you receive from your parents when you are conceived and most importantly it is the energetic connection between you and the universal lifeforce.

Formal *Gasshô*

The formal *gasshô* is commonly used on a daily basis in Japan and is used when entering a temple and before eating. It aids in retaining an alert mind. Place the hands together, palm-to-palm in front of the face. The fingers are straight and palms are slightly pressed together. The elbows are not touching the body and the forearms not quite parallel to the ground. There is one fist's distance from the fingers to the tip of the nose.

Seiza

Seiza, or correct sitting, is a traditional Japanese style of sitting on top of the ankles, with the legs folded underneath and the back erect. When sitting in *seiza* correctly, it is comfortable and easy to maintain.

To sit in *seiza* the legs bend at the knees and the left knee is placed on the floor. The right knee is placed about 20cm from the left. Now the feet are positioned onto the floor so that the big toes just touch each other. The buttocks are lowered until they rest on or between the heels. If the legs tire or fall asleep then the practitioner must slightly rise up off the knees to allow better circulation. A pillow can also be placed behind the knees to help lift the pressure off the heels. The more it is practiced the easier it becomes and the longer the *seiza* position can be sustained.

The motivation behind sitting in *seiza* is that the leg that has contact with the floor along to the toes is representative of a large foot. When standing, the body's weight is on the balls of the feet rather than the soles. This is the perfect posture of balance. So the same can be said for sitting on the ground as the weight is forward rather than on the ankles.

From this position the body must feel relaxed. Relaxation should be refreshing. Relaxation is when the body is supported permitting the circulation of blood, oxygen and energy to flow with ease. The Ancient Chinese believed that energy entered the body with the breath and moved through the body in the blood. When all three are free to move with ease – breath, energy and blood – the practitioner becomes relaxed, strong and healthy.

The spine is slightly s-shaped in a natural position. To support the head it must be balanced on the top of the spine. The chin pulled in slightly and the back of the neck stretched. It should feel as if someone has taken a strand of hair from the crown and is pulling it up, stretching the spine. Sitting supported releases stress from the body keeping it light and buoyant.

To check that the posture is relaxed – the practitioner can imagine a string attached to the crown on the inside of the head. This string drops down through the neck and torso and is attached to a weight approximately 3 inches (8cm) below the navel inside the body – this area is called the lower *hara*. By sitting too far forward or backward this string will touch the insides of the body.

The practitioner relaxes the body. Shoulders and arms are relaxed with the palms of the hands facing downward onto the knees. The eyes are either closed or gazing gently at the floor 3 feet (1 metre) in front of the body.

Quiet sitting is something that is practiced when in *seiza*. A different reading of the word *seiza* actually means to sit still. This particular *kanji* is used by a student of Mikao Usui in a 1933 book describing the technique **hatsurei hô*. What follows is a simple introduction to this practice.

The practitioner breathes slowly, naturally not forcing the breath. Breathing in through the nose. The lungs fill naturally in relaxation and the *hara* in the lower abdomen also responds. Releasing the breath. Breathing out until the need to breathe in takes over once again. The chest and shoulders are relaxed throughout. The body is imagined as a glass and a carafe of water is being poured down into it. The body begins to fill from the lower torso with life giving air and energy. It is said that each person has a limited number of breaths in this lifetime. By breathing slowly and calmly ancient Taoists believed the length of a lifetime could be extended.

While following the breath, the practitioner counts both inhalations and exhalations. Later the exhalations only are counted and finally the practitioner just sits, without counting at all. Count from one to ten and then begin again from one. If the count is lost begin again at one. Don't try to remember the last number; that is not what is important. Just count.

The practitioner relaxes the mind. All thoughts that enter float past as clouds in the sky. There is no resistance or energy put into following the thought's journey – the practitioner remains focused solely on the action of the breath. If the mind follows these thoughts the practitioner most not berate one's self. Simply bring it back and focus breathing in and out. Be aware of the movement of energy in and around the body. Keep the memory of the sense of wholeness and light that is felt. It is there to be taken and drawn on each moment of the day. It will always be there. To help bring the practitioner back into the body, the hands can be shaken from the wrist a couple of times.

People's Names

Name Order

In Japan the first name follows the family name. For example 'Mikao' is a first name and 'Usui' is a surname, therefore he would traditionally be called 'Usui Mikao'.[63]

Family Names

Most Japanese family names consist of two *kanji*. The meanings of many of the *kanji* used in family names are related to nature, geographical features or locations.

First Names

Japanese first names commonly consist of two *kanji*. The meanings of these *kanji* are generally positive characteristics such as intelligence, beauty, love or light, names for flowers, the four seasons and other natural phenomena. They may also name the order of birth like first son, second son etc … Not only are they chosen for their meaning but also for their sound.

Often, the gender of a person can be guessed by the ending of the first name. First names ending with -ro, -shi, -ya, or -o are typically male first names, while names ending in -ko, -mi, -e and -yo are typically female first names.

---

[63] *The Reiki Sourcebook* has taken the Western perspective of writing the surname last and the first name first throughout the book eg. Mikao Usui.

Titles

The Japanese commonly address each other by their surname. Only very close friends and children are usually addressed by their first name. An appropriate title is also attached to a name. These titles depend upon the gender and social position of the person being addressed. They are added to the end of the surname. Some of the most frequently used titles are:

> *san*: This is a neutral title, and can be used in most situations. In formal situations it may not be polite enough.
>
> *sama*: This is a more polite version of *san* and is commonly used in formal situations or when writing letters. It may be too polite in a casual context.
>
> *kun*: This title is informal and is used for boys and men that are younger than the speaker.
>
> *chan*: This title is informal and used for young children and very close friends or family members.
>
> *sensei*: This title is used for teachers, doctors and other people with a higher education and from whom the speaker receives a service or instructions. It may also be used on its own. See the next section for more clarification of the term *sensei*.

Sensei

A number of Reiki teachers in the West are calling themselves *sensei* – this is an incorrect use of the word. They may have picked it up from hearing practitioners say the words Usui Sensei when talking about Mikao Usui.

Sensei is, in fact, an honorific title given to a teacher by students out of respect. That is why students will say Usui Sensei but Mikao Usui would never have called himself that.

In the Japanese language ways of referring to one another depend on the context, i.e. the position of someone in comparison to the person they're talking to. So a student will call their teacher *sensei* but that same teacher might be called by their surname by a colleague.

It is always about how much respect the person talking owes to the recipient, never the other way around. *Sensei* is often used in the

West to propound the mystical qualities of the teacher. In reality, there are many people besides teachers whose position calls for the use of *sensei* as a form of address. Doctors are always addressed as *sensei* as are lawyers and politicians. There is no mystical element in the use of the term *sensei*. If a teacher in the system of Reiki wished to appoint a Japanese name to reflect one's title, *kyoshi* would be appropriate. This translates as 'one who teaches' and refers to the function of teaching without any honorific aspect.

No one can claim a sign of respect; it is given to those who deserve it.

Etiquette in Japan

If it is a practitioner's fortune to visit Japan to see sites or to make acquaintance with Japanese practitioners it is advisable to have a basic understanding of what will be expected of them. Fortunately for foreigners it is anticipated that they will not be able to follow all of these customs but it is respectful to at least attempt to do so.

- Stand outside the entrance to a house and call a formal greeting to announce one's self. Then slide the door open and wait inside the door. If invited in to the house, take off the shoes and enter. Use the indoor slippers where provided.
- When walking on tatami mats remove the indoor slippers (remaining barefoot or in socks).
- Bathrooms will generally also have special slippers to be worn.
- *arigatô gozaimasu* is thank you.
- A bow instead of a handshake indicates hello and goodbye.
- People of a lower status must bow lower.
- Instead of directly saying 'no' the Japanese may sound indecisive or unassertive. This must be accepted as a 'no'.
- It is polite to present a business card in a formal situation otherwise the other person does not understand one's status. This card is offered with both hands, bowing slightly.
- A small gift or souvenir should be offered from one's

country when visiting with Japanese people. Gifts are given and received with both hands.

- When dining out the bill is usually split. If change is offered it must not be counted in front of the other diners.
- Sit in *seiza* when on the ground. If this becomes uncomfortable a man may sit cross-legged and a woman may sit on the ground with her calves out to the side.
- Turn chopsticks upside down when eating from a communal bowl.
- Do not stick chopsticks into food so that they are standing up – this indicates someone has died.
- Do not pass food from chopstick to chopstick (this is traditionally done at cremations with charred bones only).
- Slurping is normal in Japan.
- Do not pour soy sauce over white rice.
- Always wash with soap and rinse the body off before entering a Japanese bath.
- Never blow one's nose in public.

Good Luck!

7   Reiki in the West

Hawayo Takata (1900–1980) [1]

> Just do it! Do Reiki, Reiki, Reiki and then you shall know!
>
> (Quote by Hawayo Takata from *Hawayo Takata's Story* by Helen Haberly.)

Her Early Life

Hawayo Takata came into this world, early in the morning, on Christmas Eve in 1900 at Hanamaulu on the island of Kauai, Hawaii. A midwife patted her on the head three times proclaiming that this first generation American would be a success.[2] Hawayo Takata honoured that prophecy by introducing the system of Reiki to the Western world and practicing it until the day she died in 1980. Hundreds of thousands of practitioners exist today thanks to the persistence and strong character of Hawayo Takata.

Mr and Mrs Otogoro Kawamura, Hawayo Takata's parents, had emigrated from Japan to Hawaii. This, their second daughter, was

---

[1] Information about Hawayo Takata is abundant. For this chapter, autobiographies, personal interviews and tape recordings have been drawn from to recreate her life and teachings. Unfortunately history has an inherent contradictory nature and therefore there are many inconsistencies in some of this material. These irregularities might also be relegated to the fact that Hawayo Takata was an excellent storyteller.

[2] 'Mrs Takata and Reiki Power', interview with Mrs Takata, *Honolulu Advertiser,* 25 February 1974.

to be named after their new homeland. On the morning of her birth she was held up to the rising sun and christened Hawayo.

Hawayo Takata grew up in a simple Hawaiian village where her father worked as a cane cutter. From the age of 12 she became an assistant teacher with the first grade as well as a shop assistant. Though working, she continued her studies at the Japanese school. An invitation from a wealthy woman to work in her household took her to a local sugar cane plantation. Hawayo Takata left school and remained with the family for 24 years. Here, she was eventually promoted to head housekeeper with the responsibility of supervising the 21 staff members. It was also here that she met her husband, Saichi Takata, who worked as the plantation's bookkeeper. They were blessed with two daughters before he died at the young age of 34.[3]

By 1935, five years after her husband's death, Hawayo Takata's health was at a low point. She was suffering from asthma and abdominal problems and even found it difficult to walk. For a number of reasons she decided to return to Tôkyô and it was here she went to undergo surgery for a tumour, gallstones and other physical problems.[4]

Discovering her Life's Purpose

Lying on the operating table in Japan, Hawayo Takata heard a voice. It told her that the operation was unnecessary. She was instructed to ask the surgeon, Dr Maeda, if there wasn't another option for her apart from surgery. Dr Maeda thought about her unusual request then called for his sister, Mrs Shimura, the hospital dietician.[5] Mrs. Shimura guided Hawayo Takata to Chûjirô Hayashi's drugless treatment clinic.

The clinic's receptionist was Chûjirô Hayashi's wife, Chie Hayashi. She welcomed Hawayo Takata and led her into the clinic. Here eight clients were lying with two practitioners per person. One practitioner began at Hawayo Takata's head while the other placed his hands on her abdomen.[6] She sensed the heat and vibrations from

[3] *Hawayo Takata's Story*, Helen Haberly, Archedigm Publications, 1990.
[4] *The Blue Book – Reiki*, Paul Mitchell and Phyllis Furumoto, 1985.
[5] 'Mrs Takata opens minds to Reiki', interview with Hawayo Takata, Vera Graham, *The Times*, San Mateo, California, 17 May 1975.
[6] *Hawayo Takata's Story*, Helen Haberley, Archedigm Publications, 1990.

their hands throughout the treatment.

Returning for treatment the following day Hawayo Takata checked to see if any electrical machinery was being operated to create the heat that she had felt. Nothing. To quieten her curiosity, Chûjirô Hayashi explained the basic concepts of his system to her. After three weeks of daily treatments Hawayo Takata felt much better and enquired about becoming a student. This technique was not taught to foreigners, she was told. Though she looked Japanese she had been born and educated in America. Fortunately, Chûjirô Hayashi eventually relented and allowed her to study his teachings as an honorary member.

For six months Hawayo Takata received treatments. At the end of that period she moved in with the Hayashi family and spent another year studying and practicing. In the mornings she was a practitioner at Chûjirô Hayashi's clinic and in the afternoons she set out on house calls. At the end of this period she progressed to the *okudan* level.[7] The terms 'shodan' and 'okudan' were written in Hawayo Takata's diary notes.[8]

Hawayo Takata claimed that Chûjirô Hayashi had been Mikao Usui's number one disciple before his death in 1926.[9]

Today it is known that there is an association called the Usui Reiki Ryôhô Gakkai, which states that Mikao Usui was their first President. The second President wrote the brushstrokes for the memorial stone that stands at the Saihôji Temple in Tôkyô. If Chûjirô Hayashi was the 'number one' student then he would have been the follow-up President to Mikao Usui and would probably have been, in part, responsible for the text on the memorial stone. Chûjirô Hayashi eventually started his own school in 1931, which he called the *Hayashi Reiki Kenkyû Kai* or Hayashi Spiritual Energy Research Center.

Introducing the System of Reiki to America

Once Hawayo Takata finished her practitioner training in 1937, she returned to Hawaii. Chûjirô Hayashi and his daughter followed a few weeks later and stayed for six months helping her to build her prac-

---

[7] *The Gray Book – Reiki*, Alice Takata Furumoto, 1982.
[8] For more information about Japanese Reiki Levels see page 131.
[9] Transcript of a tape of Hawayo Takata talking about Mikao Usui, 1979.

tice in Honolulu. On his departure, Chûjirô Hayashi announced publicly that Hawayo Takata had become a Master of the Usui System of Natural healing.[10] She was his thirteenth, and last, Master student. It is interesting to note that Chûjirô Hayashi did not use the name of his school but that of Mikao Usui's, on her certificate. Hiroshi Doi explained that in this way honour is given to Mikao Usui by crediting his original system. At the same time it was also appropriate for Chûjirô Hayashi to have his own name for his school as he had changed its teachings to some extent.[11]

For Hawayo Takata to receive this appointment, a student of hers claimed she had had to sell her house.

At no point did Hawayo Takata ever call herself, her teacher or Mikao Usui a Grandmaster. It was not until after she passed away that terms such as this came into use in the system of Reiki.

In Chicago, 1938, Hawayo Takata took classes in anatomy and various other therapies before continuing with her practice in Honolulu.

Hilo, on the Big Island of Hawaii, became her new home and practice in 1939. Here she built treatment rooms, a waiting room and private apartments for her family. Her practice was almost an instantaneous success and she soon became renowned as Mrs Takata or just Takata.[12]

Treatments by Hawayo Takata were performed for as long as a couple of hours and continued from one or two days up to as long as a year. She would give treatments sitting cross-legged on the ground.[13] In Helen Haberly's book, *Hawayo Takata's Story*, many individual cases treated by Hawayo Takata are recorded, including facts about the illnesses and length of treatments. This includes the story of a woman who had died. Hawayo Takata placed her hands on the woman's solar plexus and she came back to life after 5½ hours treatment. She was a great practitioner with extensive experience. As far as payment went she appears to have been very flexible and charged those who could afford it and simply helped those who couldn't.

[10] *The Blue Book – Reiki*, Paul Mitchell and Phyllis Furumoto, 1985.
[11] Information supplied by Robert Fueston from URRI, 2002.
[12] *Hand to Hand*, John Harvey Gray, Xlibris Corporation, 2002.
[13] *Hand to Hand*, John Harvey Gray, Xlibris Corporation, 2002.

Her practical approach meant that she often had suggestions for her clients as to how they could improve their health apart from having treatments or learning the system of Reiki. She was always very interested in diet, though little of this has been passed down in the Western branches of the system. She had begun working with nutrition at Chûjirô Hayashi's clinic in Japan (perhaps influenced by the dietician Mrs Shimura). There is no mention of diet in either Chûjirô Hayashi's teachings or in those taught by the Usui Reiki Ryôhô Gakkai. One level 1 student of hers in California remembers her turning up to a class with what she called a 'Reiki salad'.[14] Some of her recommended recipes for better health included sunflower seeds, red beet, grape juice and almonds.[15] Two students of Virginia Samdahl's[16] wrote a book in 1984 called *The Reiki Handbook*, which includes Reiki recipes. Hawayo Takata called herself a vegetarian and yet occasionally enjoyed lamb kidneys sautéed in gin.[17]

Her Teacher's Passing

On 1 January 1940 Hawayo Takata had a premonitory dream about Chûjirô Hayashi, her teacher in Japan. It puzzled her and though the Hayashi family assured her that all was well she decided to travel to Japan in April of that year. Once there, she found out that Chûjirô Hayashi had decided to end his time in this world. He was concerned that when Japan went to war against America (as he was sure it would) he would be forced to fight as an officer in the Japanese Navy killing many people. On 10 May 1940 Chûjirô Hayashi passed away from a self-induced stroke with his friends and family around him.[18]

There are a number of different accounts about Chûjirô Hayashi's death. His student, Chiyoko Yamaguchi, has said that he killed himself by breaking an artery. Others say that as he was a military man the honourable method of death would certainly have been *seppuku* (the cutting of the *hara* or abdomen).

[14] Author's interview with Exie Lockett, student of Hawayo Takata.
[15] 'Mrs Takata opens minds to Reiki', interview with Hawayo Takata, Vera Graham, *The Times*, San Mateo, California, 17 May 1975.
[16] Virginia Samdahl was Hawayo Takata's first trained Reiki Master in 1976.
[17] *Hand to Hand*, John Harvey Gray, Xlibris Corporation, 2002.
[18] Transcript of a tape of Hawayo Takata talking about Dr Hayashi, 1977.

One of the World's Reiki Masters

Before he passed on he said, 'my wife and five other people in Japan and yourself, that makes us seven ... will be the teachers that we will have in all Japan, including my wife.'[19]

Some of Hawayo Takata's advertising and interviews in America claimed that she was the only living Reiki Master in the world.[20] This has been proven incorrect by recent knowledge in the West of the existence of the *Usui Reiki Ryôhô Gakkai* and living students of Mikao Usui. Even Hawayo Takata herself talked about the other teacher students of Chûjirô Hayashi in interviews.

On one of about 20 audiotapes that John Harvey Gray had made during her classes, Hawayo Takata discusses meeting practitioners of Mikao Usui's teachings in Japan. She said that she actually went to Japan to teach her system of Reiki and while there spoke to these practitioners. What they taught, she explained, was highly complex and required years of training and was closely intertwined with religious practices. She felt that their approach was inappropriate for the West.[21]

Chiyoko Yamaguchi, a living student of Chûjirô Hayashi, says that Chie Hayashi continued to teach after Chûjirô Hayashi's death.[22] Some of Hawayo Takata's advertising asserted, more reasonably, that she was the only Reiki Master in America. Though this too is apparently untrue. Tatseyi Nagao completed Levels 1 and 2 with Hawayo Takata in Hawaii and while in Japan in 1950 received *Shinpiden* (Master or teacher level) from Chie Hayashi. He returned to Hawaii to teach the system of Reiki to students and died in 1980, the same year as Hawayo Takata.[23] Hawayo Takata knew both Chie Hayashi and Tatseyi Nagao.

Hawayo Takata had been left the Hayashi practice and home in Tôkyô. She accepted it but returned to America leaving it in the widow, Chie Hayashi's, hands.

---

[19] Transcript of a tape of Hawayo Takata talking about Dr Hayashi, 1977.

[20] 'Mrs Takata opens minds to Reiki', interview with Hawayo Takata, Vera Graham, *The Times*, San Mateo, California, 17 May 1975.

[21] *Hand to Hand*, John Harvey Gray, Xlibris Corporation, 2002.

[22] Information supplied to the authors by Chiyoko Yamaguchi.

[23] *The Spirit of Reiki*, Walter Lübeck, Frank Arjava Petter, William Lee Rand, Lotus Press, 2001.

Around this particular period of world history it was not a favourable time to be of Japanese origin in America. Especially after December 1941 when Japan bombed Pearl Harbor. American Japanese were even being placed in internment camps. Chûjirô Hayashi had told Hawayo Takata, before he died, that she would need to keep her 'mouth shut' or she, too, might end up in a concentration camp.[24] It is not believed that Hawayo Takata was ever placed in an internment camp.

Returning to Japan 14 years later, Hawayo Takata found the house and practice she had been left by Chûjirô Hayashi to be full of refugees. Chie Hayashi had apartmentalized the buildings to help those without any shelter, post World War II. At this point Hawayo Takata officially handed the house and clinic back to Chie Hayashi knowing that her own true place was in America.

The Growth of the System of Reiki in America

For the next 30 years Hawayo Takata worked from a base in Honolulu in Hawaii. She traveled regularly around the islands teaching. There are few accounts by others of Hawayo Takata in America leading up to the 1970s. Initially it seems she worked mainly with American-Japanese people in Hawaii as a Reiki practitioner, not as a teacher. Gradually her popularity increased and she has claimed to travel with Barbara Hutton[25] and Doris Duke (the richest woman in the world at that time) around the globe as a private healer.[26] She said that she was even set up in a private spa in Palm Springs working with Hollywood celebrities such as Danny Kaye.[27]

Through her hard work and a successful practice, her wealth increased. As she grew older she lived well and included a daily nine holes of golf into her morning routine.[28] In 1973 she also began teaching on the mainland of America and Canada. Now that she was in her seventies she decided it was time to begin training her successor/s.

---

[24] Transcript of a tape of Hawayo Takata talking about Dr Hayashi, 1977.
[25] Information supplied by a student of Hawayo Takata.
[26] *Hand to Hand*, John Harvey Gray, Xlibris Corporation, 2002.
[27] Information supplied by a student of Hawayo Takata.
[28] 'Mrs Takata and Reiki Power', interview with Hawayo Takata, *Honolulu Advertiser*, 25 February, 1974.

In 1974 Hawayo Takata told a reporter that she planned to teach until 24 December (her birthday) 1977 and that she wished to build a Reiki center on three acres of land in Olaa, Hawaii. If she could not find a replacement for herself then the property would be turned over to the county of Honolulu.[29]

Only the first two of the three levels of the system of Reiki were taught by Hawayo Takata, until she taught her first Master student at the age of 76. To become a Reiki Master, Hawayo Takata charged US$10,000 from 1976 until 1980. Her Level 1 was US$100 in 1975 and increased to US$125 in 1976. The second level was US$400.[30]

Hawayo Takata used two moving anecdotes (one about her own family and the other known as 'the beggar story') to explain why it was necessary to pay large amounts of money to become a Reiki practitioner and eventual Master. Both anecdotes were based on the principle of respect. Students would feel more responsible and have more respect for the system once they had paid their hard-earned money to receive it.

Wanja Twan wrote in her book, *In the Light of a Distant Star: a spiritual journey bringing the unseen into the seen,* that she was allowed to deduct the amount she raised from bringing Hawayo Takata new students from her Master's fee. Unfortunately, she didn't raise enough and ended up using the money she'd saved to feed her family for the coming winter. This, she believed, was an example of trusting the universe to provide for her.

In 1976, Hawayo Takata (though born a Buddhist) became an honorary Minister for the Universal Church of the Master, a metaphysical church founded in 1908. Her student, Reverend Beth Gray, ordained her on the basis of the spiritual nature of her teachings. After this, she began to sign her notes and certificates as Reverend Hawayo Takata.[31]

In 1975 Hawayo Takata suffered a heart attack in Honolulu and began preparations for her retirement.[32]

---

[29] 'Mrs Takata and Reiki Power', interview with Hawayo Takata, *Honolulu Advertiser,* 25 February, 1974.

[30] Information supplied by a student of Hawayo Takata.

[31] Information supplied to the authors by Fran Brown, a teacher student of Hawayo Takata. Fran Brown also became a Minister in Beth Gray's church in 1977.

[32] *Hand to Hand,* John Harvey Gray, Xlibris Corporation, 2002. Rather than tell John Harvey Gray that she had a heart attack she told him she had fallen off a ladder.

In a letter to a student wishing a 'Happy Prosperous 1977' she wrote that she had 'created' three Reiki Masters to carry on her 'noble work'. They were John Harvey Gray, Virginia Samdahl and Ethel Lombardi. In fact, on the transcript of the tape of Hawayo Takata telling the life history of Chûjirô Hayashi, she appears to say goodbye to all of her students. This was her seventy-seventh year and she was planning to retire at the end of it on her birthday.

The two students of Hawayo Takata who claimed to be her successors once she died were Barbara Weber Ray (Master in 1979) and Phyllis Lei Furumoto (Master in 1979). Neither of them was from these initial three. It's said she tried to set up her granddaughter, Phyllis Lei Furumoto, with classes on the mainland before she died.[33]

Retirement was obviously not on the agenda as Hawayo Takata taught the majority of her 22 Reiki Masters (16 of them) after 1977. In 1978, even though she was failing in health, she participated in Virginia Samdahl's class and was still teaching all levels of her system.[34]

Hawayo Takata's Master Students

Below are listed the 22 Master students of Hawayo Takata in order of their year of training (where known). Hawayo Takata gave a list of the 22 students to her sister before she died.

1. Virginia Samdahl 1976
2. Ethel Lombardi 1976
3. John Harvey Gray October 1976
4. Dorothy Baba 1976
5. Bethel Phaigh (it is not verified that she was fifth)
6. Harry Kuboi 1977
7. Fran Brown January 1979
8. Barbara McCullough (it is not verified that she was eighth)
9. Kay Yamashita (one of Hawayo Takata's sisters)
10. Iris Ishikuro
? Phyllis Lei Furumoto April 1979
? Shinobu Saito May 1980

---

[33] Information supplied by a student of Hawayo Takata.
[34] Information supplied by a student of Hawayo Takata.

? Barbara Weber Ray September 1979
? Beth Gray October 1979
? Paul Mitchell November 1979
? Rick Bockner 1980
? Barbara Brown 1979
? Wanja Twan 1979
? George Araki 1979
? Patricia Ewing
? Ursula Baylow
? Mary McFadyen

Though it took three years for Hawayo Takata to become a Reiki Master, she did not have a required waiting period between levels for her own Reiki Masters.

Rick Bockner completed Level 1 on 10 October 1979, Level 2 on 20 October 1979 and Master Level on 12 October 1980. Bethal Phaigh wrote in her unpublished book *Journey into Consciousness*: 'The lessons (in life that I needed to learn) may have been particularly painful because my initiations had been timed so closely together. I had left Hawaii that spring not knowing of Reiki. I return this winter as a Reiki Master, a very green one.'[35]

Hawayo Takata was known to have limited the number of Masters that one Reiki Master could teach. Iris Ishikuro stated that she was asked to teach just three Reiki Masters and no more in her lifetime.[36]

Hawayo Takata's Teachings

Oral Tradition

Exactly what Hawayo Takata taught her Level 1, 2 and Master students has always been contentious. The system of Reiki, she professed, was an oral tradition. As such, she could teach what she wished. Fortunately some students did take notes after her classes and these verify that her teachings were often at variance with one another. This may

---

[35] Information supplied to the authors by Robert Fueston from his research about Hawayo Takata and her students.
[36] Information supplied to the authors by Robert Fueston from his research about Hawayo Takata and her students.

well have been because there was a large lapse of time between her learning the system and her teaching it. There may have been up to 30 years in this gap.

The Usui Reiki Ryôhô Gakkai uses a manual called the *Reiki Ryôhô Hikkei*. It has a section where Mikao Usui answers questions about Reiki. It contains *waka* (poems) by the Meiji Emperor, the five Reiki precepts and hand positions to be used for specific illnesses.

Hawayo Takata had a copy of Chûjirô Hayashi's *Ryôhô Shishin*. Its front cover read *Healing Method's Guidelines*, explaining that it had been set up for American distribution. The branch name on the cover was the *Hayashi Reiki Kenkyû Kai* or Hayashi Spiritual Energy Research Society. It also stated that it was not for sale and was a printed copy of the original. Written in Japanese, Hawayo Takata is known to have handed it to a number of her students including Harue Kanemitsu. John Harvey Gray also received a copy from Alice Takata Furumoto, Hawayo Takata's daughter.[37]

Hawayo Takata did teach what she felt was appropriate at the time. This means that no two teachings were identical.

The Five Precepts

Hawayo Takata taught a simple version of the five precepts to all of her students.[38] This is one aspect of the system of Reiki that has been passed from teacher to student with regularity.

Hand Positions

There has been controversy in the system of Reiki since Hawayo Takata's death regarding the hand positions that she taught. Some students say she started at the abdomen and others say the head. Perhaps her own experience taught her that both methods were valid. Her teachings about the abdomen or *hara* were, 'Spend half your treatment time here because this is the main factory. It processes the fuel taken in and delivers it to the places it is needed.'[39] Hawayo Takata is often accredited with 12 hand positions, which she called the Foundation Treatment. This was made up of four positions on

---

[37] *Hand to Hand*, by John Harvey Gray and Lourdes Gray.
[38] For a simple version of the precepts see page 30 and for the traditional version see page 66.
[39] *Living Reiki – Takata's Teachings*, Fran Brown, Life Rhythm, 1992.

the head, front and back of the torso. At the end of the treatment she would often perform the *finishing treatment or *nerve stroke.

It is believed that Mikao Usui did not use any hand positions when he first began teaching.[40] This developed into five hand positions for the head.[41] Chûjirô Hayashi's school used five head positions or seven positions including the head.[42]

Hawayo Takata stressed that students should treat themselves first and then their family and friends. This way, the student becomes whole and is also surrounded by harmony.[43]

Mantras and Symbols

The symbols taught by Hawayo Takata were once again not completely regimented. Yes, there were three mantras and symbols used for the second level and one for the Master level but they did vary slightly (or at least the versions that her Master students used were varied). Students were not allowed to keep copies of these mantras and symbols.

The first meeting of the Master students was in 1982 – just over a year after Hawayo Takata's death. Here the Masters compared the teachings and symbols that Hawayo Takata had given them. Each Master drew their symbols and were shocked to find that they were different 'similar in some respects and different in others'.[44]

There are a number of possible reasons for this: Hawayo Takata taught that Reiki was an oral tradition therefore no one had original copies of the symbols. It is easy to unintentionally change something that may not have been memorized completely or perhaps correctly. Two of the four symbols are in fact Japanese *kanji*. If the student, a Westerner, is not aware that the symbol is *kanji* it may be drawn in an incorrect manner.

---

[40] Information supplied to the authors by Andrew Bowling's website www.usuireiki.fsnet.co.uk.

[41] Information supplied to the authors by the *Reiki Ryôhô Hikkei*.

[42] Information supplied to the authors by Chûjirô Hayashi's *Ryôhô Shishin* and Dave King's website www.usui-do.org respectively.

[43] Information supplied from the tapes of Hawayo Takata's teachings, compiled by John Harvey Gray.

[44] Letter written by Carrell Ann Farmer on 31 December 1997 (she was the fourth Master initiated by Phyllis Lei Furumoto and was present at the first Reiki Masters meeting in 1982).

This particular group of Masters, not all were present (though all were invited), decided to standardize the symbols. As a result no one was ever really sure if they were using the correct symbols or not.

Attunements

Hawayo Takata practiced four attunements for Level 1, two or three for Level 2 and one for Level 3. She taught the first level over four evenings and students received one attunement on each of these evenings.

It has been suggested that the four are representative of the four levels of proficiency of *shoden* practiced by the Usui Reiki Ryôhô Gakkai.[45]

The actual attunement process is so varied throughout the West that it is almost impossible to even track back to what Hawayo Takata taught. It is feasible though to pinpoint where components were added (chakras, repetition of movement etc …) by either Hawayo Takata or her students (or their students and so on).[46] There is also the chance that she may have varied processes according to students' abilities.

Student accounts relate that there were sometimes up to 30 students in a Level 1 course. For the attunement, four students would be taken into a separate room where they would sit in a row. One student said that she was asked to remove her watch as the 'teacher's power' (Hawayo Takata's) would damage the watch.[47]

She is also known to have taught the second level in just two hours to a group of 10 students. The reason for the short length of the course, she told the group, was because they were exceptionally gifted.[48]

Techniques

In the traditional teachings of Mikao Usui there are a number of techniques practiced. These consisted of practice on others as well as meditative methods to build the practitioner's energy.

[45] *The Spirit of Reiki*, Walter Lubeck, Frank Arjava Petter, William Lee Rand, Lotus Press, 2001.

[46] For more information about additions to the system of Reiki see Part IV – Reiki Branches on page 257.

[47] Student notes from a Level 1 class with Hawayo Takata.

[48] Information supplied by a student of Hawayo Takata.

Hawayo Takata used some traditional techniques or at least versions of some of them: *ketsueki kôkan hô* (she called it the *finishing treatment or *nerve stroke), *nentatsu hô* (*deprogramming technique), *byôsen reikan hô* (*scanning) and *shûchû* Reiki (*group Reiki). In her diary she wrote that Chûjirô Hayashi had bestowed upon her the secret of *shinpiden*, Kokiyu hô (either *koki hô* or *kokyû hô*) and the Leiji hô (*reiji hô*).[49] She also wrote that before beginning a treatment a student should 'close your hand together'.[50] This is a traditional way to begin all treatments using the *gasshô*.[51] When she wrote about the *hara*, she said that to work with it would help one to concentrate, to purify one's thoughts and to meditate letting the true energy from within come out.[52] This is the basis of traditional Japanese Reiki techniques such as *hatsurei hô*.

These techniques were not passed on systematically to all of her students. Some were taught them, others not.

There is no evidence that Hawayo Takata taught the chakra system and instead spoke of the 'true energy' in the body that 'lies in the bottom of the stomach about 2 inches below the naval'.[53] This is a reference to the *hara*.[54]

The New Age Movement became increasingly popular throughout the world during the 1970s. Modifications made to the Indian chakra system by many New Age practitioners during this time made it an easily accessible system. Western teachers perhaps found comfort in using a 2000-year-old established tradition rather than following Hawayo Takata's words, 'Reiki will guide you. Let the Reiki hands find it. They will know what to do.'[55]

John Harvey Gray[56] did teach the chakra system and admitted that Hawayo Takata did not. Fran Brown[57] agrees that Hawayo Takata did not teach the chakra system.[58] Other Master students of Hawayo Takata's began to use the chakra system in their teachings. It was

---

[49] *The Gray Book – Reiki*, Hawayo Takata's Diary Notes, Alice Takata Furumoto, 1982.
[50] *The Gray Book – Reiki*, Hawayo Takata's Diary Notes, Alice Takata Furumoto, 1982.
[51] For more information about the *gasshô* see page 136.
[52] *The Gray Book – Reiki*, Hawayo Takata's Diary Notes, Alice Takata Furumoto, 1982.
[53] *The Gray Book – Reiki*, Hawayo Takata's Diary Notes, Alice Takata Furumoto, 1982.
[54] For more information about the *hara* system see page 135.
[55] *Hawayo Takata's Story*, Helen Haberly, Archedigm Publications, 1990, p. 58.
[56] John Harvey Gray became Hawayo Takata's third Reiki Master in 1976.
[57] Fran Brown became a Reiki Master through Hawayo Takata in 1979.

said that Phyllis Lei Furumoto, Hawayo Takata's granddaughter who became a Master student in 1979, introduced the chakra system into the attunement process – but she denies this.[59] Chakras have been included into the system of Reiki in many creative ways: One Western branch professes that with each attunement a separate chakra is focused on. Another Western branch has broken the system of Reiki into seven levels focusing on a different chakra for each level.

Hawayo Takata Tells the History of Mikao Usui

Since the mid-1990s, the West has gained more knowledge and insight into the life of Mikao Usui. This has occurred largely through the discovery of the Mikao Usui Memorial Stone in Tôkyô and through research completed by various practitioners.[60] Up until her late 70s Hawayo Takata popularized a history of Mikao Usui and his teachings. Her manner was entertaining and her stories seemed aimed more at getting a point across rather than having a strong base in reality. One of her Master students wrote, 'Her retelling of his story was a long, involved, dramatically highlighted, and somewhat speculative third- or fourth-hand account.'[61]

Hawayo Takata taught that Mikao Usui, or Dr Usui as she called him, was the principal of the Doshisha University in Kyôto. On Sundays he also became the University's minister. She called him a 'full-fledged Christian Minister'. She also credited him with having traveled to America to study at the University of Chicago. Chûjirô Hayashi, Hawayo Takata claimed, told her this particular history of Mikao Usui. Her story went on to recount that Mikao Usui studied many religions.

The focus on Mikao Usui as a Christian may well have been a clever way for Hawayo Takata to introduce a Japanese system, initially created by a Buddhist, to America during World War II. To create a credible story she included in it convincing names such as the

[58] Information supplied to the authors by Robert Fueston from his research into Hawayo Takata and her students.

[59] Information supplied to the authors by Robert Fueston from his research into Hawayo Takata and her students.

[60] For more information about research into the system of Reiki in Japan see page 113.

[61] *The Reiki Factor*, Barbara Weber Ray, Exposition Press, 1983, p. 49.

Doshisha University in Kyôto and the University of Chicago. We now know that neither of these universities knew Mikao Usui as lecturer, principal, minister or student.[62] She called Mikao Usui a 'Doctor', which has often been misinterpreted in the West as a physician. 'Doctor' may simply have been her translation for the respectful Japanese term *sensei* used for one's teacher.[63] It may also have been an excellent back-up to Hawayo Takata's story that Mikao Usui had received a Doctorate in Theology at the University of Chicago.

A certain freedom of interpretation was natural for Hawayo Takata and it was not unusual for her to use the words 'church' and 'temple' when talking about identical subjects. In this same way Mikao Usui no longer solely filled the 'Christian Minister' role but is actually described as a Zen monk in some of her advertising in the 1970s. In contrast to the system of Reiki's first introduction to America in the 1940s and 1950s Zen Buddhism had become a popular trend. It may even have added an attractive element to her advertisements.

Yes, Hawayo Takata told stories that changed with each telling but her nature may simply not have found these semantics important. Her words appeared randomly chosen depending on the moment itself. This eccentricity was accepted by most who knew her perhaps because of her dedication to her topic and the strict manner in which she taught.

It does not seem that Hawayo Takata's Master students could grasp her ease of changing the facts. After her death most clung tightly to the 'full-fledged Christian Minister' belief – this was probably what she had spoken of most convincingly. Even Helen Haberly's biography neatly sidelines writing the words 'monk', 'Zen' or 'Buddhism' in combination with Mikao Usui himself – though she was certain to have read the transcripts where Hawayo Takata talks about Mikao Usui the 'Buddhist monk'.[64]

End of an Era

There have been dogmatic claims from Reiki practitioners the world

---

[62] *The Spirit of Reiki*, Walter Lübeck, Frank Arjava Petter, William Lee Rand, Lotus Press, 2001.

[63] For more information about the term *sensei* see page 140.

[64] Transcript of a tape of Hawayo Takata talking about Mikao Usui, 1979.

over that they only teach the system of Reiki that was taught by Hawayo Takata. Interestingly they all teach something different. There is no consistency between those asserting to be the 'original' or 'traditional' method. The subjects of the contentions all differ and are as small as how to spell the word 'Reiki'[65] or as integral as how to perform an attunement.[66] Due to the multitude of unreliable reports it is almost impossible to evaluate exactly what Hawayo Takata did teach.

Hawayo Takata invented tenets that may also have created dogma. Rules such as 'if you teach this method to anyone you will lose your healing power' are recorded as having been taught in a Level 1 course. There is nothing to substantiate this claim but it does leave the door open for further unsupported statements to be made on behalf of other Reiki Masters.

Additions to her teachings can be seen in the number of branches of Reiki that exist today. It can also be seen that charging US$10,000 for Reiki Mastership to retain control over her system did not work. In fact it led to rebellion. Diane Stein's book, *Essential Reiki*, published in 1995 was a revolt against the 1980s system of Reiki and the elitism that was being practiced under its name.

Hawayo Takata died of a heart attack on 11 December 1980. Her remains were placed at a Buddhist temple on the island of Hawaii.[67]

The Evolution of Reiki in the West

Hawayo Takata's Successors

Directionless. This appeared to be the emotion that most of Hawayo Takata's 22 Master students felt after she died. Their Master was gone and most were not sure what was to happen next. Hawayo Takata had talked for years of naming a successor/s who would continue in her steps but no one had officially been recognized. Many practitioners today believe that if Hawayo Takata had wanted a successor she would have named one.

---

[65] Posters advertising her teachings in the 1970s are written as Reiki – one word.
[66] For more information about attunements see page 97.
[67] *Hand to Hand*, John Harvey Gray, Xlibris Corporation, 2002.

The 1980s saw the creation of a systemized Western Reiki. A meeting was called for the Masters to come together in 1982 to discuss the future of this system. Not one of them knew that there were still traditional practitioners living, and practicing Mikao Usui's teachings, in Japan. They therefore assumed that what they decided would regulate the way the modern teachings would be practiced throughout the world for all time. This great responsibility was in their hands. What a great shock it was for them when they decided to compare their symbols to find that they were, to some extent, different. Regulation began here when the Masters present decided upon which symbols were to become the standard Western symbols.[68] The initial meeting may also have been held as a reaction to a stand taken by one of Hawayo Takata's Master students, Barbara Weber Ray. In 1979 she had become a Reiki Master and was now claiming to be Hawayo Takata's successor. Barbara Weber Ray did not attend this meeting.

Most of the Masters who came together felt that Phyllis Lei Furumoto, Hawayo Takata's granddaughter, was the natural successor. Phyllis Lei Furumoto had already trained Master students by the meeting in 1982 and appeared confident in the role. Phyllis Lei Furumoto was said to be open to becoming Hawayo Takata's successor and the others at the meeting were happy for her to do so.[69]

This group eventually became known as The Reiki Alliance (teaching Usui Shiki Ryôhô) with the first of its inaugural meetings held in Canada in 1983. Phyllis Lei Furumoto also became known as the lineage bearer of the system of Reiki (by The Reiki Alliance) and gained their official 'title of holder' of the 'Office of the Grandmaster'. This was the first time that either term had been used in the system of Reiki.

It is good to remember that today there are many, many more non-Alliance Master teachers than Alliance Masters. These non-Alliance members do not generally consider Phyllis Lei Furumoto to be their lineage bearer or Grandmaster. The Reiki Alli-

---

[68] Letter written by Carrell Ann Farmer on 31 December 1997 (she was the fourth Master intiated by Phyllis Lei Furumoto and was present at the first Reiki Masters meeting in 1982).

[69] Letter written by Carrell Ann Farmer on 31 December 1997 (she was the fourth Master initiated by Phyllis Lei Furumoto and was present at the first Reiki Masters meeting in 1982).

ance claims to have a membership of over 700 Reiki Masters. It can be guessed that there are hundreds of thousands of practitioners throughout the world – perhaps more. A recent Internet survey that has been held by the International Center for Reiki Training had 8000 contributors (a drop in the Western Reiki system ocean) and, of these, 43 per cent had taken a Master training course somewhere on this planet. To even raise the percentage higher, 13.5 per cent of those who filled in this survey had not even completed a Reiki course.[70] It is always difficult to know how accurate these unsupervised surveys are but it is still an indication that there are a great many people who have technically become Reiki Masters.

Meanwhile, Barbara Weber Ray was publishing what she called the first ever Reiki book. Little did she know that there had already been a number of books published in Japan from as early as 1930 by students of Mikao Usui.[71] The first edition of her book connects Reiki with ancient Tibet and the Aquarian New Age. It is true that Hawayo Takata once mentioned that Reiki is spoken of in the ancient history of Japan and the Buddhist sutras.[72] She was never known to have elucidated on this nor taught any information about Tibet etc. This may very well have been her manner of restating that Reiki 'can stem from the sun, or moon or stars' and that it 'is nature, it is God'.[73] Barbara Weber Ray asserts that she had been carefully instructed in the advanced levels of the system of Reiki by Hawayo Takata and yet only goes on to explain the same three levels that Usui Shiki Ryôhô teaches.[74] In later editions these three levels are extended to the seven levels that are taught today. It has been suggested that she changed the number of levels after a Japanese student of hers met a member of the Usui Reiki Ryôhô Gakkai in Japan who explained that there

---

[70] If you would like to contribute to this Internet survey you can find it at www.reiki.org/#survey.

[71] *Te No Hira Ryôji Nyûmon (Introduction to healing with the palms)*, Toshihiro Eguchi and Kohsi Mitsui, 1930; *Te No Hira Ryôji Wo Kataru (A story of healing with the palms)*, Toshijiro Eguchi, 1954; *Reiki To Jinjutsu – Tomita Ryû Teate Ryôhô (Reiki and Humanitarian Work – Tomita Ryû Hands Healing)*, Kaiji Tomita, 1933.

[72] 'Mrs Takata opens minds to Reiki', interview with Hawayo Takata, Vera Graham, *The Times*, San Mateo, California, 17 May 1975.

[73] 'Mrs Takata opens minds to Reiki', interview with Hawayo Takata, Vera Graham, *The Times*, San Mateo, California, 17 May 1975.

[74] *The Reiki Factor*, Barbara Weber Ray, PhD., Exposition Press, 1983.

were different stages within the three levels. Today The Radiance Technique official website actually denies there was a split after Hawayo Takata died. That, their website states, is impossible as there is only one true authentic system of Reiki. Anything else is 'an imitation, a copy, a part and a fabrication'.

Only one of the 22 Reiki Masters (Virginia Samdahl)[75] is known to have followed Barbara Weber Ray while many joined The Reiki Alliance. Virginia Samdahl actually joined both The Radiance Technique and The Reiki Alliance. She may have been hoping to be a sensible go-between though eventually she left The Radiance Technique. One of the reasons given was that Barbara Weber Ray had told her she would have to re-train with her as a Reiki Master.[76]

Standardization

The Reiki Alliance quickly created an elite standardized system. Course costs became identical across the board without room for individual assessment. The amounts of US$150 for Level 1, US$500 for Level 2, and US$10,000 for the Master Level are still being charged by them today. The Master student is required to complete an apprenticeship (not full time) with their Master for a period of at least one year. Once the new Master begins to teach, it is under their Master's supervision, and the Master receives all course fees. This continues for at least one year. The new Master may not train a Master themselves for three years. Hawayo Takata said that the fees she charged were the same as when she trained in 1936–38. She asked her Masters not to increase the fees even though the value of the dollar would change.[77] According to a poster advertising her courses in 1975, she charged $100 for her Level 1, which went up to $125 ($25 less than The Reiki Alliance claimed) in 1976. Her Level 2 cost just $400[78] in comparison to the Alliance's $500.

---

[75] Virginia Samdahl was Hawayo Takata's first Reiki Master and trained in 1976.
[76] Information supplied to the authors by Robert Fueston from his research about Hawayo Takata and her students
[77] Information supplied to the authors by Robert Fueston from his research into Hawayo Takata and her students.
[78] Information supplied by a student of Hawayo Takata.

There is a major problem with charging $10,000 for the Master Level. The Reiki Alliance claims that a large amount of money helps separate those who really want to do it from those who don't. Consequently what has happened is that instead of teaching those who sincerely wish to learn – rich people (the term rich being relative) end up being taught. Of course, there will always be exceptions to this rule, but an average person in India or Africa (even after selling their house!) could not raise this amount of money. On the other hand a well-to-do Westerner would not think twice about paying it if they so wanted. The dogma may have been well intentioned as a means to protect the system of Reiki but this is not what has happened. Throughout the 1980s there were struggles within the community. The Reiki Alliance was soon 'undermined' by a number of Hawayo Takata's Reiki Masters who did not wish to conform to their, or The Radiance Technique's, rulings.

New Branches of Reiki

Mari-EL, created by Ethel Lombardi in 1983, though based on the system of Reiki, was filled out with her own interpretations. She did not wish to be a member of either of the post-Hawayo Takata organizations.

Around the same time Iris Ishikuro and Arthur Robertson began teaching Raku Kei Reiki. Iris is said to have asked Arthur Robertson not to charge $10,000 for Reiki Mastership as she considered it unfair for those sincerely wanting to become Reiki Masters but who could not afford it.[79] Raku Kei Reiki appears to have included a number of techniques that are commonly taught today by many Independent Reiki Masters as well as the 'Tibetan' symbols. These techniques are; *breath of the fire dragon or *violet breath; the Johrei symbol (Iris Ishikuro was a member of the Johrei Fellowship)[80]; and the *hui yin breath.

Other branches began to use these techniques too (some still use variations of them) including Tera Mai Reiki, Ichi Sekai Reiki, Usui/

---

[79] Information supplied to the authors by Robert Fueston from his research into Hawayo Takata and her students.
[80] Information supplied to the authors by Light and Adonea's website: www.angelfire.com/az/SpiritMatters/contents.html.

Tibetan Reiki, Johrei Reiki, Karuna Reiki, Karuna Ki, Seichim and Reiki Jin Kei Do. Diane Stein wrote about many of these techniques in 1995 and this has popularized them even further.

Something was missing from the system of Reiki in the West after Hawayo Takata died. Her personality, strength of character and depth of healing knowledge were sorely missed. There seemed to be a void that needed to be filled. And people were filling it!

Reiki Plus was a system started in 1981 by David Jarrell, a student of Phyllis Lei Furumoto. David Jarrell's teachings were influenced by a spiritual initiation into the mystical energy of Reiki from a Tibetan Master. Tibet was definitely 'in' in the 80s.

Seichim evolved through the system of Reiki and was being taught by 1984. It was originally a mixture of Egyptian and Sufi initiations and knowledge within the Reiki system's framework. This took off and has too many variations today to mention. There's also an influence here from Raku Kei Reiki with techniques like *breath of the fire dragon or *violet breath being practiced.

The 1980s was full of upheaval for the system of Reiki. In 1988, a book that listed some of Hawayo Takata's teachers was recalled due to objections. The relevant pages were cut out and the book was re-issued. From those closed-door attitudes the system of Reiki then entered the rebellious 1990s. With it followed many new lineages and globalization – primarily due to the success of the Internet. Today almost every Western Reiki website has a list of Hawayo Takata's 22 Master students. How quickly things change.

Independent Reiki Masters emerged in the 90s. This is a generic term for a branch that doesn't really exist, as it has no underlying foundation. Independent Reiki Masters can come in two categories: The first type of Independent Reiki Masters is one that teaches from a number of different lineages and offers these to students. Such teachers call themselves Independent Reiki Masters and clearly show the lineages and branches that they teach from.

The second are individuals who claim to teach 'Usui Reiki' or something that sounds vaguely familiar to another branch of Reiki. They do not align themselves with a definitive school of Reiki but instead teach bits and pieces from various branches. Once one of these Independent Reiki Masters teaches a teacher, who teaches a teacher, who then teaches a teacher (and so on …) the teachings can become very unclear. This is unless a comprehensive understanding of the background of the teachings is held by the teacher and passed on.

Tera Mai Reiki was taught in the early 90s by Kathleen Milner and exists today along with its counterpart, Tera Mai Seichem. Extra symbols were intuited by a number of practitioners with the belief that there had been symbols missing from the system of Reiki and that the attunement process was also incomplete.[81] Karuna Reiki became a registered system in 1995 and evolved from a mix of schools. One school was Sai Baba Reiki that held aspects of Raku Kei Reiki and the other was Tera Mai Reiki. Tera Mai Reiki in turn had elements of Seichim in it. Both Raku Kei Reiki and Seichim are offshoots of Usui Shiki Ryôhô. Sai Baba Reiki soon disappeared after Sai Baba (Indian guru) found out that there was a profit-making system using his name.[82]

Channeling has also been a popular way to create a new branch of Reiki in the West. The Ascended Masters, Egyptian gods, Archangels and even Mikao Usui himself is said to have been channeled offering new (and of course 'better') information about the system of Reiki.

Conflict in the New Age

With these new lineages came lawsuits that no one wishes to talk about. The problem with the creation of new branches is that, often, it is no longer understood what is 'original' any more and no clear boundaries remain intact. The answer to this has been trademarking. Barbara Weber Ray had already complained that the system of Reiki could be used 'by anyone for anything' and has trademarked a whole bunch of names. Reiki Plus, another early branch of Reiki, trademarked their name. Tera Mai and Tera Mai Seichem, Karuna Reiki, Vajra Reiki, Sekhem and so on followed in this trend. A breath of fresh air (perhaps) was the statement made by Seichim's founder, Patrick Zeigler, who said that he does 'not wish to control the name, as anyone is still free to use it and any of the teachings. I encourage you all to share all information and allow it to grow with you.'

---

[81] *Reiki and Other Rays of Touch Healing*, Kathleen Milner, 1995.
[82] *Reiki News*, Center for Reiki Training, Spring 1995.

The next great trademarking escapade was in the mid-90s when Phyllis Lei Furumoto (The Reiki Alliance's Grandmaster) attempted to trademark Reiki itself. This was a worldwide effort. In Germany the words 'Reiki', 'Usui' and 'Usui Shiki Ryôhô' were attempted. In America it was 'Usui System' and 'Usui Shiki Ryôhô' and in Canada, 'Usui System of Reiki Healing', 'Usui Shiki Ryôhô' and 'Usui System of Natural Healing'. Almost every other country followed. It was stated in America that 'she could not identify or distinguish her goods from those of others nor do they indicate their source'.[83] As Frank Arjava Petter pointed out, it would be impossible to trademark the word Reiki in Japan. This would be like taking a shot at trademarking the word 'milk' in the West. It is understood, though, that in South America the trademarks were granted.

The West Visits Japan

In the late 90s Japan was back in the picture. Frank Arjava Petter was researching the system of Reiki in Japan, coming up with some interesting facts and making them public. Dave King coincidentally met another Japanese Reiki Master, Tatsumi – a student of Chûjirô Hayashi, while traveling in Japan. The most surprising fact may well have been that the Usui Reiki Ryôhô Gakkai existed – trained teachers originating directly from Mikao Usui in a closed society that wanted nothing to do with the West.

A Japanese manual was translated and published in book form with the title *The Original Reiki Handbook of Mikao Usui*. The Usui Reiki Ryôhô Gakkai possesses the manual that was collated by Kimiko Koyama for the society's fiftieth anniversary but no one knows when the actual information first came into use. The Usui Reiki Ryôhô Gakkai uses only parts of the manual. The excitement of finding out that the system of Reiki may not have been an 'oral' tradition (as strongly purported by The Reiki Alliance) meant that the West was zealously rushing two steps forward while having to take another step back. Small pieces of the puzzle were coming together though. Moving into the new millennium, progress is gradually being made in the connection of these methods between the West and Japan.

---

[83] Information supplied to the authors by the The International Center for Reiki Training's website: www.reiki.org.

Large gatherings for Reiki practitioners have been held annually since 1999. These are called URRI (Usui Reiki Ryôhô International) projects, where Japanese teachers (Hiroshi Doi and Hyakuten Inamoto, for example) have been invited to various countries to teach what they practice.

With this current intense focus on Japan there has been an increase of 'new' Reiki stories over the last few years. Some are completely inaccurate while others are quite fascinating. Verification is the only way to know whether something originates from Mikao Usui's teachings or not. In what could almost be called 'a true western Reiki tradition' some of these unverified teachings have already been added to and altered by Reiki Masters in the West. To stop this happening those with the information need to meet to piece together the teachings and make them available to all, rather than a select few.

Modern Influences

This century has introduced the concept of spiritual energy to more people than ever.

The Internet has successfully allowed people from every culture to access teachings. Reiki practitioners are communicating with ease across continents via e-mail, msn, ICQ or forums and chat programs.

The concept of distant attunements, once controversial, is by and large accepted today. Just log onto the Internet at the appropriate time and follow the Reiki Master's directions.

Initiatives such as free Reiki courses are another Internet speciality. Free courses are offered (with distant attunements, of course) plus communal websites, forums and chat programs for members.[84]

The anonymity that the Internet provides can also lead to a misuse of its astonishing powers. People gossip or create smear campaigns – all the while operating under a pseudonym and signing off with the Western Reiki signature of 'Love and Light'.

The system of Reiki is also reaching people through the greater infrastructure that is evolving from within its ranks. Apart from

---

[84] For more information see Part IV – Directory, Reiki Internet Resources on page 297.

the URRI mentioned earlier, Mari Hall, an American Reiki Master living in Prague, plans to organize large Reiki conferences around the world.

The Future

Looking to the future, some questions will invariably be asked. What will happen to The Reiki Alliance and its Lineage Bearer, Phyllis Lei Furumoto? With fewer and fewer people willing to pay $10,000 to become Reiki Masters (there are many other options today) will it continue to exist? The fee of $10,000 may include approximately five days of one-on-one teachings between the student and teacher and continued support. This (and sometimes more) can be found in other branches or schools of Reiki for a lot less money. The Reiki Alliance may already be reviewing its price structure to accommodate the changes that have taken place.

In the mid-1990s The Reiki Alliance began an inner struggle. Their 1996 newsletter read, 'Does The Reiki Alliance want to follow the evolving teachings of the Office of the Grand Master?' To discuss the shift in teachings The Reiki Alliance offered US$25,000 to Phyllis Lei Furumoto and Paul David Mitchell (Head of the Discipline) to be key presenters at The Reiki Alliance annual meeting. Questions relating to why members' dues would be raised by an extra $25 each to support the Office of the Lineage Bearer (Phyllis Lei Furumoto) were also discussed in the article. In the end, Phyllis Lei Furumoto and Paul David Mitchell did not attend the conference as speakers even though, as Phyllis said, 'the money and the commitment' had been offered. Today The Reiki Alliance still honours the Office of the Bearer of the Lineage but neither Phyllis Lei Furumoto nor Paul David Mitchell are members of The Reiki Alliance.

Many associations are available today for Reiki practitioners to join.[85] Some are open only to practitioners from a particular lineage while others are open to all. Neil Anthony, co-founder of the UK Reiki Federation, is one of its forward moving and thinking representatives. He has managed to bring practitioners from all lineages throughout the UK together with one voice. The UK Reiki

---

[85] For more information about associations see page 291.

Federation has achieved a great many successes for Reiki with the general public. A main accomplishment is the initiation of an effective Reiki Awareness Week. This week is kicked off with a gathering of Reiki practitioners in a festival called, 'Our Celebration of Energy'. During Reiki Awareness Week publicity stunts take place such as Reiki practitioners entering the Houses of Parliament and giving sample treatments to the Members of Parliament. On one occasion some of the UK Reiki Federation members were invited to Kensington Palace by Prince Charles to mingle and meet the CEOs from UK hospitals and other health industries. The success of this association reflects on all Reiki practitioners throughout the world. This particular organization is also setting a European precedent by pioneering voluntary self-regulation in the UK.

The system of Reiki continues to intrigue people from all countries and its number of practitioners is growing daily. Reiki is truly a miracle and yet, it is a fact, that as humans we wish to control this magic, this beauty and keep it for ourselves. Sharing the wonder of this system and this spiritual energy, can only bring joy to the world.

8 Characteristics of Reiki Branches

The river flows on, but something remains from the past, leading us through the present, and into the future, if we but step into the clear waters for a drink.

(Excerpt from 'What is a Ryû?' Wayne Murumoto. Issue 8, *Furyu – The Budo Journal*.)

Which elements denote that a branch of healing or energetic work has its foundations in Mikao Usui's teachings?

Mikao Usui was born into a *samurai* family and appears to have been heavily involved in martial arts as a practitioner.[1] Elements of Mikao Usui's teachings therefore can be found to have a foundation in martial arts both energetically and spiritually. There has always been a link in Japan between spirituality and martial arts. Lao tzu is quoted as saying, 'He who excels in combat is one who does not let himself be roused.' Warriors would train in peaceful hermitages to practice their fighting and meditative skills.

Shûgyô, the training that Mikao Usui is said to have completed on *kurama yama*[2] is both a martial art and an esoteric Buddhist term. To elucidate on the concept of lineage and branches in the system of Reiki, traditional Japanese viewpoints from both backgrounds have been utilized.

In traditional Japanese martial arts the founder of a style must first have received a divine understanding through a spiritual experience – not unlike Mikao Usui's experience. A traditional style is

---

[1] Information supplied to the authors by Chris Marsh.
[2] Mikao Usui's experience on *kurama yama* is described on the memorial stone, see Appendix B on page 339.

then begun with this simple divine understanding. It is from this seed that the founder of a style creates a method. If this method is to remain divinely inspired then it must always flow back to the founder. This is a traditional belief in Japan.

Unless it can be claimed that one has the pure source and the direct teachings from the founder (who initially received the divine guidance) then what is practiced is considered a degeneration. This does not mean that the true method should remain stagnant. Teachers are expected to be able to teach using their own personal methods to support the original teachings. Often these teachings are called 'outside' teachings. This creates clarity as to what the original teachings are and where they have been added to. Remember that the method flows from the source. Innovative attempts to make a method 'better' cut off links to its divine origins. In maintaining the method's integrity the proximity to its origins must be close. Otherwise the teachings need to be given a new name unrelated to the original method.[3]

In this context, all branches of Mikao Usui's teachings would need to retain the original methods while teaching their personal add-ons openly. This is not always the case and one of the reasons for this is that, unfortunately, no one is certain what the original system entails any more – even though many may claim this right.

A branch is generally created in the system of Reiki when teachers change what they have been taught. At first they may call themselves Independent Reiki Masters or they create a new, more apt, name to work under that is added to the word 'Reiki'. Once this new name is passed on to a student, written on certificates, it becomes a new branch of the system of Reiki.

One suggestion by Reiki Master Vincent Amador[4] as to why there are so many branches of Reiki is that in the West it is unclear whether people are teaching 'Reiki' as in 'Mikao Usui's teachings' or 'Reiki' as in 'spiritual energy'. If it is understood that it is a set of teachings then there are certain guidelines for the system to adhere to *but* if it is solely the energy then any 'system' or 'teachings' can be applied to it. This is extremely confusing for the general public and practitioners alike.

[3] 'What is a Ryû?' Wayne Murumoto, Issue 8 of *Furyu – The Budo Journal*.
[4] Vincent Amador hosts an extensive Reiki website: http://angelreiki.nu.

Vincent Amador also states that the confusion created by this misunderstanding or the use of the word 'Reiki' can be deliberate by those wishing to create their own system and yet give the impression that it is the system of Reiki that is being taught.

Seichim (and its variations) has deliberately not included Reiki in the system's name. The founder, Patrick Zeigler, believes that his first initiation took place in an Egyptian pyramid by a spiritual Egyptian energy force. It was not till later that Patrick Zeigler became a Reiki Master. Seichim's complete system though (which was created *after* he studied the system of Reiki) appears to have benefited from its energetic link to Reiki as well as drawing on the technicalities of the Reiki system. Most practitioners appear to believe that the two systems are interlinked with Seichim being an offshoot of the system of Reiki. Some Reiki Masters teach a mixed Reiki/Seichim Master Level.

Apart from the continuity of teaching, a shared lineage is the other major requirement for all Reiki branches.

Lineage

Lineage must be able to be traced back to Mikao Usui. Reiki is a Japanese system and has developed from Mikao Usui's teachings.

Some branches claim that Mikao Usui created his teachings from a far older and, often, 'more powerful' system. Egyptian, Tibetan and inter-galactic origins are often suggested. Some of the branches that make these statements are Raku Kei Reiki, Reiki Jin Kei Do, Jinlap Maitri Reiki, Seichim (and its variations), The Radiance Technique, Tera Mai, Wei Chi Tibetan Reiki and Usui/Tibetan Reiki. Many of these lineages mentioned are offshoots from one another, simply carrying the story along and occasionally adding to it.

From Part II – Reiki History it can clearly be seen that Reiki grew out of a Japanese culture. The mantras and symbols have Japanese origins (some are *kanji*) and therefore do not link in to any of these so-called histories. The traditional techniques are also specifically Japanese, originating from Shintôism, Tendai Buddhism and Japanese martial art practices. It is curious that this interest in alternative histories occurred only a few short years after Hawayo Takata's death in 1980. Perhaps the trend of 'all things Tibetan' or 'mystical Egypt' at the time influenced the sellability of the system of Reiki to the general public? The New Age Movement also introduced channeling as an acceptable form (in some circles) of acquiring information. Channeled information often appears to have no lineage. In such cases Reiki Masters, preferring to use their guides as the higher authority, relegate their lineage as unimportant. In most cases though, the teacher was a Reiki Master before the channeling took place and it is the system of Reiki that forms the solid foundation for the branch's existence.

Founder

The founder of a branch of Reiki is not necessarily Mikao Usui. He is the founder of his teachings but not of a branch where an individual has deliberately altered the teachings. That person then becomes the founder, as it is a new or different approach to the original system. Traditionally a branch must still hold the original essence of the teachings and in some of the Reiki branches this might not be the case.

Some founders claim to be the lucky recipient of new texts or channeled knowledge. In this way they do not take personal responsibility for the changes that they make to the teachings. Their sources may be Buddha, Mikao Usui, Angels, Ascended Masters, etc…

Some of the channeled teachings are Angelic RayKey, Ascension Reiki, Blue Star Reiki, Brahma Satya Reiki, Medicine Dharma Reiki, Shamballa Reiki, Tummo Reiki and Wei Chi Tibetan Reiki. Often these channeled teachings allege to provide new information about Mikao Usui's teachings.

Verification as an issue has been discussed at length throughout *The Reiki Sourcebook*. To seriously search for verification can mean turning up many questions and receiving few answers. Even some of the historical information that is accepted as 'true teachings' today has not been fully verified – simply accepted. Since the 1980s there have been many beliefs as to what the correct teachings are, or are not. The Radiance Technique asserts it teaches Hawayo Takata's original system (though it appears to be based on Barbara Weber Ray's understanding of the New Age).[5] In a similar fashion, The Reiki

[5] *The Reiki Factor*, Barbara Weber Ray, Exposition Press, 1983.

Alliance (who teach 'traditional Western' Usui Shiki Ryôhô) is said to have quietly standardized Hawayo Takata's teachings to create a system that was acceptable to her Master students after her death.[6] Today the Method to Achieve Personal Perfection offers teachings from living students of Mikao Usui but this has not as yet been totally verified. The same can be said of Usui Dô. An interesting point here is that through all of the systems that claim to have the true or original teachings there are some parallels but also major differences. How then does one know what the original teachings were?

Other founders are happy to disclose that they are fully aware of the alterations they have made to the system they teach. The creation of a more 'powerful' system than the one that was already in place is generally the root cause of these changes. Tera Mai Reiki, the Seven Level System and Prema Reiki all belong to this category.

A number of the Japanese branches teach a mixture of both Japanese and Western Reiki and claim to have the best of both worlds. Such branches are Gendai Reiki Hô, Reido Reiki and the Vortex school.

Levels

Many different names exist for the levels that one will go through to receive the highest teachings available in that branch. They might be called facets or degrees or carry Japanese names such as *shoden*, *okuden* or *shinpiden*. The levels begin at 1 and can be ongoing (without end in some cases).

It is said today that Mikao Usui initially taught without levels.[7] Once he began working with lay students with varying abilities he then came to the conclusion that a more formalized system with levels was valuable. Most 'traditional' Western and modern Japanese branches today teach three levels. These correspond to a beginner, practitioner and teacher level. Level 3 is sometimes called the Reiki Master level, the Reiki Master/Teacher level or *shinpiden*.

---

[6] Letter written by Carrell Ann Farmer on 31 December 1997 (she was the fourth Master initiated by Phyllis Lei Furumoto and was present at the first Reiki Masters meeting in 1982).

[7] Information supplied to the authors by Chris Marsh.

In the West and modern Japan the first level generally consists of self-treatment, treatments on others, hand positions, history and four attunements. The second level commonly teaches three mantras and three symbols, techniques such as *distant Reiki and two or three attunements. The third level teaches one more mantra and symbol, how to perform attunements and one attunement.

Various branches will use the first two levels in a more 'traditional' manner and then divide the third level up into two or even five separate levels. All three levels have had information, mantras and symbols added to and taken away from them. They have been broken up to create more levels (the more levels generated – the more financially lucrative teaching can become) or condensed to help impatient students cram their experiences into a shorter timeslot.

Closely linked to the different levels is the number of attunements[8] that are performed. Those branches that have extended their number of levels often base each level around the receiving of the attunement. Each attunement generally has a separate function and ritual. In the traditional Japanese Usui Reiki Ryôhô Gakkai the *reiju*[9] are performed repeatedly at their weekly or monthly meetings.

Different branches perform an assortment of attunements and these are generally influenced by the origins of the branch. If the system is a channeled form then the founder may have received, through guides, new information about the attunement process. Tibetan attunements may include Tibetan sounds, symbols/mantras, deity connection or bells. An Egyptian system of Reiki may include attunements based around an Egyptian god or entity. A teacher's lack of faith in their own ability may mean that they repeat parts of the attunement endlessly in the hope that it will prove more 'powerful'. The length of time that an attunement takes can be from a couple of minutes up to 45 minutes.[10]

---

[8] For more information about attunements see page 97.

[9] *Reiju* is a Japanese name for attunement and is performed without mantras and symbols. For more information see page 97.

[10] If you are interested in this topic then Vincent Amador at www.angelReiki.nu sells an e-book with at least 20 diverse attunements in it.

Mantras and Symbols

The terms 'traditional' or 'non-traditional' mantras and symbols[11] are used in *The Reiki Sourcebook*. This term is simply a yardstick for mantras and symbols and is based on information about the four mantras and four symbols practiced in Japan and initially in the West. These are not exactly the same. It is impossible to know precisely what Hawayo Takata taught when she brought Chûjirô Hayashi's teachings to the West. It is well known that after her death her Reiki Master students came together (the founders of The Reiki Alliance) only to discover that their mantras and symbols differed.[12]

Hawayo Takata had never let students keep written copies of their mantras and symbols. Therefore, it is uncertain whether Hawayo Takata taught variations on them or whether the students had remembered them incorrectly. It could even be a mixture of both. The Reiki Alliance consequently decided how the standard four traditional Western mantras and symbols should be identified.

As Reiki is passed from one teacher or Master to another there have naturally been alterations made in the drawing of the symbols (especially as no copies were kept). In the West there has been such little understanding of the mantras and symbols and their Japanese origins that it is easy for them to be drawn incorrectly. Once incorrect symbols are taught and passed on to others the flawed cycle continues.

In Japan, students traditionally copied their teacher's symbols on paper.[13] Today such copies still exist from teachers such as Chûjirô Hayashi via Tatsumi.[14] Some traditional Japanese based branches of Reiki (several of these have been influenced by the West) like Satya Reiki (Pune school), Usui Reiki Ryôhô, Gendai Reiki Hô, and Usui

---

[11] For more historical information about mantras and symbols see page 82.

[12] Letter written by Carrell Ann Farmer on 31 December 1997 (she was the fourth Master initiated by Phyllis Lei Furumoto and was present at the first Reiki Masters meeting in 1982).

[13] There were no photocopy machines available in the early 1900s. It is still traditional in Japan to respect sacred teachings by not taking photos or copying them thoughtlessly by machine.

[14] Dave King copied these symbols from Tatsumi's notes in Japan. These are considered to be traditional symbols.

dô use Tatsumi's and other traditional hand-drawn copies to teach from.

As the West veers further away from Mikao Usui's teachings, more and more symbols are appearing. Westerners see the symbols as the 'energy'; therefore if more symbols are used they believe that the 'energy' will become stronger. In traditional Japan it is not believed that the symbols are the power – they simply invoke certain energy.

These new symbols are either channeled (such as those used in Tera Mai Reiki) or taken from existing religions and cultures. The symbols Hrih, Houng, Ah and Om are Tibetan and/or Indian in origin and can be found in Usui/Tibetan Reiki or Tera Mai Reiki. Our own collective symbology provides new symbols such as the infinity symbol (used in the Seven Level System and Seichim).

As long as there are attempts to make the system of Reiki 'bigger and better' more symbols will continue to be added.

Branch Claims

'Traditional' and 'non-traditional' branches are descriptions occasionally used by Reiki practitioners. There is no real defining line between the two because, as mentioned earlier, no one is entirely sure what Mikao Usui taught.

Some of the Reiki branches have influenced one another, i.e. the majority of the 'Tibetan' techniques are linked to Arthur Robertson and his branch called Raku Kei Reiki. William Lee Rand's Usui/Tibetan Reiki has gone on to popularize some of these techniques and concepts. Many smaller branches have further evolved calling themselves Tibetan Reiki, or Tibetan/Usui Reiki.

Seichim is perhaps not considered to be a Reiki branch by its founder, Patrick Zeigler, but it has certainly become entangled with Reiki branches along its journey. Today the major extensions to it are Tera Mai Seichem, Sekhem, Seichim, SKHM, Newlife Reiki Seichim, Isis Sekhem, Renegade Seichim, Seichim-Sekhem-Reiki (SSR) and Seven Facet Seichim.

9   Scientific Studies on Reiki

Mikao Usui is quoted saying in the *Reiki Ryôhô Hikkei* that the mind and body are one. Recent studies in the world of science are beginning to finally comprehend that statement. Brainwaves and body pulses and their role in stimulating healing can all be measured today allowing the concept of Reiki, as spiritual energy, to be more widely understood by the medical community. The growth of the system of Reiki is benefited by this community awareness and acceptance.

The introduction of 'therapeutic touch' by Dolores Krieger into nursing in the 1970s has increased interest in other energetic systems such as Reiki. This in turn has boosted the amount of research that has recently been undertaken using Reiki and other forms of energetic work.

The system of Reiki is also being accepted into hospitals across the world. Patients can often either bring their Reiki practitioner with them or Reiki is made available to them.

The article 'The first Reiki Practitioner in our O.R.' by Jeanette Sawyer in 1988 in the *AORN Journal* describes the steps that were taken to allow a Reiki practitioner into the theatre at the request of a patient during a laparoscopy.

Also in 1988, patients were given the opportunity to experience a 15-minute pre- and post-surgery Reiki treatment. More than 870 patients took part and as a result there was less use of pain medication, shorter stays in hospital and increased patient satisfaction. This was discussed in the article, 'Using Reiki to Support Surgical patients' by Patricia and Kristin Aladydy in the *Journal of Nursing Care Quality.*

Heart surgeon, Dr Mehmet Oz, has worked with Julie Motz who

used Reiki on his patients. These patients had received heart transplants and had experienced open-heart surgery. She treated 11 patients in total and none of them had the usual post-operative depression. The bypass patients had no post-operative pain or leg weakness and the transplant patients experienced no organ rejection. Julie Motz has written about this experience in her book, *Hands of Life*. Listed below are a number of trials tested on Reiki. For more research details there are some Reiki books with relevant research material, or personal observations, that have been written by both doctors and nurses. *Spiritual Healing* by Daniel J. Benor has listed a number of Reiki trials as well as some very interesting trials on distant healing and healing through touch in general.

There are many aspects of Reiki that are being researched today. Some to see if Reiki speeds up healing, others to see if, how and whom it relaxes, to measure biomagnetic fields and to verify the concept of distant healing.

Here is a well-known trial completed using Reiki to examine its effect on human blood levels:

Human Hemoglobin Levels and Reiki
Reiki Healing: a Physiologic Perspective

Wendy Wetzel.
Published in *Journal of Holistic Nursing*, 7 (1), pp. 47-54 (1989).
Purpose: The purpose of this study is to examine the effects of Reiki on human hemoglobin and hematocrit levels.
Procedure: The hemoglobin and hematocrit levels of 48 adults participating in a Level 1 course were measured. Demographics and motivation were also examined. An untreated control group was used to document the changes in hemoglobin and hematocrit under normal circumstances.
Findings: Using a t-test there was a statistically significant change between the pre- and post-course hemoglobin and hematocrit levels of the participants at the $p > 0.01$ level. 28 per cent experiencing an increase and the remainder experiencing a decrease. There was no change for the untreated control group within an identical time frame.

Conclusions: That Reiki has a measurable physiologic effect. The data supports the premise that energy can be transferred between individuals for the purposes of healing, balancing, and increasing wellness. Some individuals found that their blood levels went up while others went down which is consistent with the concept that Reiki is balancing for each individual.

This trial tests Reiki on patients with chronic illnesses using electrodermal screening:

The Efficacy of Reiki Hands on Healing: Improvements in Adrenal, Spleen and Nervous Function as Quantified by Electro-Dermal Screening

Betty Hartwell and Barbara Brewitt.

Published in *Alternative Therapies Magazine*, 3 (4), p. 89 (July 1997)

Purpose: The purpose of this study is to evaluate the therapeutic effects of Reiki treatments on chronic illnesses using electrodermal screening.

Procedure: This study was carried out on five patients with life-threatening and chronic illnesses: lupus, fibromyalgia, thyroid goiter, and multiple sclerosis. Eleven one-hour Reiki treatments using 4 different Level 2 practitioners and one Reiki Master were performed over a ten-week period. These Reiki practitioners systematically placed their hands over the same body positions including the neurovascular regions on the cranium, neurolymphatic points on the trunk and minor chakra points on the limbs. No new conventional or alternative medical treatments were given during this period. Initially, three consecutive treatments were given and then one treatment per week for eight weeks.

Findings: The patients were tested three times during the study. 1. Before the study commenced. 2. After their third treatment. 3. After their tenth treatment.

Each individual was measured for skin electrical resistance at three acupuncture points on hands and feet. At the cervical/thoracic point the measurements went from 25 per cent below normal to the normal range. The adrenal measurements went from 8.3 per cent below normal to normal – some time between the middle and last measurements. The spleen measurements went from 7.8 per cent below normal to normal after only three sessions. All the patients reported increased relaxation after Reiki treatments, a reduction in pain and an increase in mobility.

These trials are concerned with the effect of Reiki on pain relief and other symptoms:

Pain, Anxiety and Depression in Chronically Ill Patients with Reiki Healing

Linda J. Dressen and Sangeeta Singg.
Published in *Subtle Energies and Energy Medicine Journal*, 9 (1) (1998).
Purpose: To measure the results of Reiki and its effect on pain, anxiety, and depression in chronically ill patients.
Procedure: 120 Patients who had been in pain for at least 1 year were trialed. Their complaints included: headaches, heart disease, cancer, arthritis, peptic ulcer, asthma, hypertension and HIV. Four different styles of treatment were performed on 3 groups of 20 people. The four styles of treatment were: Reiki, Progressive Muscle Relaxation, no treatment and false-Reiki. Each of the groups received ten 30-minute treatments, twice a week over five weeks. Patients were examined before and after the series of treatments. Reiki patients were examined three months after completion.
Findings: Reiki proved significantly superior (p<.0001-.04) to other treatments on ten out of 12 variables.
At the three-month check-up these changes were consistent and there were highly significant reductions in Total Pain Rating Index (p<.0006) and in sensory (p<.0003) and Affective (p<.02) Qualities of Pain.
Conclusion: Significant effects of Reiki on anxiety, pain and depression are shown here. Some possible variables were not controlled.

Using Reiki to Manage Pain: a Preliminary Report

alta.karino@cancerboard.ab.ca
Cross Cancer Institute, Edmonton, USA.

Published in *Cancer Prev. Control,* 1 (2) pp. 108-13 (1997).
Purpose: To explore the usefulness of Reiki as an alternative to opioid
    therapy in the management of pain. This was a pilot study.
Procedure: 20 volunteers experienced pain at 55 sites for a variety of
    reasons, including cancer. A Level 2 practitioner provided all Reiki
    treatments. Pain was measured using both a visual analogue scale
    (VAS) and a Likert scale immediately before and after each Reiki
    treatment.
Findings: Both the instruments showed a highly significant (p
    < 0.0001) reduction in pain following the Reiki treatments.

This trial is interested in finding out if it is possible to gauge the experience of a Reiki treatment using normal trialing procedures:

Experience of a Reiki Session

J. Engebretson and D. W. Wardell.
University of Texas Health Science Center in Houston, USA
Published in *Alternative Therapies in Health and Medicine,* 8 pp. 48-53
    (2002).
Purpose: To explore the experiences of Reiki recipients so as to
    contribute to understanding the popularity of touch therapies
    and possibly clarify variables for future studies.
Procedure: All Reiki treatments were 30 minutes long and performed
    in a sound proof windowless room by one Reiki Master. There
    were audio taped interviews immediately after the treatment in
    a quiet room adjoining the treatment room. The recipients were
    generally healthy volunteers who had not experienced Reiki
    previously.
Findings: The recipients described a conscious state of awareness
    during the treatment. At the same time, paradoxically, they expe-
    rienced sensate and symbolic phenomena.
Conclusions: Conscious awareness and paradoxical experiences
    that occur in ritual healing vary according to the holistic nature
    and individual variation of the healing experience. These find-
    ings suggest that many linear models used in researching touch
    therapies are not complex enough to capture the experience of the
    recipients.

This particular trial is not specifically about Reiki but deals with the effectiveness of *distant healing which is relevant to Reiki practitioners:

A Randomized Double-Blind Study of the Effect of Distant Healing in a Population with Advanced AIDS

Fred Sicher, Elizabeth Targ, Dan Moore II and Helene S. Smith. Published in the *Western Journal of Medicine*, 169, pp. 356-363 (December 1998).

Purpose: To find the effect of distance healing (DH) on AIDS patients during a six-month double-blind study.

Procedure: Forty patients with advanced AIDS were randomly divided into two groups. Half the patients received DH in addition to their usual medical care. They were not told they were being given DH. Forty healers from various locations throughout the US with an average of 17 years of experience were used. The healers practiced a variety of healing methods including Christian, Jewish, Buddhist, Native American, shamanism, meditative, and bioenergetics. Each of the treated subjects received DH for one hour a day for six days from each of a total of ten different healers, and this was performed over a period of ten weeks.

Findings: After six months, treated patients had significantly fewer outpatient visits and hospitalizations, less severe illnesses, fewer new illnesses, and improved mood.

Part III
Reiki Techniques

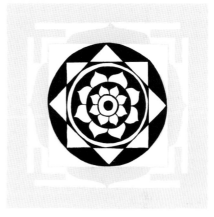

A student is poorly trained if he learns many [techniques] but only possesses a shallow understanding of performing them

(Quote by Funakoshi Gichin in 'Tapenshu' by Patrick and Yuriko McCarthy.)

There are a number of fixed components that make up the complete system that has evolved from Mikao Usui's teachings. These include:

- *Reiju* or attunements[1]
- The physical practice on one's self or others for the purpose of healing[2]
- The spiritual and mental connection using precepts and/or *waka*[3]
- Mantras and symbols[4]
- Techniques.

Part II – Reiki History covered the first four components. The last, techniques, is a large and integral part of the system of Reiki as it stands today.

The term technique can be qualified here to include exercises that aid the development of the individual's personal practice and methods of using Reiki to achieve certain ends.

There are some similarities between techniques used in Japan and the West while the differences often lie in the point of focus.

The majority of Japanese techniques aid the practitioner's own self-development by building energy in the *hara*, clearing the meridians and teaching sensitivity to energy. It seems that many of the Japanese techniques have their roots in traditional Eastern energy work such as *ki ko* (Japanese Qi Gong), Tendai Buddhism, Mikkyô, martial arts and Shintôism.

Techniques that have been used in the West since Hawayo Takata's arrival in Hawaii, and especially since her death, are often

---

[1] Attunement is the Western term for the Japanese word *reiju*. For more information about *reiju* or attunements see page 97.

[2] For more information on hand positions see page 77.

[3] For more information about the five precepts see page 66 and for *waka* see page 74.

[4] For more information about mantras and symbols see page 82.

of a different nature. Some still have their origins in the Japanese techniques while others are obvious add-ons from individuals and the New Age movement. Many claim to have their foundation in Tibetan, Indian or Egyptian origins. The Indian chakra system became incorporated into the system of Western Reiki by some of Hawayo Takata's students. It is now almost inseparable from a Reiki course in the West and, even, modern-day Japan. Some techniques center on various ways of using Reiki to achieve an end result with the use of *talismans or *manifesting grids. The more complex and dramatic additions to Reiki may lessen the connection with Reiki itself though provide a connection to other forms of esoteric arts.

Overlapping techniques between Japan and the West include *enkaku chiryô hô* and *distant Reiki; *shûchû* Reiki and group Reiki; *ketsueki kôkan hô* and the *nerve stroke; *byôsen reikan hô* and *scanning and *gedoku hô* and the x-ray technique.

As practitioners progress through the various levels of the teachings new techniques are learnt. Included in this sourcebook are techniques from each level. The catalogue of techniques is from the major Japanese and Western branches. Today the system of Reiki is so diverse that it would be almost impossible to list all the variations on each technique. Therefore the included techniques are merely representative of what is taught in a branch or branches. They are also written in a summarized form yet aim to be as succinct and accurate as possible. To achieve optimal results from any technique it is best to practice with the assistance of a teacher. The authors do not accept any liability for the use or misuse of any techniques in this book.

10 Japanese Reiki Techniques

Mikao Usui's teachings were initially created as a form of self-development for his students. The Japanese techniques are based on building the energy flow through the meridians and strengthening the *hara* center using Reiki. This, in turn, clears the body emotionally, physically, mentally and spiritually thus raising our vibration level until we become lighter and lighter. We shed our human ties and bonds and become One with the natural energetic flow of life.

But where exactly did these techniques come from?

Mikao Usui's teachings appear to have been developed rather than 're-discovered' as previously believed in the West. This indicates that it was an evolving process and leaves open the possibility that his 21 teacher students may have been taught slightly different techniques to work with depending upon when they were taught.

The teachings were broken up into three major divisions.[1] This ensured that those with different capabilities worked with the appropriate energetic techniques. Each of the three divisions was created to achieve the same outcome. The three approaches are listed below:

1. Experienced practitioners such as advanced meditators were taught meditation techniques that belonged originally to forms of Buddhism such as Tendai.

2. Experienced practitioners who were martial arts practitioners and Shintô followers were taught four mantras without any symbols. The mantras are chanted in a different manner to that in the third approach.

---

[1] Information supplied to the authors by Chris Marsh.

3. Lay people like farmers or naval personnel (this would have included Chûjirô Hayashi and possibly Usui Reiki Ryôhô Gakkai members)[2] were taught four mantras and four symbols. The focus of these teachings was to aid those who were unfamiliar with energy work.

Techniques listed in this section of *The Reiki Sourcebook* were either taught by Mikao Usui or are practiced in Japanese branches of Reiki that claim to teach in a traditional manner.[3] These include the Usui Reiki Ryôhô Gakkai, Gendai Reiki Hô, Komyo Reiki, Method to Achieve Personal Perfection, Usui dô, Usui Reiki Ryôhô and Jikiden Reiki. Some of the Japanese techniques are no longer taught while some were introduced after Mikao Usui's death. It is noted beside each technique whether it is still practiced today or not and what its origins are where known. Many of the Japanese techniques train the mind that energy or *ki* is entering the body through breath. By breathing in this manner access to *ki* becomes unlimited.

Some of the Japanese branches today practice Western techniques alongside more traditional ones.[4] Since Mikao Usui's death in 1926 his teachings were not always practiced in an overt manner. Once these teachings made their way to America in the late 1930s the system of Reiki became very popular and swept around the world finally finding its way back to its land of origin. Mieko Mitsui took a branch of Reiki called The Radiance Technique to Japan in 1986 and began teaching the first and second degree to the Japanese.[5] Western styles of Reiki quickly gained in popularity in Japan due to their ease of availability. The actual system though was different and techniques had been altered and added to. With the return to Japan of some of Mikao Usui's teachings there has definitely been a crossover and any obviously Western techniques have been listed under that heading rather than Japanese techniques.

---

[2] The Usui Reiki Ryôhô Gakkai claims to have been created in 1922 and yet some researchers today claim that it did not begin until after Mikao Usui's death.

[3] Mikao Usui's teachings were re-introduced to Japan from the West in the 1980s. This has influenced many modern schools of Japanese Reiki.

[4] An example is Gendai Reiki Hô as it practices a mixture of both Western and Japanese techniques.

[5] 1986 article 'Mysterious Report 28' from *The Twilight Zone* by Shiomi Takai – translated by Shiya Fleming for Rick Rivard's website: www.threshold.ca/reiki.

Some of the branches taught by Hawayo Takata still retain the few original techniques she taught. Generally, techniques introduced by Hawayo Takata and teachers in her lineage have not been included in this section.

The Hara Center[6]

For an understanding of how the Japanese consider energy and the body to work together information has been included on the *hara* center and two other main centers of the body.

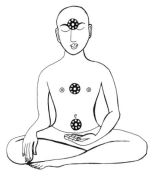

1. *Hara* or lower *hara* (approximately 3 inches (8cm) below the navel)
   In this center, the Original Energy is stored. This is the energy you are born with, the energy that is the essence of your life and gives you your life's purpose. The Original Energy is not only the energy you receive from your parents when you are conceived but most importantly it is the energetic connection between you and the universal life force. When the singular term *hara* is mentioned it is the lower *hara* that is being discussed.

2. Middle *hara* (at the heart center)
   The energy in this center is connected with emotions. It is 'human' energy connected with human experience. Through this center you learn your life's process. From childhood through to adulthood and back to being a child. When you are a child you are without experience and as you grow older you become a child with experience.

3. Upper *hara* (third eye area)
   This is the energy connected with your spirit. When you are connected with this center you may see colours or you might have psychic ability. It is important for you not to become unbalanced and keep yourself centered. If you can use this energy in a balanced way, you can see beyond the immediate.

---

[6] For more information about the *hara* see page 135.

Practicing the techniques

Each of the techniques described in this chapter includes the Japanese *kanji* and its literal meaning for a deeper understanding of the purpose of the technique.

Listed are the levels that the techniques may be taught in and the specific branches that practice them. This is just a guideline and may alter depending upon the school that teaches them.

Any historical information relating to each technique is included and any important points relating to the practice of the technique.

The particular technique is then explained in detail. Within one branch a technique may be approached from different viewpoints and therefore the details may not be matching.

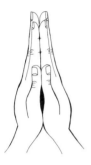

The techniques as described generally all use the *gasshô* position. This is where the palms of both hands are placed against one another, with thumbs closest to the body and fingertips facing upwards. It is often called the 'prayer position' or 'namaste position' in English as it is commonly used in many cultures. When practiced in conjunction with Mikao Usui's teachings it represents the balance of the body; harmony; respect for the energy, practitioner and client and humility. It is also an aid in setting intent clearly. *Gasshô* is used before and after all Japanese techniques and before and after treating clients.[7]

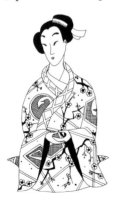

When practitioners are asked to sit while practicing a technique they can either sit in *seiza*[8] or on a chair with feet flat on the ground.

The techniques may also ask that practitioners close their eyes. The eyes may be fully closed or partially. Partially closed eyes means that the practitioner is in fact gazing in an unfocused manner at the ground about 3 feet (1 meter) from the body. The advantage of partially closed eyes is that the practitioner is more likely to retain awareness of the practice.

[7] For more information about *gasshô* see page 136.
[8] For more information about *seiza* see page 137.

Byôsen Reikan Hô 病腺霊感法

Sensing imbalances

byôsen 病腺 – illness, disease
reikan 霊感 – inspiration, sacred
  intuition
hô 法 – method

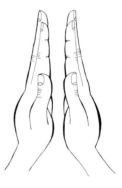

- *Shoden* or *okuden* technique
- Practiced by the Usui Reiki
  Ryôhô Gakkai, Usui Reiki
  Ryôhô, Gendai Reiki Hô and
  once practiced by Chûjirô
  Hayashi and Hawayo Takata

To be used on yourself or others to sense imbalances in the body.
1. *Gasshô* – to center the mind and set intent.
2. Move the hands approximately 2 to 6 inches (5-15 cm) over the sitting, standing or lying body looking for a sensation in your hands.
3. When you sense *hibiki* (heat/cold/tingling/pain/itchiness/pulsating, etc…) in your hands place your hands on that part of the body.
4. Wait until the *hibiki* has passed before moving on.
5. *Gasshô* – to give thanks.

Enkaku Chiryô Hô 遠隔治療法

Remote healing

enkaku 遠隔– distant, remote
chiryô 治療 – treatment, cure, remedy
hô 法– method

- *Okuden* technique
- Taught originally by Mikao Usui in a
  different format and practiced today in all
  Japanese branches of Reiki

This technique can be practiced in a number of different ways.
  Traditional Japanese teachings do not believe that you *send* Reiki or even need to connect to another person – instead you become One with that person. The concept is that we are already One and do not need to make this connection happen.

Some say Mikao Usui used a photograph to practice *enkaku chiryô hô*. Photography was not as common as it is today and therefore it is likely that they also focused on their intent alone.

The system using a photograph is commonly practiced today.

1. Obtain a photo of the person; write their name, age, location and condition on the back. If you cannot get a photo write the name, age, location and condition of the person on a piece of paper. This is to help you focus on the person. If it is someone you know, you can simply visualize the person between your hands.
2. *Gasshô* – to center the mind and set intent.
3. Hold the photograph in your hands and raise your energy level.
4. Focus on the person you wish to help.
5. Visualize or draw the symbols 3, then 2, then 1 with their accompanying mantras.
6. Continue focusing on the person for as long as you feel the energy moving.
7. *Gasshô* – to give thanks.

Gasshô Kokyû Hô 合掌呼吸法 (see *seishin toitsu*)

Gasshô Meditation 合掌瞑想

A meditation method concentrating on the hands

gasshô 合掌 – to place the two palms together
meditation 瞑想 – meditation, contemplation

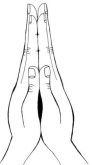

- *Shoden* technique
- This technique is taught by Frank Arjava Petter and is claimed to be a traditional Japanese Reiki technique

This is a meditation technique to calm and focus the mind.

1. Sit and gasshô to center the mind and set intent. Close your eyes.
2. Breathe in naturally focusing on the point where your two middle fingers come together. When your mind wanders use this physical point as your focus to bring yourself back to this single pointed meditation.
3. Continue the meditation for up to 30 minutes.
4. *Gasshô* – to give thanks.

Gedoku Hô (see *tanden chiryô hô*)

Gyôshi Hô 凝視法

A method of healing by staring

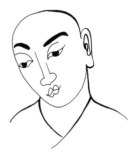

gyôshi 凝視 – stare, eye-focus

hô 法– method

- *Shoden* or *okuden* technique
- Taught in Usui Reiki Ryôhô, Komyo Reiki, Gendai Reiki Hô and Reido Reiki and once practiced by the Usui Reiki Ryôhô Gakkai

In the *Reiki Ryôhô Hikkei* it states that Reiki emanates from all parts of the body and is strongest in the hands, eyes and the breath. *Gyôshi hô* is a technique for sending Reiki with the eyes. This is a useful technique when working with people you may not be able to touch. It may be used during a treatment in conjunction with hands-on practice or simply on it's own.

1. Gaze with soft, defocused eyes and intent at the area on the body.
2. Visualize the energy moving from your eyes to that place.
3. Continue until you are ready to finish or move on to the next position.

Hadô Kokyû Hô 波動呼吸法

A method of vibrational breathing

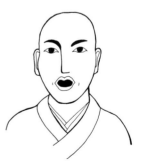

hadô 波動– wave, vibration

kokyû 呼吸– breathing

hô 法– method

- *Shinpiden* technique
- Taught in Gendai Reiki Hô and used in some traditional Japanese Reiki schools

The 'Haa' sound brings us to a different vibration level. The breathing improves the functioning of the immune system and detoxifies the blood and body tissues. It raises your level of energy and brings about relaxation and calm. Various Japanese schools use different versions of this technique. According to the school it is not always taught in *shinpiden*. This technique is practiced in traditional Japanese *ki* schools[9] and in some Buddhist traditions[10] as well.

1. Sit and *gasshô* – to center the mind.
2. Place your hands on your knees, facing upwards with eyes closed.
3. Breathe in and then breathe out from mouth with a 'haa' sound and hold it as long as you can. The out breath will gradually lengthen as you become more practiced. The final aim is to hold the 'haa' sound for approximately 40 seconds. Focus solely on the 'haa' sound as you breath out until you reach your limit.
4. When you finish the sound you release the tension in your abdomen. This creates a natural inhalation.
5. Repeat steps 3 and 4 with the aim of creating a free-flowing breath without tension.
6. *Gasshô* – to give thanks.

Hadô Meisô Hô 波動瞑想法

A method of vibrational meditation

hadô 波動 – wave, vibration
meisô 瞑想 – meditation, contemplation
hô 法 – method

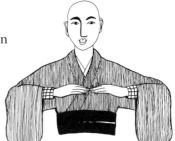

- *Shinpiden* technique
- Introduced by Hiroshi Doi and taught in Gendai Reiki Hô

This technique can bring you into a deep state of meditation.

1. Sit and *gasshô* – to center the mind and set intent. Close your eyes.
2. Reach your hands up to the sky with both hands facing each other (forming a funnel shape). Feel the connection to Reiki. Once you feel the energy moving down through your hands and into the body bring your arms out to the side until they are parallel to the ground. Palms facing the ground.
3. Bend your elbows and move the hands in front of the chest, fingertips touching, palms still facing the ground.
4. Breathe out doing the *hadô* breath of 'haa' with the hands pushing down to the ground.
5. Move your hands up to the forehead as you breathe in. Move the hands slowly down while breathing out with the *hadô* breath with palms facing the body.

---

[9] *Ki – A practical Guide for Westerners*, William Reed, Japan Publications Inc. 1986.
[10] Information supplied by Hiroshi Doi.

6. Complete step 5 three times. Now feel the energy move throughout the body. You can repeat step 5 as often as you want.
7. *Gasshô* – to give thanks.

Hanshin Kôketsu Hô 半身交血法
(see *ketsueki kôkan hô* and *zenshin kôketsu hô*)

Half body blood exchange or cleansing

hanshin 半身 – half body
kôketsu 交血 – blood exchange
hô 法 – method

- *Okuden* or *shinpiden* technique
- Taught in Usui Reiki Ryôhô, Komyo Reiki, Gendai Reiki Hô, Reido Reiki, Jikiden Reiki and once practiced by the Usui Reiki Ryôhô Gakkai, Chûjirô Hayashi and Hawayo Takata

If the client has diabetes then reverse the direction of the sweeps beginning at the base of the spine and working up toward the neck.

1. *Gasshô* – to center the mind and set intent.
2. Begin at the top of the spine and sweep (with one hand on either side of the spine) out to the side of the body. Work down the back, one hand width at a time, until you reach the coccyx. Repeat ten to 15 times.

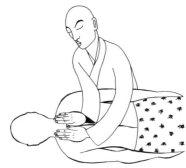

3. Place index and middle fingers at the base of the neck on either side of the spine. Hold the breath and press down sweeping to the base of the spine. Press fingers into the bottom of the spine and breathe out. Repeat ten to 15 times.
4. Place the hands about 1 to 2 inches (3 to 5 cm) above the neck. Hold the breath and sweep down the back to the coccyx. At the coccyx separate the hands and move them towards the feet.
5. *Gasshô* – to give thanks.

Hatsurei Hô 発霊法

A method for generating greater amounts of spiritual energy

hatsu 発 – to generate

rei 霊 – spirit

hô 法 – method

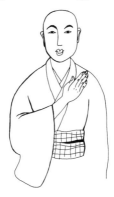

- *Shoden* or *okuden* technique
- Practiced by the Usui Reiki Ryôhô Gakkai and versions of it are taught in Gendai Reiki Hô, Usui Reiki Ryôhô, Komyo Reiki and Reido Reiki

Method 1

This method cleanses the body using energy, in turn allowing for a greater flow of energy through the body. In some schools *hatsurei hô* is initially broken into different techniques and taught separately. These are *kenyoku hô, *jôshin kokyû hô* and *seishin toitsu*. This particular version is based on one taught by Hiroshi Doi. He also states that *reiju* is performed during *jôshin kokyû hô*. When practiced in the West the five precepts and the *waka* are generally not included.

1. Sit in *seiza* and *gasshô* – to center the mind and set intent. Close your eyes.
2. Recite *waka* written by the Meiji Emperor.[11]

   kenyoku hô
3. a) Place your right hand on the left shoulder (where collarbone and shoulder meet). Breathe in and on the out breath sweep diagonally down from the left shoulder to right hip.
   b) On the in breath place your left hand on the right shoulder and on the out breath sweep down diagonally from right shoulder to left hip.
   c) Breathe in returning your right hand to the left shoulder and on the out breath sweep diagonally down from left shoulder to right hip.
4. a) With the left elbow against your side and with your arm horizontal to the ground, place your right-hand on the left forearm. Breathe in and on the out breath sweep downward along the arm to the fingertips.
   b) With the right elbow against your side and with your right arm horizontal to the ground, place your left hand on the right

---

[11] For more information about *waka* see page 74.

Japanese Reiki Techniques   199

forearm. Breathe in and on the out breath sweep down along the arm to the fingertips.

c) Breathe in and with the left elbow against your side and with your arm horizontal to the ground, place your right hand on the left forearm. On the out breath sweep down along the arm to the fingertips.

jôshin kokyû hô

5. Place your hands in your lap, palms facing upwards.
6. With each in breath feel the energy coming in through the nose, moving down to the *hara* and filling the body with energy.
7. On the out breath expand the energy out of the body, through your skin and continue to expand the energy out into your surroundings.
8. Repeat steps 6 and 7 until finished. The exercise may take anywhere from five minutes to half an hour. If you begin to feel dizzy then finish the exercise and slowly build on the amount of practice time.

seishin toitsu

9. Place your hands in the *gasshô* position. Focus on your *hara*. On the in breath begin to bring the energy into your hands. Feel the energy move along your arms, down though your body and into the *hara*.
10. On the out breath visualize energy moving from the *hara* back up through the body and then to the arms and out through the hands.
11. Repeat steps 9 and 10 until finished. The exercise may take anywhere from five minutes to half an hour. If you begin to feel dizzy then finish the exercise and slowly build on the amount of practice time.
12. Recite the five precepts.[12]
13. *Gasshô* – to give thanks.

Method 2

This method is a translation of an exercise called *hatsurei hô* from a 1933 book by a student of Mikao Usui. His name was Kaiji Tomita and he became a well-known healer in his own right. The book's name is *Reiki To Jinjutsu – Tomita Ryû Teate Ryôhô* meaning *Reiki and Humanitarian Work – Tomita*

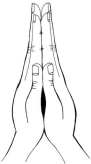

[12] This is understood to be included when the Usui Reiki Ryôhô Gakkai practice *hatsurei hô*. For more information about the five precepts see page 66.

Ryû Hands Healing. Kaiji Tomita considered this technique to be the fundamental technique for working with spiritual energy. First sit down and try to concentrate (unify) the mind and body. Choose a quiet place or somewhere comfortable where you can relax. Included in the text are two different readings of the word *seiza*. One means to sit still and is the first part of the technique the other relates to the physical action of sitting in *seiza*.

Seiza (lit. Japanese) to sit still

1. Sit in the *seiza* position and *gasshô* with the objective to gather/concentrate the energy from the heart into the palms of the hands. Hold the hands together without using force from the arms or the shoulders. Drop the shoulders and clasp the hands, joining the fingers lightly and feel the alignment of the posture. Close your eyes.

Jôshin hô (Mind purification method)

2. The aim of *jôshin hô* is to unify and purify the mind. Once the sitting upright is achieved, recite (in your head) some *waka* poetry and feel at One with its meaning.

    Following is an example of poetry that be used for *jôshin hô*:
    あさみどり澄みわたりたる大空の
    広きおのが心ともがな　　（天）
    Asamidori sumiwataritaru ohzorano
    　hiroki onoga kokoro to mogana (Ten)
    As a great sky in clear light green
    　I wish my heart would be as vast. (Sky)

*hatsurei hô

3. If you have followed the previous steps and stayed focused on the palms of your hands they start to become warm. This is (what *Tomita ryû* calls) *reiha* 霊波 (wave of *rei*). It describes the tingling sensation that is comparable to an electrical current. The heat created and the wave of *rei* are what constitute spiritual energy. Even if the sensations are weak at first, they should become stronger as you keep concentrating.

Five-day plan

4. Repeat the above steps for five consecutive days, and concentrate for at least 30 minutes (progressively increasing eventually reaching an hour)

Heso Chiryô Hô 臍治療法
A method of healing at the navel

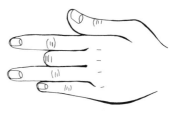

heso 臍 – navel

chiryô 治療 – treatment, cure, remedy

hô 法 – method

- *Okuden* technique
- Taught in Usui Reiki Ryôhô, Komyo Reiki, Gendai Reiki Hô and Reido Reiki and once practiced by the Usui Reiki Ryôhô Gakkai

This method works on the umbilical connection and therefore the practitioner's connection to mother. It also strengthens the kidneys as the hand on the back is placed on an important kidney acupuncture point.

1. This can be practiced on yourself or others.
2. Sit or stand and *gasshô* – to center the mind and set intent.
3. Place one hand flat over the navel area or place the middle finger gently in the navel, feeling the pulse. Place the other hand flat on the back over the corresponding area.
4. Hold until you feel that the body is balanced.
5. *Gasshô* – to give thanks.

Hikari No Kokyû Hô 光の呼吸法 (see **jôshin kokyû hô*)

Jakikiri Jôka Hô 邪気きり浄化法

A method for energetically cleansing and enhancing inanimate objects

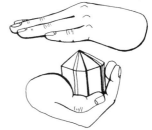

jaki 邪気 – bad, negative energy

kiri きり – cut

jôka 浄化 – purification, cleansing

hô 法 – method

- *Shoden* technique
- Taught in Usui Reiki Ryôhô, Gendai Reiki Hô and Reido Reiki and once practiced by the Usui Reiki Ryôhô Gakkai

This technique is only to be used on inanimate objects such as crystals, stones, jewellery, furniture, houses, etc … Not to be practiced on humans, plants or animals. While 'chopping' with the

hand focus on your *hara* and hold the breath.
1. Sit or stand and *gasshô* – to center the mind and set intent.
2. Hold the object in your non-dominant hand.
3. Place your dominant hand over the object approximately 2 inches (or 5 cm) with your palm facing the object. Chop three times in the air above the object. Hold the object and use Reiki.
4. Chop three times above the object to seal the energy in.
5. *Gasshô* – to give thanks.

Jiko Jôka Hô 自己浄化法

A method of self-purification

jiko 自己 – self
jôka 浄化 – purification
hô 法 – method

- *Okuden* technique
- Introduced by Hiroshi Doi and taught in Gendai Reiki Hô

1. Stand with your feet shoulder-width apart. Knees slightly bent.
2. *Gasshô* – to center the mind and set intent. Close your eyes.
3. Reach your hands up to the sky with both hands facing each other (forming a

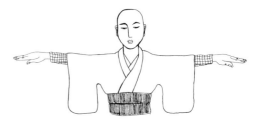

funnel shape). Feel the connection to Reiki. Once you feel the energy moving down through your hands and into the body bring your arms out to the side until they are parallel to the ground. Palms facing the ground.
4. Bend your elbows and move the hands in front of the chest, palms still facing the ground with fingertips touching.
5. Push both hands down toward the ground while doing *hadô kokyû hô. Feel imbalances leaving the body as you do this. Repeat again.
6. On the in breath move arms out to the side of the body and up with palms facing down. Bring the energy up with the movement of the hands. When hands are high above the head, face hands palm to palm and then open them up to the sky.

Release the energy upwards. Feel energy coming down through your fingertips and hands into the body.

7. Now breathe out doing the *hadô kokyû hô* turning palms downward and moving hands over your head. Bring them down the front of the body.
8. Repeat steps 5, 6 and 7 a number of times.
9. *Gasshô* – to give thanks.

Jôshin Kokyû Hô 浄心呼吸法
(also called *hikari no kokyû hô*)

Focusing the mind on one thing with breath

jôshin 浄心 – pure mind

kokyû 呼吸 – breath, respiration

hô 法 – method

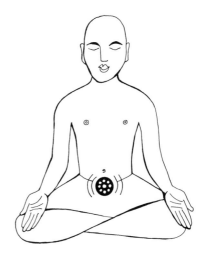

- *Shoden* technique
- Practiced by the Usui Reiki Ryôhô Gakkai as a part of *hatsurei hô* and taught as a separate exercise in Gendai Reiki Hô, Usui Reiki Ryôhô, Komyo Reiki, Method to Achieve Personal Perfection and Reido Reiki

It is used to focus the mind, clear the meridians and to build energy in the *hara*.

1. Sit and *gasshô* – to center the mind and set intent. Close your eyes.
2. Place your hands in your lap, palms facing upwards.
3. With each in breath feel the energy coming in through the nose, moving down to the *hara* and filling the body with energy.
4. On the out breath expand the energy out of the body, through your skin and continue to expand the energy out into your surroundings.
5. Repeat steps 3 and 4 until finished. The exercise may take anywhere from five minutes to half an hour. If you begin to feel dizzy then finish the exercise and slowly build on the amount of practice time.
6. *Gasshô* – to give thanks.

Kenyoku Hô 乾浴法

A method of dry bathing or brushing off

kenyoku 乾浴 – dry bath

hô 法 – method

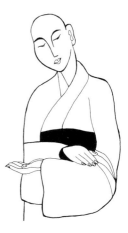

- *Shoden* technique
- Practiced by the Usui Reiki Ryôhô Gakkai as a part of **hatsurei hô* and taught as a separate exercise in Gendai Reiki Hô, Komyo Reiki, Usui Reiki Ryôhô, Method to Achieve Personal Perfection and Reido Reiki

This is a practice to purify the body, the heart and spirit. This technique is generally used before and after the practice of any energy work. It is based on a Shintô *misogi* technique.[13]

You clear the tension of the shoulders, the heart, the stomach and liver with stroke 1. Stroke 2 clears the tension of the shoulder, heart, stomach and spleen. Strokes along the arms specifically clear the arm and hand meridians.

1. *Gasshô* – to center the mind and set intent while standing or sitting.
2. a) Place your right hand on the left shoulder (where collar bone and shoulder meet). Breathe in and on the out breath sweep diagonally down from the left shoulder to right hip.

   b) On the in breath place your left hand on the right shoulder and on the out breath sweep down diagonally from right shoulder to left hip.

   c) Breathe in returning your right hand to the left shoulder and on the out breath sweep diagonally down from left shoulder to right hip.
3. a) With the left elbow against your side and with your arm horizontal to the ground, place your right hand on the left forearm. Breathe in and on the out breath sweep downward along the arm to the fingertips.

---

[2] *Misogi* is a purification rite and these are a vital part of Shintôism. Shintô priests practice **kenyoku hô* or the dry bath method. One Shintô practitioner said that he performed a similar ritual with a group of men from his village where they wore only a red loincloth at the *hekogaki* festival (putting on the loincloth festival).

b) With the right elbow against your side and with your right arm horizontal to the ground, place your left hand on the right forearm. Breathe in and on the out breath sweep down along the arm to the fingertips.

c) Breathe in and with the left elbow against your side and with your arm horizontal to the ground, place your right hand on the left forearm. On the out breath sweep down along the arm to the fingertips.

4. *Gasshô* – to give thanks.

Ketsueki Kôkan Hô 血液交換法

(also called *kôketsu hô* see variations *hanshin kôketsu hô* and *zenshin kôketsu hô*)

Blood exchange method

ketseuki 血液 – blood

kôkan 交換 – exchange

hô 法 – method

This technique is described in detail under its different variations. It is to be practiced by the practitioner on the client's bare back and massage oil may be used. If the client has diabetes then reverse the direction of the sweeps beginning at the base of the spine and working up toward the neck. This technique is mentioned in the *Ryôhô Shishin* or *Healing Method's Guidance* in the *Reiki Ryôhô Hikkei* as well as in Chûjirô Hayashi's *Ryôhô Shishin*. Western variations are the *finishing treatment or *nerve stroke.

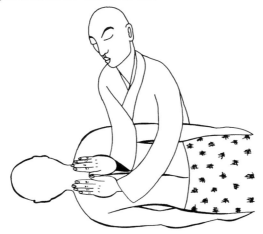

Kôketsu Hô 交血法 (see *ketsueki kôkan hô*)

Koki Hô 呼気法

A method of sending *ki* with the breath

koki 呼気 – exhaled air

hô 法 – method

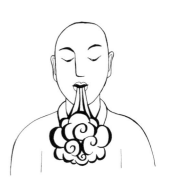

- *Okuden* technique
- Taught in Usui Reiki Ryôhô, Komyo Reiki, Gendai Reiki Hô and Reido Reiki and once practiced by the Usui Reiki Ryôhô Gakkai

You can incorporate this technique into a regular treatment or use it on its own. It is useful in situations where you cannot touch.

1. *Gasshô* – to center the mind and set intent.
2. Breathe in through your nose, focus on the *hara*, feel the lungs filling with this energy.
3. Blow the energy out through your 'O' shaped mouth to the area.
4. *Gasshô* – to give thanks.

Nadete Chiryô Hô 撫手治療法

A method of stroking with the hands

nadete 撫手 – stroking with the hands

chiryô 治療 – treatment, cure, remedy

hô 法 – method

- *Okuden* technique
- Taught in Usui Reiki Ryôhô and Gendai Reiki Hô and once practiced by the Usui Reiki Ryôhô Gakkai

You can incorporate this technique into a regular treatment or use it on its own.

This technique stems from Traditional Chinese Medicine and has its roots in *Qi Gong* and Chinese Massage (*tui-na*). The most important thing in stroking is that you have the intent to clear the energy of meridians and organs. You stroke with the palm of your hand, either with one hand or with both hands on top of each other.

Emotional links of the organs:

Heart – hurt, pain, joy, excitement, shock

Stomach – sadness, worry

Liver – anger

Spleen – depression, frustration, resentment, pensiveness

Kidneys - fear

Front of the body:

1. Start at the heart (middle of chest) then move to the stomach, on to the liver and all the way down the outside of the leg and flick off the energy at the toes. In one long stroke.
2. Start at the heart (middle of chest) then move to the stomach on to the spleen and all the way down the out side of the leg and flick off the energy at the toes. In one long stroke.
3. Begin at the heart on to the shoulders and down the arm, flick off energy at the fingers.
4. Put your index and middle fingers of both hands just between the eyebrows, finger tips touching and hold there for about 20 seconds. Then stroke slowly towards the temples along the eyebrows, hold the fingers at both temples for another 20 seconds. Stroke further till the ears and flick off energy.
5. Put your index and middle finger of both hands on either side of the nose just below the eyes and hold there for about 20 seconds. Follow the cheekbones till your hands reach the ears and flick off the energy.

The areas to stroke on the back of the body:

1. Start at the base of the neck and stroke along the spine all the way down to the tailbone. This will clear the heart, kidneys and spinal meridians.

Nentatsu Hô 念達法 (a variation is also called *seiheki chiryô hô*)

A method of sending thoughts

nen 念 – thought

tatsu 達 – reach, attain, notify

hô 法 – method

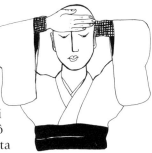

- *Shoden* technique
- Taught in Usui Reiki Ryôhô, Komyo Reiki, Gendai Reiki Hô, Jikiden Reiki, Reido Reiki and once practiced by the Usui Reiki Ryôhô Gakkai, Chûjirô Hayashi and Hawayo Takata

The five precepts are a form of positive affirmation. *Nentatsu hô* also uses affirmations with the aim of changing one's set behavioral beliefs. It is valuable for achieving goals, overcoming set beliefs and for ridding one's self of bad habits. In *seiheki chiryô hô* the symbols and mantras are also used.

1. Create the affirmation you wish to use. To make affirmations always set your sentence in the present. Keep the sentence positive by focusing on what you want in your life instead of what you don't want.
2. Sit or lie down and close your eyes, breathing regularly.
3. *Gasshô* – to center the mind and set intent.
4. Place one hand on your forehead and the other hand on the back of the head at the medulla oblongata.
5. Repeat your affirmation for as long as five minutes saying it out loud or to yourself.
6. Remove the hand from forehead while keeping other hand in place and relax for up to five minutes. You may wish to place the hand that was on your forehead next to or on to the body.
7. *Gasshô* – to give thanks.

Oshite Chiryô Hô 押手治療法

A method of using pressure with the hands

oshite 押手 – hand pressure

chiryô 治療 – teatment, cure, remedy

hô 法 – method

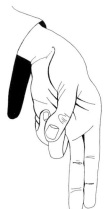

- Okuden technique
- Taught in Usui Reiki Ryôhô and Gendai Reiki Hô and once practiced by the Usui Reiki Ryôhô Gakkai

This technique is useful for areas of the body that are experiencing pain or stiffness. You can incorporate this technique into a regular treatment or use it on its own.

1. *Gasshô* – to center the mind and set intent.
2. Push the area of pain or problem with your fingertips sending Reiki through to the area you are focusing on.
3. *Gasshô* – to give thanks.

Reiji Hô 霊示法

A method of being guided by spirit

rei 霊 – spirit
ji 示 – show
hô 法 – method

- *Okuden* technique
- Taught in Usui Reiki Ryôhô Gakkai, Usui Reiki Ryôhô, Gendai Reiki Hô and once practiced by Chûjirô Hayashi and Hawayo Takata[14]

Once a student is confident working with **byôsen reikan hô* then **reiji hô* is taught. This technique guides your hands like magnets to the places on the body that are in need of treatment. Practicing **reiji hô* will heighten your sensitivity to energy work. It can be practiced on yourself or others. The hands are placed in *gasshô* in front of the upper *hara* thus stimulating the intuitive center, which helps to sense the body's imbalances.

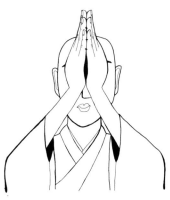

1. Sit or stand and *gasshô* – to center the mind and set intent.
2. Move your hands maintaining them in the *gasshô* position up to your forehead, in between your eyes (upper *hara*).
3. From this position allow the Reiki to draw your hands like magnets to the areas of the body that need it.
4. Hold your hands there until you feel that that part of the body is balanced.
5. Move on to the next position that draws your hands.
6. Continue to allow the hands to be drawn to the different parts of the body until it is no longer necessary and then let the hands relax onto your lap or to the sides of the body.
7. *Gasshô* – to give thanks.

[14] Hawayo Takata wrote in her diary in May 1936 that Chûjirô Hayashi had granted and bestowed on her *Leiji hô* (this is a spelling mistake and was probably meant to read *reiji hô*).

Reiki Mawashi 霊気回し

A current of spiritual energy

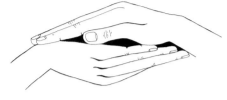

rei 霊 – spiritual
ki 気 – energy
mawasu 回す – pass on

- *Shoden* technique
- Practiced in Gendai Reiki Hô, Usui Reiki Ryôhô, Komyo Reiki and Reido Reiki

This technique helps to sensitize practitioners to feel energy flow. A group of practitioners make a circle, hold hands and allow Reiki to flow first to the right and then to the left.

1. Practitioners sit in a circle and *gasshô* – to center the mind and set intent. Close the eyes.
2. Everyone's left palm faces up and right palm faces down, hands out to the side of the body. This way your right hand is on top of your neighbors left and so on around the circle. Though the palms are facing each other they do not touch.
3. The teacher begins sending Reiki to the right. This increases in strength as it passes from one student to another. Practice this for a couple of minutes.
4. Now swap your hands and place the right palm facing upwards. Once again the teacher sends Reiki through the circle though this time from the other direction.
5. *Gasshô* – to give thanks.

Reiki Undô 霊気運動

Movement of spiritual energy

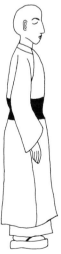

rei 霊 – spiritual
ki 気 – energy
undô 運動 – movement

- *Shoden* technique
- Practiced in Usui Reiki Ryôhô and Gendai Reiki Hô and was introduced by previous Usui Reiki Ryôhô Gakkai President Kimiko Koyama

This technique uses physical movement to cleanse and release the body's energy. The energy will guide the physical body once we totally let go. For each person the movement will be completely unique – release may be expressed through movement, sound, breathing or silence. This is originally a *Qi Gong* practice.

1. Stand with your feet shoulder-width apart. Knees slightly bent.
2. *Gasshô* – to center the mind and set intent. Close your eyes.
3. Reach your hands up to the sky with both hands facing each other (forming a funnel shape). Feel the connection to Reiki. Once you feel the energy moving down through your hands, in-between your hands and onto your head then let your arms flop relaxed to the side.
4. With each in breath feel the energy coming in through the crown on top of the head, moving down through the body and filling the *hara*.
5. On the out breath send the energy through your whole body from the top of the head to the tips of the fingers and toes. While still on the same out breath, move the energy out of the physical body into the energetic body and continue to expand the energy until it reaches infinity.
6. Repeat steps 4 and 5 until there is a strong flow of energy.
7. Now let the body totally relax and breathe normally. You will want to move with the energy that is pulsing through the body. Let go but don't force yourself to move either.
8. Take as long as you feel you need. At each practice session you will find yourself giving over to the energy more and allowing it to move the body as it feels the need.
9. *Gasshô* – to give thanks.

Saibo Kassei Kokyû Hô 細胞活性呼吸法

A method of vitalizing the cells through breath

saibo 細胞 – cell
kassei 活性 – activate, vitalize
kokyû 呼吸 – breathing
hô 法 – method

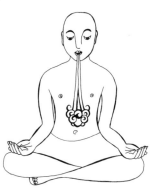

- *Okuden* technique
- Introduced by Hiroshi Doi and taught in Gendai Reiki Hô

1. Sit or stand and *gasshô* – to center the mind. Close the eyes.
2. Reach your hands up to the sky with

both hands facing each other (forming a funnel shape). Feel the connection to Reiki by sensing the vibrations of light. Once you feel this move your hands down and onto your head then place your hands on your knees, facing upwards.

3. Slowly scan down the body with your mind's eye.
4. Where you sense an imbalance breathe in and on the out breath send Reiki to that area. Talk to the area showing your gratefulness for the insight that you receive and for the balance that is currently taking place in your life. After a while you can just say 'thank you' and then eventually there will be a natural gratefulness attached to this technique and it will not be necessary to voice these words at all.
5. *Gasshô* – to give thanks.

Seiheki Chiryô Hô 性癖治療法 (see *nentatsu hô*)

Seishin Toitsu 精神統一
(also called *gasshô kokyû hô*)

Creating a unified mind

seishin 精神 – spirit, mind, soul, intention
toitsu 統一 – to unite, unify (to make one)

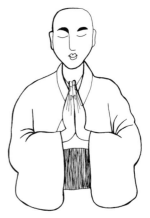

- *Shoden* technique
- Practiced by the Usui Reiki Ryôhô Gakkai as a part of *hatsurei hô* and taught as a separate exercise in Gendai Reiki Hô, Usui Reiki Ryôhô and Reido Reiki

It is used to clear your mind, to develop sensitivity in the hands and strengthen the *hara*. In Japanese schools slightly different versions of this technique are practiced.

1. Sit and *gasshô* – to center the mind and set intent. Close your eyes.
2. Place your hands in the *gasshô* position. Focus on your *hara*. On the in breath begin to bring the energy into your hands. Feel the energy move along your arms, down though your body and into the *hara*.
3. On the out breath visualize energy moving from the *hara* back up through the body and then to the arms and out through the hands.

4. Repeat for as long as you wish.
5. *Gasshô* – to give thanks.

Sekizui Jôka Ibuki Hô 脊髄浄化息吹法

A method of cleansing the spinal cord with breath

sekizui 脊髄 – spinal cord
jôka 浄化 – purification, cleansing
ibuki 息吹 – breath
hô 法 – method

- *Shinpiden* technique
- Introduced by Hiroshi Doi and taught in Gendai Reiki Hô

In Japan it is said that the spinal cord records our karma.[15] This technique works solely on the spinal cord, rebalancing it and consequently balancing the rest of the body.

1. Sit and *gasshô* – to center the mind and set intent. Close your eyes.
2. Reach your hands up to the sky with both hands facing each other (forming a funnel shape). Feel the connection to Reiki. Once you feel the energy moving down through your hands, in-between your hands and onto your head then place your hands on your knees, facing upwards.
3. Imagine that your spine is a pipe from the crown of your head down to the coccyx. As you breathe you practice the *hadô* breathing cleaning the dirt out of the body from the crown to the coccyx.
4. Breathe in through your nose and at the same time imagine pure water entering your coccyx and going up the pipe to the area in between the eyes on the forehead.
5. On the out breath feel the water leaving the coccyx.
6. Repeat steps 4 and 5 seven times and counting five breaths in one cycle.
7. *Gasshô* – to give thanks.

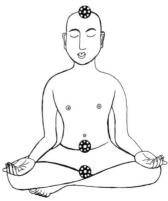

---

[15] *Modern Reiki Method for Healing*, Hirosho Doi, Fraser Jounal Publishing, 2000.

Shûchû Reiki 集中霊気 (also called *shûdan Reiki*)

Concentrated spiritual energy

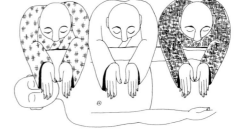

shûchû 集中 – concentrated
rei 霊 – spiritual
ki 気 – energy

- *Shoden* technique
- Practiced in most Japanese schools especially those that are influenced by Chûjirô Hayashi and taught by Hawayo Takata

This is a technique where several practitioners work on one person. Often practiced during a *shoden* class or at meetings and share evenings. *Shûchû* Reiki is generally performed over a shorter time frame than a regular treatment due to the intensity of working together with other practitioners.

1. *Gasshô* – to center the mind.
2. Each practitioner places hands on the body of the person lying down.
3. The practitioners cover the main parts of the body and any imbalances.
4. *Gasshô* – to give thanks.

Shûdan Reiki (see *shûchû reiki*)

Tanden Chiryô Hô 丹田治療法 (also called *gedoku hô*)

A detoxifying and purifying method

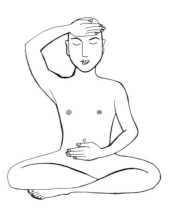

tanden 丹田 – the point below the navel where all the body's energy concentrates, also called *hara*
chiryô 治療 – treatment, cure, remedy
hô 法 – method

- *Okuden* technique
- Taught in Usui Reiki Ryôhô, Komyo Reiki, Gendai Reiki Hô and Reido Reiki and once practiced by the Usui Reiki Ryôhô Gakkai

This technique is used to purify and clear the body. The hand on the lower *hara* is connecting to your original nature. Meanwhile the hand on the upper *hara* makes the connection with the mind. When you bring the hand from the upper *hara* down to join the hand at the lower *hara* you are reminding your consciousness about your original nature. There is a similar de-toxifying technique called **gedoku hô* where one hand is placed on the front and the other on the back of the *hara*.

1. Sit and *gasshô* – to center the mind and set intent. Close your eyes.
2. Place one hand on the *tanden* or lower *hara* and the other hand on the forehead.
3. Connect with the energy of the upper *hara* at the forehead. Hold this position for approximately five minutes.
4. Remove your hand from the upper *hara* and now place it on top of the hand at the lower *hara*. Hold for approximately 20 minutes.
5. *Gasshô* – to give thanks.

Uchite Chiryô Hô 打手治療法

A method of patting with the hands

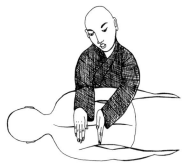

uchite 打手 – patting with the hand

chiryô 治療 – treatment, cure, remedy

hô 法 – method

- *Okuden* technique
- Taught in Usui Reiki Ryôhô, Gendai Reiki Hô and once practiced by the Usui Reiki Ryôhô Gakkai

You can incorporate this technique into a regular treatment or use it on its own. It is used to encourage the flow of energy. This technique stems from traditional Chinese medicine and has its roots in Qi Gong and Chinese Massage (*tui-na*).

There are four different ways to pat with the hand:
- with the palm of the hand
- with the back of the hand
- with the side of the hand
- with the fingers.

The most important thing in patting is that you have the intent to clear the energy of either the organs or the meridians.

The areas to pat on the front of the body:
On the front you only pat with the back of the hand, as this is the softest way to pat.
Pat from the wrist and not with the force of the whole arm.

1. Start at the heart (middle of chest) then in a straight line down to the pubic bone. Be careful not to pat too hard on the abdomen.
2. Begin just below the collar bone and then move up to the shoulder and then down along the inside of the arm – again you pat with the back of the hand.
3. Start just above the hip bone and follow the outside of the leg till the knee, then move to the inside of the leg till the feet and flick off the energy at the toes.
4. Or start just above the hip bone and follow the outside of the leg till the knee, then move to the front of the leg till the feet and flick off the energy at the toes.

The areas to pat on the back of the body:
On the back you can pat either with your palm, side of hand or the back of the hand as the back is not as sensitive as the front of the body.

1. Begin at the base of the neck and pat all the way down to the tailbone, on the spine. This helps to clear out the meridians that travel alongside the spine.

Zenshin Kôketsu Hô 全身交血法
(see *ketsueki kôkan hô* and
***hanshin kôketsu hô*)**

Whole body blood exchange or cleansing

zenshin 全身 – whole body
kôketsu 交血 – blood exchange
hô 法 – method

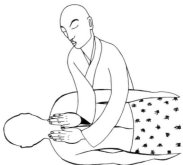

*   *Okuden* or *shinpiden* technique
*   Taught in Usui Reiki Ryôhô, Komyo Reiki, Gendai Reiki Hô, Reido Reiki, Jikiden Reiki and once practiced by the Usui Reiki Ryôhô Gakkai, Chûjirô Hayashi and Hawayo Takata

If the client has diabetes then reverse the direction of the sweeps beginning at the base of the spine and working up toward the neck.

1. *Gasshô* – to center the mind and set intent.
2. Complete a full treatment covering head, lungs, heart, stomach and intestines.
3. Begin at the top of the spine and sweep (with one hand on either side of the spine) out to the side of the body. Work down the back, one hand width at a time, until you reach the coccyx. Repeat ten to 15 times.
4. Place index and middle fingers at the base of the neck on either side of the spine. Hold the breath and press down sweeping to the base of the spine. Press fingers into the bottom of the spine and breathe out. Repeat ten to 15 times.
5. Place the hands about 1 to 2 inches (3 to 5 cm) above the neck. Hold the breath and sweep down the back to the coccyx. At the coccyx separate the hands and move them towards the feet.
6. Rub and sweep both arms from the shoulder to the tips of the fingers several times.
7. Sweep down from the thighs to the toes.
8. *Gasshô* – to give thanks.

11 Western Reiki Techniques

Western Reiki techniques have been sourced from many fields. Naturally, some are variations on the more traditional Japanese Reiki techniques while others are obvious imports. As seen in the previous section there are numerous Japanese techniques so it is a wonder that it has been necessary to include new techniques at all.

The teacher, Chûjirô Hayashi, taught only four or five of the Japanese techniques to his students Hawayo Takata and Chiyoko Yamaguchi. This may mean that Chûjirô Hayashi did not know them to pass on, did not place an emphasis on them, or the other techniques were not introduced till a later date. Hawayo Takata was not known to add any new techniques to the teachings during her lifetime, though she may have approached the techniques in a unique way.

The aims of the techniques used in the West are varied. These include methods to clear the meridians and chakras allowing the body to heal and become One with the universal energy – not unlike the Japanese techniques. Enhancing existing energetic modalities is also a common method used in Western Reiki as in the examples of *crystal grid work or *talismans. Other techniques are said to, themselves, enhance Reiki such as the *hui yin breath and *antakharana meditation. Western techniques can also focus on the achieving of a specific result; for example using Reiki as a tool for manifestation (this may sometimes have a materialistic aim).

Not only have techniques been added to the system of Reiki but, as seen in *The Reiki Sourcebook*, so have mantras, symbols, hand positions, beliefs and attunement methods. Why have there been so many add-ons? What is the motivation for changing the system of Reiki?

Humans continually attempt to improve and do their best. Though what one thinks is the best could be quite different as to what another's view is of the best – it's relative to one's own experiences in life and knowledge gained from within that. One practitioner may believe that the system works best when it includes a favourite breathing technique or physical movement. That practitioner tells their student that this is in fact the best way to do it and then that student tells their student and … this pattern repeats itself over and over again and is in fact the game commonly known as Chinese Whispers. It can make humans feel powerful to have changed an existing system 'for the better'; it can also reflect an attitude of knowing better than any existing system.

Reiki techniques are technically valuable in helping the individual continue to develop their connection to the energy. They sensitize practitioners offering them deeper insights into their true nature. The techniques are also valuable as a means to stimulate intent. When a technique is practiced with dedication a very clear intent is set. This intent affects the practitioner's ability to perform the exercise and that strength of character thus dominoes into every aspect of life. When these techniques started to disappear from Mikao Usui's teachings it is no wonder that new techniques have replaced them.

New Age Additions to Techniques

A most beautiful facet of this energy is its ability to adapt to any situation.

The New Age has been a period of the rediscovering of ancient ways. Egyptian, Tibetan, South American, Indian, Celtic and Chinese cultures have had many of their mysteries extracted for use by New Age individuals.

Mikao Usui's teachings were not New Age based though mystical and energetic elements of the New Age have been included into what is now known as the system of Reiki today. This has naturally weakened the connection to the original teachings while redirecting practitioners into New Age practices. Some of these are:

- Talismans – originating from the Western magical tradition.

- Energy bodies and auras – adapted from either Victorian spiritualism or Theosophy or from Eastern yogic practices – or all of these.
- Spirit guides – definitely shamanism and yet witches were also known to have familiars. Mystics, too, have been guided throughout the centuries by angelic beings – so the concept of spiritual guidance is quite broad based.
- Chakra system – is yogic in nature and the New Age has adapted it from the energetic system written about in the Indian Vedas. Traditionally the chakras or energy centers are pictured as multi-petalled lotus flowers, each associated with different deities, symbols, colours, syllables and animals. Today it is taught that there are seven major chakras and they begin at the base of the spine with the root chakra and work their way up to the crown chakra on top of the head.

Listed below are some of the basic qualities of chakras as written about by the medical intuitive, Caroline Myss:

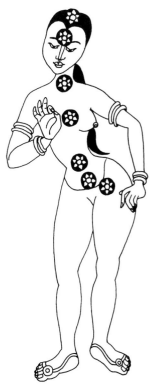

Root Chakra – groundedness, family identity, bonding

Sacral Chakra – creativity, survival instincts, sexuality

Solar Plexus Chakra – self respect, self esteem, ethics

Heart Chakra – love and compassion

Throat Chakra – choice, faith, personal authority

Third Eye Chakra – wisdom, intellectual skills, inspiration

Crown Chakra – inner divinity, inner guidance

Mikao Usui did not teach the chakra system instead using the Japanese *hara*[1] method. Hawayo Takata was aware of the *hara* method and is not known to have taught the chakra system in the West. A number of her students included the chakra system into the modern teachings of Reiki, including them in the techniques and the attunement process.

> It [Reiki] is nature's greatest cure, which requires no drugs. It helps in all respects, human and animal life. In order to concentrate, one must purify one's thoughts in words and to meditate to let true 'energy' come out from within. It lies in the bottom of the stomach about 2 inches below the naval
>
> (Excerpt from Hawayo Takata's diary writing about the hara, 10 December 1935.)

Practicing the techniques

Each of the technique descriptions consists of the levels that the techniques may be taught in and the specific branches that practice them. There are so many split-offs from branches as well as vague groupings, such as Usui Reiki, that it is often impossible to know what one school teaches in comparison with other schools even if they do belong to the same branch.

Historical information relating to where a technique originates is included where possible. Many of these are New Age additions and do not have a specific background. Any important points relating to the practice of the technique are also cited.

The particular technique is then described in detail. Mantras and symbols are linked as one in the West (unlike Mikao Usui's traditional teachings) therefore, unless noted, the word 'symbol' will stand for both. Symbol 1, Symbol 2, Symbol 3 and Symbol 4 have been used to represent both the mantra and the symbol.

---

[1] For more information about the *hara* see the Japanese Techniques on page 135.

Antakharana

A non-traditional Reiki healing symbol

- Level 3a (or Advanced Reiki Training) technique
- Introduced to the system of Reiki in Raku Kei Reiki and practiced in Usui/Tibetan Reiki and by various Independent Reiki Masters

In Sanskrit it is said to mean 'internal instrument such as mind, intellect, ego and the subconscious mind'. The antakharana is a two dimensional cube with three 7s on its face surface. Myth has it that this symbol originated from Tibet and China. Apart from being a cure-all if you meditate on the antakharana you will connect the physical brain with the Higher Self.

Meditation 1

1. Simply gaze at the antakharana symbol drawn on a piece of paper or make a 3-dimensional cube and draw 7s on it.
2. Meditate on the image and experience the energy

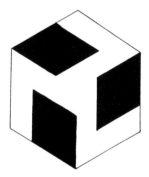

Meditation 2

1. Place the antakharana symbol under your feet.
2. Do a healing attunement on yourself.
3. Place your hands on your thighs and relax experiencing the energy.
4. Draw Symbol 4 in the air before you and repeat its mantra three times and meditate on the symbol.
5. Gaze at the antakharana symbol and repeat its name three times and meditate on the symbol.
6. Visualize the symbols, sending them to the light.
7. Perform the *hui yin breath
8. Visualize Symbol 1 clearing each chakra from the sacral chakra up and down the body.

Anti-Clockwise Energy Spirals

To ease the client into a change that is about to happen

- Level 1 technique
- Introduced to the system of Reiki by the West and practiced in Satya Reiki

It is easy to become very relaxed during a Reiki treatment. This method is used to bring someone's awareness back to the treatment room gently.

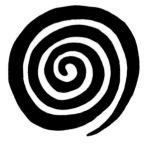

1. Draw anti-clockwise spirals with the tip of the index finger just touching the client's skin from the shoulder down to the feet and from the shoulders to the fingers.

Blue Kidney Breath (see *breath of the fire dragon)

Breath Of The Fire Dragon
(also known as *blue kidney breath, *Reiki breathing)

Non-traditional breath technique used with non-traditional attunement process

- Level 3 technique
- Introduced to the system of Reiki in the West and different variations are practiced in Tera Mai, Ichi Sekai Reiki, Johrei Reiki, Karuna Reiki, Karuna Ki, Seichim and Reiki Jin Kei Do

A variation of this technique is the *violet breath.

1. Begin the *hui yin breath
2. While you hold the contractions begin by breathing blue into your kidneys and white out. Repeat three times.
3. Visualize that there is a white mist cloud above your head. Breathe the white light in, all the way down to your root chakra.
4. Hold your breath.
5. The energy comes up the center of your spine and when it

reaches your brain it then turns white, sapphire blue, royal purple and gold.

6. Draw each symbol once and repeat their mantras. Breathing the symbols out.

Chakra Balancing

Balancing the chakras with each other

- Level 1 technique
- Introduced to the system of Reiki by the West and practiced in Satya Reiki and by various Independent Reiki Masters

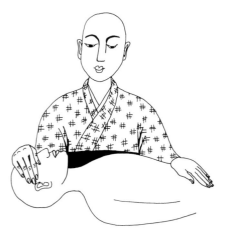

This chakra balancing technique may be used on yourself or on another person. Remember never touch a person's private parts. If necessary, place your hands a couple of inches/centimeters above the body – this is just as effective as hands on. This technique takes up to 15 minutes to execute and the crown chakra is not used. The crown chakra will naturally fall into line if the other chakras are balanced. Do feel free to use different combinations with all seven chakras if you intuitively feel this is appropriate.

The chakra system was incorporated into the system of Reiki by a number of Hawayo Takata's students but was not taught by her.

1. Lie on your back and place one hand on your third eye and one on your root chakra.
2. Leave your hands here until you feel that the energy has been absorbed into the body or up to five minutes.
3. Place one hand on your throat chakra and one on your sacral, your lower abdomen. Leave your hands here until you fell that the energy has been absorbed into the body or up to five minutes.
4. Place one hand on your heart chakra and one on your solar plexus. Once again, leave your hands here until you feel that the energy has been absorbed into the body or up to five minutes.

Chakra Kassei Kokyû Hô
Breathing method to activate the chakras

- Reiki 1 technique
- Introduced to the system of Reiki by Hiroshi Doi and practiced in Gendai Reiki Hô

kassei 活性 – active or activate

kokyû 呼吸 – breath, respiration

hô 法 – technique, method or way

Hiroshi Doi's technique has been added under Western techniques, as the chakra system is not used in traditional Japanese techniques. This is a product of the modern interest in the chakra system in the West and in Japan.

Set up

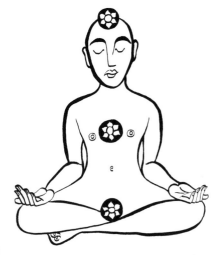

1. Sit and *gasshô* – to center the mind and set intent. Close your eyes.
2. Reach your hands up to the sky with both hands facing each other (forming a funnel shape). Feel the connection to Reiki. Once you feel the energy moving down through your arms and onto your head place your hands on your knees, facing upwards.
3. With each in breath feel the energy coming in through the crown chakra (top of the head), moving down through the body and filling the body with energy. On the out breath the body relaxes.

Basic Exercise Pattern: Root – Heart – Crown

4. a) Breathe in through the root chakra (base of spine), bring the energy to the heart, pause, and breathe out through the heart chakra (center of the chest).
   b) Breathe in through the heart chakra, take the energy to the crown, pause, and breathe out through the crown chakra.
   c) Breathe in through the crown, take the energy back to the heart, pause, and breathe out through the heart chakra.

d) Breathe in through the heart chakra, take the energy to the root chakra, pause, and breathe out through the root chakra.
e) Repeat this exercise a number of times.
f) *Gasshô* – to give thanks.

It is possible to work with all the chakras individually by replacing them, one by one, with the heart chakra using steps a) to f) e.g. Root – Sacral – Crown.

Chanting

Enhancing the qualities of symbols with the sound of mantras

- Level 2 technique
- Introduced to the system of Reiki by the West and different variations are practiced in Karuna Reiki and Karuna Ki Reiki

Chanting mantras is a technique used throughout the world in many cultures. This specific technique uses non-traditional symbols and non-traditional mantras. Chanting is used at any time during a treatment or during meditation and is preferably practiced out loud. It intensifies the flow of energy in the top chakras while protecting the body allowing it the space to heal.

1. Start the treatment with your hands on the temples of the client's head.
2. Chant 'Om' seven times then wait for the energy to move.
3. Continue with the rest of the treatment.

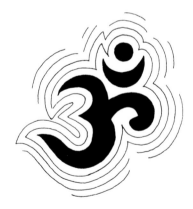

Communicating with your Higher Self
Re-connecting with the Higher Self

- Level 3 technique
- Introduced to the system of Reiki by Hiroshi Doi and practiced in Gendai Reiki Hô

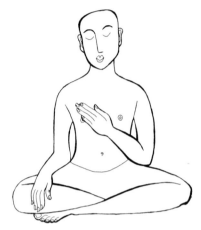

The system of Reiki has been re-imported into Japan from the West and therefore even the more traditional teachers may use Western material such as this.

1. Sit and *gasshô* – to center the mind and set intent. Close your eyes.
2. Draw Symbol 4 in the air and say the mantra three times.
3. Reach your hands up to the sky with both hands facing each other (forming a funnel shape). Feel the connection to Reiki.
4. Place your dominant hand on the center of your chest. Repeat 'My higher self, my soul' to yourself three times. Note any sensation.
5. Repeat step 4 with the non-dominant hand.
6. Communicate with the higher self through the hand on the chest.
7. *Gasshô* – to give thanks.

Crystal Healing With Reiki

Crystals are renowned as excellent healers. There are so many versions of crystal healing being used in the Western system of Reiki that it is hard to decide which one to print. It is advisable to clear and charge crystals before using them in any of the following techniques.[2]

Method 1
Crystal Chakra healing – helps people who have very low energy

- Level 1, 2 or 3 technique

---

[2] For clearing and charging crystals see *jakikiri jôka hô* in the Japanese Reiki Techniques on page 201.

- Introduced to the system of Reiki by the West and practiced by various Independent Reiki Masters

For this technique you will need ten crystal quartz stones, preferably rose quartz.

1. Place one on each of the seven chakras (be aware of people's boundaries), and in the palms (minor chakra) of the hands and one on the ground in between the feet chakras.
2. Perform a complete one-hour Reiki treatment, starting with the head, working your way down the body. Also treat the hands and the feet.

Method 2

Crystal Grid – sending continual energy to a person, place or event

- Level 3a (or Advanced Reiki Training)
- Introduced to the system of Reiki in the West and practiced in Usui/Tibetan Reiki and by various Independent Reiki Masters

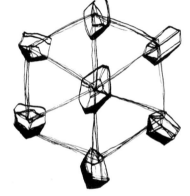

1. Choose eight similarly sized quartz crystals. From these have one as a center quartz crystal (sphere, cluster or multi-terminated).
2. Cleanse all the crystals.
3. Pick up each crystal, empowering them with all three of the symbols. Set the intention that the crystal's abilities are enhanced with Reiki.
4. Find a special place for the grid.
5. Place the center crystal in the middle.
6. From the rest of the crystals, intuitively choose one that feels like it has strong energy as the 'charging crystal'.
7. Place the six remaining crystals (points facing inward toward the center crystal) in a circle, evenly distributed like the numbers on a clock.
8. Pick up the charging crystal and place it in your dominant hand, point downwards over the grid of crystals. Place the point of the charging crystal over the center crystal and draw pie-shaped triangles over each of the crystals in a counter-clockwise direction. Draw a line from the center crystal out to one of the crystals, then move counter-clockwise to the next crystal, then

back to the center, then back out to the crystal you just left, and
move counter-clockwise to the next crystal, moving around
the circle several times, until you feel that the grid is strongly
empowered.

9. The intent is to charge this grid with Reiki. Every couple of days
you can re-charge the grid by repeating step 8.

10. Now place your list of persons, places or things to be healed
into the center of the grid with the intent to send it to every
individual on the list.

De-Programming Techniques

There are two traditional Japanese techniques that work on releasing
set mental patterns. One is *nentatsu hô* and the other is *seiheki chiryô
hô*. They are the same technique except that the latter is practiced
in *okuden* (or Level 2) and uses mantras and symbols. In the West
a number of variations of these techniques are practiced. Chûjirô
Hayashi and Hawayo Takata taught these traditional techniques, as
do some other traditional Japanese branches.

To make affirmations always set your sentence in the present.
Keep the sentence positive by focusing on what you want in your life
instead of what you don't want.

Method 1

Works on the removal of bad habits

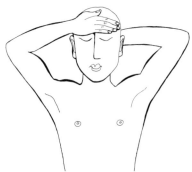

- Reiki 2 technique
- Variations are practiced in The
  Radiance Technique, Usui Shiki
  Ryôhô, Tera Mai Reiki, Gendai
  Reiki Hô and various Independent
  Reiki Masters

Create an affirmation for the habit
you wish to work with.

1. Place one hand on the back of
the head.
2. Draw Symbol 3, Symbol 2, and
Symbol 1 on the head with the other hand and chant the mantra.
3. Now place one hand on the forehead and one on the back of the
head with the intent that light is filling up the head.
4. Repeat the affirmation for the bad habit three times in your
mind.
5. Repeat this exercise everyday for six days.

Method 2
A method for changing mental patterns

- Reiki 2 technique
- Practiced in Seichim by Diane Shewmaker

Create the affirmations you wish to use together with your client.

1. The client sits and closes the eyes, breathing regularly.
2. Do Symbol 1 over the client's head and repeat the mantra three times.
3. Place your left hand on the back of the head where the skull has a bump just above the neck.
4. With your right hand do Symbol 2 over the crown or third eye and repeat its mantra three times.
5. Place your right hand across the crown or forehead of the client.
6. Call the client's name in your mind three times then repeat the affirmations silently or aloud. The client may also repeat the affirmations at the same time. Stay with your hands in that position for as long as you feel that it is necessary.
7. Give a written copy of the affirmations to the client and ask them to repeat them several times a day.

Distant Healing (also called *distant Reiki)

Send Reiki to a person, place or thing in the past, present or future

- Level 2 technique
- Practiced in the West and originally taught by Chûjirô Hayashi and Hawayo Takata (based on the traditional Japanese Reiki technique *enkaku chiryô hô*)

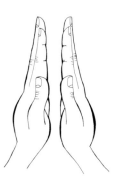

There are many, many versions of this technique. Some people hold a teddy bear and pretend that the bear is the client to whom the Reiki is being sent. Some pretend that their thigh is the body of the client. Others have the intent that their own bodies are representative of the person they are sending Reiki to and simply do Reiki on themselves.

Below is a simple version of distant healing:

1. Hold a photo of the person, place or event you wish to send Reiki to in between your hands.
2. Focus on the photo.

3. Visualize or draw the Symbols 3, 2, 1 with their accompanying mantras onto the photo with your finger.
4. Allow the energy to move through the body until you feel that it is finished.

Distant Reiki (see *distant healing)

Finishing Treatment (also called the *nerve stroke)

Blood cleansing method

- Level 2 technique
- Practiced in the West and originally taught by Chûjirô Hayashi and Hawayo Takata (based on the traditional Japanese Reiki technique *ketsueki kôkan hô*)

Hawayo Takata used the finishing treatment at the end of a treatment. Chûjirô Hayashi often recommended the blood exchange technique, as he called it, for various diseases.[3]

1. Place fingers from both hands on either side of the spine. In one fluent stroke move your hands from the neck to the coccyx. For diabetes always move from the coccyx upwards.
2. Place hands flat on shoulder blades, palms facing down and do circular movements anti-clockwise. Move hands down a hand width and repeat until the coccyx is reached.
3. Place one hand on the tailbone and one on the back of the neck.
4. Use one fluid stroke from the shoulder to the hand on both arms. Stroke down from the hip to the feet. For diabetics stroke towards the heart.

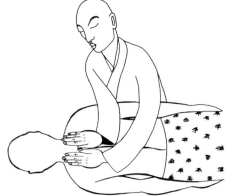

[3] Information supplied by Chûjirô Hayashi's *Ryôhô Shishin*.

Grounding

A method of connecting to the center of the earth energetically

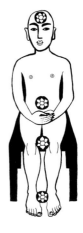

- Level 1, 2 or 3 technique
- Practiced throughout the world in many cultures

Grounding techniques energetically center a person by connecting to the earth's energy. Most of these techniques can easily be practiced within the system of Reiki. Below is just one of the many grounding techniques used within this system. Level 1 practitioners can practice it without using the symbols.

1. Sit calmly with your hands relaxed in your lap and your eyes closed.
2. Visualize Symbol 3, Symbol 2 and Symbol 1 and repeat each appropriate mantra three times.
3. Place your hands on the forehead and the back of your head and intend to send Reiki.
4. Place your hands on your sacral and send Reiki.
5. Place your hands over your knees and send Reiki.
6. Place your hands over your feet and send Reiki.

Group Distant Healing

A method where a group of Reiki practitioners send Reiki to a person, place or event

- Level 2 technique
- Introduced to the system of Reiki by the West and practiced by various Independent Reiki Masters

This is one variation of *distant healing in a group:

1. Practitioners sit in a circle facing each other.
2. Visualize Symbol 3, Symbol 2 and Symbol 1 and repeat each appropriate mantra three times.

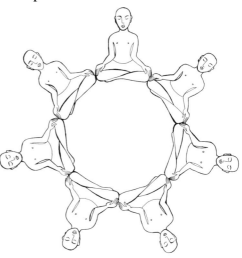

3. The name, age and any other information about the person to be treated are read out.
4. The practitioners send Reiki to the person who is then visualized in the center of the circle.

Group Reiki

Healing with Reiki in a group

- Level 1 technique
- Practiced in the West stemming from Chûjirô Hayashi and Hawayo Takata (based on traditional Japanese technique *shûchû Reiki*)

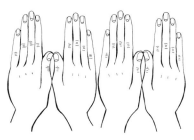

This is a technique where several practitioners practice on one person. Often practiced during a Level 1 course or at Reiki meetings, Reiki circles and share evenings. Group Reiki is generally performed over a shorter time frame than a regular Reiki treatment due to the intensity of working together with other practitioners. Chûjirô Hayashi had two people working on one client at the same time in his clinic.

1. Each practitioner places hands on the body of the person lying down.
2. The practitioners cover the main parts of the body and any imbalances.

Guide Meditation

Meet your Reiki Guide

- Level 3a or Advanced Reiki Training technique
- Concept introduced to the system of Reiki by the West and popularized by Diane Stein, William Lee Rand and Walter Lubeck and now practiced by various Independent Reiki Masters

Guide work is used in Shamanic traditions throughout the world. Here it has been adapted to be used with Reiki. Unlike Reiki, with guide work it is traditional to use protection before undertaking such methods. Protection can be as simple as visualizing yourself surrounded by protective white light.

1. Sit and close your eyes.

2. Imagine yourself engulfed by Reiki and divine light.
3. See a figure coming towards you through this light.
4. As the figure comes closer you have a clearer image of what the figure looks like.
5. To begin to connect ask some simple questions and listen to the answers. Know that you will remember these answers. What is the name, gender, appearance or even smell of your Reiki guide.
6. Take the hand of the figure and see if you recognize it. Feel the energy of the Reiki guide.

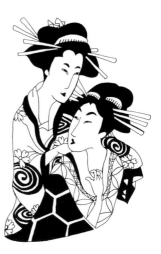

7. Now ask why this guide has come to you and what its message is for you.
8. Ask the Reiki guide how you will recognize it in the future and if you may call on it at any time you need assistance.
9. Know that the guide will always be there for you.
10. Come back to the room and open your eyes.

Healing the Past and the Future

Send Reiki to yourself to heal your past, present and future

- Level 2 technique
- Introduced to the system of Reiki by the West as an extension to *distant Reiki and practiced by various Independent Reiki Masters

1. Begin on Day 1 (after completing your regular treatment on yourself) by visualizing yourself in your mother's womb. Were you feeling happy, fearful, relaxed? Try to imagine exactly how you felt. Hold that image.

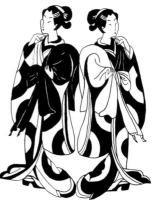

2. Now, imagine yourself in the future, choose a date 10, 20, 30, years from now and visualize how you would like to be. Are you a fit and healthy 80-year old with a passion for life? Choose an image that will be the ideal you.

3. Now, attempt to visualize the older you making contact with the past you. It is a beautiful meeting and now you are going to send Reiki to the image.
4. Use Symbol 3 and its mantra repeated three times.
5. Then Symbol 2 with its mantra also repeated three times.
6. Mentally draw Symbol 1 saying its mantra three times.
7. Wait peacefully as the energy is sent.
8. On Day 2 visualize yourself as a 1-year-old and see if you can remember back to events happening within that year. Perhaps someone has told you about yourself at this age, use this information as well. Then visualize that the 1-year-old you, will meet the future you.
9. On Day 3 visualize yourself as a 2-year-old etc... etc...
10. Continue until you reach your present age.
11. Repeat this technique as often as you wish beginning from in the womb.
12. Try to remember both good and bad experiences from your life and Reiki will heal all that you wish.

Hui Yin Breath

Non-traditional breath technique used with attunement process

- Level 3 technique
- Introduced to the system of Reiki in Raku Kei Reiki and practiced in Usui/Tibetan Reiki, Karuna Reiki, Karuna Ki as well as by many Independent Reiki Masters

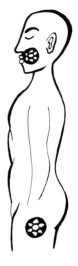

This breath technique originates from Chinese Qi Gong practices. Diane Stein uses the hui yin technique in a 'combined' attunement. According to her the use of this breath allows the teacher to perform one attunement instead of four in a Level 1 course. The hui yin technique is sometimes used in conjunction with the *breath of the fire dragon or *violet breath.

1. Contract your perineum (between your anus and genitals).
2. Place the tip of the tongue against the top soft palate (behind the upper teeth).
3. Hold the breath.

Making Contact with Higher Beings

Connecting and asking for guidance from higher beings

- Level 3 technique
- Introduced to the system of Reiki by Hiroshi Doi and practiced in Gendai Reiki Hô

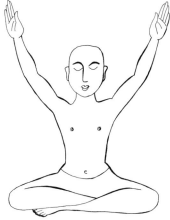

1. Close your eyes. Draw Symbol 4 in the air and say the mantra three times.
2. Reach your hands up to the sky with both hands facing each other (forming a funnel shape).
3. Feel the connection to Reiki.
4. Focus your intent on the higher being and sense its vibration. Think of your question.
5. *Gasshô* and melt into that vibration level. Your consciousness becomes One with it.
6. Now send your question to this higher being.
7. You will receive your answer in your everyday life or dreams.

Manifesting

Manifest what you need or want

- Level 2 technique
- Introduced to the system of Reiki by the West and practiced in Usui/Tibetan Reiki and by various Independent Reiki Masters

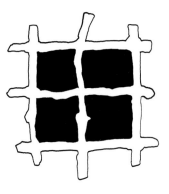

The ethics of manifesting with Reiki are simple and clear. If you must ask for something in such a way that it will deprive someone else, it is unethical. In asking for a job, for example, it is wrong to ask for someone else's job simply ask for the *best possible* employment of your own. If you want someone else's love but they are in a relationship with someone else, it is unethical to ask for this relationship to end. Ask instead for the *best possible relationship* for you, without designating who the person is. To manifest a relationship, make a list of all the qualities you wish

for in the *best possible* mate and use this list as a focal point.
1. Visualize your wish with you in it.
2. Place the earth behind you and your wish.
3. Bring a golden grid over the picture, spiraling from sky to earth.
4. Draw the Symbol 1 over the whole picture.
5. Hold the image for as long as you can, then let go.

Metta Meditation

Meditation focusing on goodwill and sending love and compassion to all beings

- Level 2 technique
- Introduced to the system of Reiki by the West and practiced in Reiki Jin Kei Do

metta – loving kindness (lit. Pali)
This technique is a well-known Mahayana Buddhist practice.
There are many Metta meditations depending on what your particular intention is. This Reiki Jin Kei Do technique is an adaptation of the Metta Golden Light meditation. You may wish to send Metta to your family, your fellow travelers, to world leaders, etc…

1. Sit in a chair with palms in the lap, right over left.
2. Focus on your heart chakra.
3. Focus on goodwill and loving kindness toward yourself and as you inhale visualize the heart area as a lotus flower opening on the in breath. Feel compassion for yourself and gently feel the energy blooming in the heart chakra.
4. As you exhale visualize compassion expanding from the heart as a beam of light. Send goodwill and loving kindness to all beings. This light expands in every direction throughout the whole universe benefiting all beings.
5. After a few minutes visualize the energy coming from the flower in the heart chakra as a silver mist. It spreads from the heart to every single cell in your body filling you with compassion and love.
6. Visualize this compassion expanding from your physical body outwards in all directions filling the whole universe benefiting all beings.

Morning Prayer

Prayer to be practiced each morning

- Level 1 technique
- Introduced to the system of Reiki by Shingo Sakuma and practiced in Satya Reiki

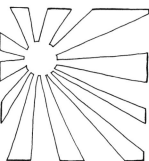

1. Make a bow to the Sun two times thanking God and existence.
2. Clap your hands two times, purifying the space around you.
3. Repeat three times.
   HARAE – TAMAE, cleanse all
   KIYOME – TAMAE, purify all
   MAMORI – TAMAE, protect all
   SAKIHAE – TAMAE, may all beings be happy
4. The Sun's Mantra.
   A-MA-TE-RA-SU OO MI-KAMI
5. Make a personal wish.
6. Repeat three times.
   KAMNAGARA - TAMACHI – HAEMASE, as the God wishes
7. Make a bow to the Sun one time and thank God.

Nerve Stroke (see *finishing treatment)

Open Heart Exercise

Creates a trusting and open relationship with others

- Level 1, 2 and 3 technique
- Introduced to the system of Reiki by the West and practiced by various Independent Reiki Masters

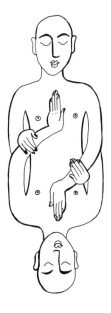

Reiki is about opening up your heart and living life in a compassionate, loving way. Here is a technique to open the students up to each other before experiencing the first Level 1 attunement.

1. Stand opposite your partner.
2. Place your palms flat against theirs (right against left).

3. Your right hand gently clasps their left wrist.
4. Make and maintain eye contact throughout the whole exercise.
5. When you feel the link is made at eye-to-eye level and you begin to feel your partner's energy place their left hand on your heart chakra.
6. Now move your hands so that you and your partner are palm to palm again.
7. Slowly bring all four hands together to form a diamond shape between index fingers and thumbs.
8. Bring this up to eye level and maintain your eye-to-eye contact through the diamond's center.
9. Raise your arms up as far as you can reach above, still maintaining eye-to-eye and palm-to-palm contact.
10. Let go of your partner and fan your arms slowly out horizontally and then embrace each other.

Power Sandwich

Increases effectiveness of hands-on or distant treatments

- Level 2 technique
- Introduced to the system of Reiki by the West and practiced in Seichim and by various Independent Reiki Masters

This technique is practiced with the belief that Symbol 1 activates the other symbols.

1. Repeat the symbols in this sequence as an alternative to using just one symbol.
2. Symbol 1, 3, 1, 2, 1

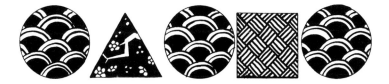

Preparative Mini Reiki Session (see *Reiki boost)

Quick Treatment (see *Reiki boost)

Reiki Aura Cleansing

Clearing the aura of heavy energy

- Level 3 technique
- Introduced to the system of Reiki in the West and practiced by various Independent Reiki Masters

This clearing technique can be used for both the client or on the self. There are many versions of this in use and below is just one example.

1. Stand and close your eyes.
2. Reach your hands up to the sky with both hands facing each other (forming a funnel shape). Feel the connection to Reiki.
3. Visualize Symbol 4, then visualize energy coming down into your body through the crown chakra filling the whole body and hands, inside and out, with a white light.
4. Now visualize Symbol 1 in three dimensions. The top of the symbol is just above the head. Let the energy spiral around you in a clockwise direction moving downward. As it spins around see Reiki removing blockages and strengthening the aura as it goes. Repeat the mantra three times.
5. Repeat step 4 nine times.
6. Visualize Symbol 4 starting above the head and going down to below the feet. Repeat the mantra 3 times. See Reiki as a white mist and breathe it in. Expand your energy out to the rest of the universe as you breathe out.
7. Open your eyes when you feel ready.

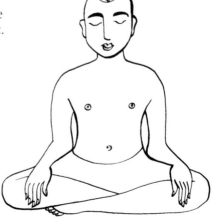

Reiki Boost
(also called the *quick treatment, *preparative mini Reiki session)

Balances and harmonizes the chakras allowing a greater flow of Reiki in the body

- Level 1, 2 or 3 technique
- Introduced to the system of Reiki in the West and variations are practiced in Tera Mai Reiki, The Radiance Technique, Reiki Jin Kei Do and by other various Independent Reiki Masters (see *seated chakra treatment for Reiki Jin Kei Do version)

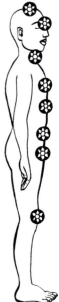

The chakra system was incorporated into the system by a number of Hawayo Takata's students but was never taught by her.

This technique can be used before a student receives an attunement. The intent is that it harmonizes the energy of the body so that the student can then receive full benefit from the attunement.

1. Stand the client sideways in front of you.
2. Place your hands on their shoulders to make an energetic connection.
3. Begin by placing your hands above their crown chakra, palms facing down and hold for 2–5 minutes.
4. Third eye chakra – palms facing each other on the front and back of the head and hold for 2–5 minutes.
5. Throat chakra – palms facing each other front and back and hold for 2–5 minutes.
6. Heart chakra – palms facing each other front and back and hold for 2–5 minutes.
7. Solar plexus chakra – palms facing each other front and back and hold for 2–5 minutes.
8. Sacral chakra – palms facing each other front and back and hold for 2–5 minutes.
9. Root chakra – palms facing each other front and back and hold for 2–5 minutes.
10. Knees – palms facing each other front and back and hold for 2–5 minutes.
11. Turn palms upward and slowly lift the energy up to the crown chakra.
12. Sweep down the aura to the knees.
13. Snap your fingers to break the energy connection.

Reiki Box

Send Reiki to a person, place or event in the past, present or future

- Level 1 or 2 technique
- Introduced to the system of Reiki in the West (popular in India) and practiced in Gendai Reiki Hô and by various Independent Reiki Masters

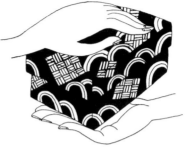

This is a technique for sending Reiki without having to use symbols or mantras. You will need a non-metallic box and paper and pen.

1. Write or draw any intentions you wish to send Reiki to on a piece of paper.
2. Put the paper in the box and keep it in a special place.
3. Send Reiki to the box every day by placing your hands on it with the correct intention.
4. Remove the paper once the intentions have been realized or you feel that it is no longer relevant.

Reiki Breathing (see *breath of the fire dragon)

Reiki Meditation

Meditation using Reiki to increase sensitivity and connection to the source

- Level 3 technique
- Introduced to the system of Reiki by Hiroshi Doi and practiced in Gendai Reiki Hô

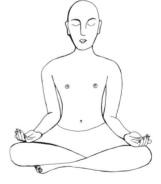

1. Close your eyes. Reach your hands up to the sky with both hands facing each other (forming a funnel shape). Feel the connection to Reiki and feel the energy moving down through your hands, in between your hands and onto your head.
2. Bring your hands down in front of your face in the *gasshô* position. Feel the energy moving through the whole body. Breathe in and out through your fingertips.

3. Raise the non-dominant hand a little higher and place your dominant hand, facing up, on your lap. Once again sense the energy running through the body. Place your dominant hand on any body areas that feel unbalanced.
4. Bring your non-dominant hand down onto the dominant hand in the lap. Relax into the energy.
5. Bring one hand to the heart and send Reiki to your higher self and say an affirmation.
6. Then bring one hand to the forehead and one to the back of the head and say an affirmation.

Reiki Shower

A cleansing technique that also increases energy flow in the body

- Level 1 technique
- Introduced to the system of Reiki by the West and variations are taught in Gendai Reiki Hô and Reiki Jin Kei Do

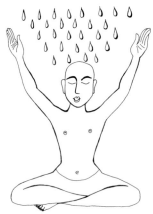

This technique has been adapted from *Qi Gong*. In another version of this you can keep your hands in the area where you feel any imbalances to rebalance the energy.

1. Close your eyes. Reach your hands up to the sky with both hands facing each other (forming a funnel shape). Feel the connection to Reiki and feel the energy moving down through your hands, inbetween your hands and onto your head.
2. Once you can sense the energy coming over and into the body like a shower bring the hands slowly down over and just off the body. Your palms are facing you with the visual idea that you are washing and cleaning yourself with energy. Move the hands over and across the body and finally down to the ground sending the 'dirty' energy down to the earth.
3. Repeat this as often as you wish reconnecting to the energy each time.

Scanning

Sensing imbalances in the energy field

- Level 1, 2 or 3
- Practiced in the West and taught by Karuna Reiki, Karuna Ki, Usui/Tibetan Reiki and various Independent Reiki Masters. A different version was originally taught by Chûjirô Hayashi and Hawayo Takata and is called *byôsen reikan hô*

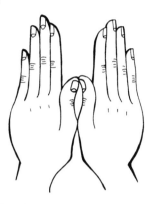

Scanning is placing your hands into a person's energy field and trying to sense energetic differences. This may be practiced on yourself or on a client before or during a treatment. In *byôsen reikan hô* as you scan you place your hands immediately on any imbalances but in scanning you first scan the whole body before placing your hands anywhere.

1. The client lies or sits and closes the eyes.
2. Stand at the crown with hands about 2 to 6 inches (5 to 15cm) above the body. Move your hands from the crown to the feet and back up again. This may take a few passes.
3. See if you can feel heat/cold/tingling/pain/itchiness/pulsating, etc… in your hands.
4. This is useful in finding places that may need extra attention before or during a healing session.

Seated Chakra Treatment

Stimulating the chakras

- Level 1 technique
- Introduced to the system of Reiki by the West and taught in Reiki Jin Kei Do (variation of *Reiki boost)

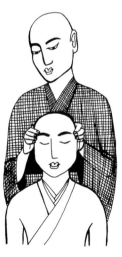

The chakra system was incorporated into the system by a number of Hawayo Takata's students but was never taught by her.

1. Seat the client and ask them to close their eyes.

2. Place your hands above the crown sensing the energy.
3. Begin to move both hands in a circular motion. After a while, begin to move your hands in an upward expanding motion. Then return to the circular movements contracting the energy.
4. Place the palms of both hands at the back of the head and bring the fingertips around to rest on the temples covering the ears to seal the energy.
5. Stand to the side of the client and move your right hand in front of the forehead and your left hand to the back of the head and repeat the motions of step 3. Seal the energy in by holding the back of the head and moving the right hand in small circular movements in front of third eye.
6. At the throat chakra repeat the motions of step 3. Then place your left hand on the back of the throat while the right hand is off the body at the front of the neck sealing the energy in in small circular movements.
7. At the heart chakra repeat the motions of step 3. Then place your left hand on the back of the heart while the right hand is off the body at the front of the heart chakra sealing the energy in in small circular movements.
8. At the solar plexus repeat the motions of step 3. Then place your left hand on the back of the solar plexus while the right hand is off the body at the front of the solar plexus sealing the energy in in small circular movements.
9. At the sacral chakra repeat the motions of step 3. Then place your left hand on the back of the sacral chakra while the right hand is off the body at the front of the sacral chakra sealing the energy in in small circular movements.
10. At the root chakra repeat the motions of step 3. Then place your left hand off the back of the root chakra while the right hand is off the body at the front of the root chakra sealing the energy in in small circular movements.
11. Stand behind the client and at the shoulders repeat the motions of step 3. Then place your hands on both shoulders to seal the energy in.
12. Stand at the side of the client again and hold the left hand above the crown and the right hand between the legs balancing the energy.
13. Stand at the front of the client and from the root chakra sweep upwards with both hands. Repeat three times.

Seventh Level Technique

Activating the gateway chakra

- Level 7 technique
- Introduced to the system of Reiki by the West and practiced in the Seven Level system (based on The Radiance Technique)

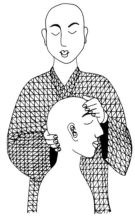

The chakra system was incorporated into the system of Reiki by a number of Hawayo Takata's students but was never taught by her.

This technique uses the gateway chakra that is situated where the neck meets the base of the skull.

1. Hold one hand over the gateway chakra and the other on the crown for five minutes.
2. Move the hand from the crown and place it over the third eye chakra for five minutes.
3. Now place one hand on the crown chakra and one on the third eye chakra for five minutes.

Six Point Meditation for Energy Awareness

Creating an even flow of energy in the body

- Level 2 technique
- Introduced to the system of Reiki by the West and practiced in Reiki Jin Kei Do

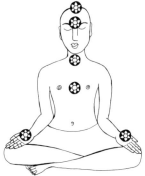

1. Center yourself by taking three breaths.
2. Bring your awareness to your crown chakra. Sense the energetic changes that may be taking place.
3. Bring your awareness to your third eye chakra. Sense any changes that may be taking place.
4. Bring your awareness to your throat chakra. Sense any changes that may be taking place.
5. Bring your awareness to your heart chakra. Sense any changes that may be taking place.

6. Bring your awareness to your palm chakras. Sense any changes that may be taking place.
7. Repeat as often as you feel necessary to create an even sense of energy flow.

Smudging

Using the vibration of smell to affect energy

- Level 1, 2 or 3 technique
- Introduced to the system of Reiki by the West and practiced by various Independent Reiki Masters

Our sense of smell is far more important than we can imagine. Smudging is used for clearing the energetic space in a room or around a person. Level 2 or 3 practitioners can draw the symbols with the incense sticks while clearing.

1. Clients stand with their feet and arms spread out while the practitioner wafts an incense stick around the front and back of the body and under their feet, encasing them in the energetic vibration.

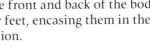

Solar Image Training

Method to lose dependency on symbols

- Level 3
- Introduced to the West by Hiroshi Doi and practiced in Gendai Reiki Hô

This technique uses images instead of symbols to help the student lose their dependency on the symbols. Symbol 1 uses the earth or red colour, Symbol 2 uses the sun or gold colour, Symbol 3 uses the moon or blue colour and Symbol 4 uses white light. Below is the technique using Symbol 2.

1. Close your eyes.

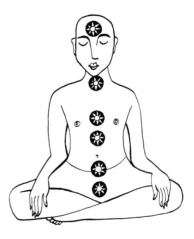

2. Reach your hands up to the sky with both hands facing each other (forming a funnel shape). Feel the connection to Reiki and its light.
3. Face your palms toward each other and visualize a golden sun in between them. Count to ten. Use a blue, cool sun if you have high blood pressure.
4. Place your hands on either side of your head at the level of the third eye chakra and visualize the sun in and around it. Count to ten.
5. Place your hands on the sides of your neck at the throat chakra. Visualize the sun having grown larger and encompassing it too. Count to ten.
6. Place your hands on the heart chakra. Visualize the sun having grown larger and encompassing it too. Count to ten.
7. Place your hands on the solar plexus chakra. Visualize the sun having grown larger and encompassing it too. Count to ten.
8. Place your hands on the sacral chakra. Visualize the sun having grown larger and encompassing it too. Count to ten.
9. Place your hands on the root chakra. Visualize the sun having grown larger and encompassing it too. Count to ten.
10. Relax and sense the sun's energy expanding from your body.

Symbol Exercises

Increase your connection to Reiki by meditating on the symbols

When students learn Level 2 they are traditionally taught three mantras and three symbols. In Level 3 they are traditionally taught one mantra and one symbol. Depending upon the branch of Reiki you practice this may vary as non-traditional schools will often teach more mantras and symbols.[4] Below are a number of methods shown to aid the student with their mantra and symbol practice.

Method 1 – Sense the energy of the symbols and mantras

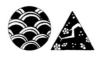

- Level 2 technique
- Introduced to Reiki by the West and practiced in Satya Reiki
1. With the palm flat and facing away from you draw the symbol. Repeat the mantra out loud. Breathe in and sense the energy.

[4] For more information about mantras and symbols see page 82.

2. Look at the symbol and whisper the mantra. Breathe in and sense the energy.
3. Now visualize the symbol in your mind and repeat the mantra to yourself while holding the breath.

Method 2 – Gain a deeper understanding of the energy of the symbols

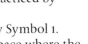

- Level 2 and 3 technique
- Introduced to the system of Reiki by the West and practiced by various Independent Reiki Masters
  1. With the palm flat and facing away from you draw Symbol 1. Repeat the mantra three times and step into the space where the symbol was drawn. Feel the energy of the space.
  2. Repeat step 1 for each of the symbols.

Method 3 – Connect with the symbols

- Level 2 or 3 technique
- Introduced to the system of Reiki in the West and practiced by various Independent Reiki Masters
  1. Seat yourself and place your hands on your knees or if you wish in your lap with the right hand over the left, palms up.
  2. Close your eyes and breathe into your sacral chakra, do not force the breath. Remember that while meditating your mind will start to wander. Do not chastise yourself or continue to put energy into these thoughts. Let them float away – you can imagine a fluffy white cloud coming along and taking them gently away. Let them go and concentrate on this specific meditation.
  3. To begin the meditation, intend that Reiki enters through your crown chakra and fills your body in a golden glow. Continue to breathe into your sacral chakra filling your organs, arteries, bones and skin with Reiki. The in breath brings the energy into you and the out breath expands it through the body. Now begin the visualization.
  4. The first symbol to visualize is Symbol 4. You can draw it in front of you or visualize it in your mind. Allow the energy to flow into you and then ask the energy for any message that this symbol might have for you. Remain focused on the symbol and allow the Reiki to flow through you showing you it's meaning. Continue for at least 15 minutes. You can now finish the meditation or continue with the three other symbols finding your personal connection with each symbol.
  5. With the Symbol 1 visualize it in a yellow colour, the Symbol 2 as

a blue colour and the Symbol 3 as a red colour. You may change these colours if you wish – just follow your intuition.

6. To finish the meditation draw your symbols while saying their mantras and thank the energy.
7. It might be necessary to ground yourself after this meditation. You can do whatever it is that is appropriate for you. You can place your hands on your sacral chakra and send energy there, drink a glass of water, stand solidly on the ground with your feet slightly apart and wring your hands or lie down and feel the root of a tree growing downwards from your sacral chakra into the earth.

Talismans

A method of manifesting using an image as the focus

- Level 2 technique
- Introduced to the system of Reiki by the West and practiced by various Independent Reiki Masters

You can use a talisman to manifest and to send distance healing. The time and energy spent on making a talisman may strengthen your intent. Once the talisman is finished hang it, or place it (in an envelope so that it is private) somewhere where you see it often e.g. in the kitchen or next to your bed. Every time you look at the talisman you are sending energy to that person, place or wish. Replace it with a new talisman when you feel the need. Some people burn the old talismans after seven days and make new ones.

1. On a sheet of paper write down the person, place or wish in detail in violet.
2. In the corners draw Symbol 1s in yellow.
3. Top and bottom, either side of the page draw Symbol 2s in blue.
4. Over your wish draw one large red Symbol 3.
5. These are just suggested colours; you may also make a talisman completely in gold or black if you wish.

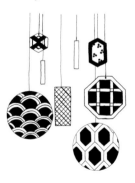

Toning

A method of using the voice as a healing tool

- Level 3 technique
- Introduced to Reiki in the West and variations are practiced in Karuna Reiki and Karuna Ki

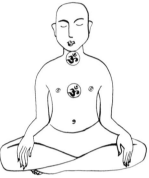

This technique is used to amplify the Karuna energies and can bring you to higher levels of energy. Toning is not like singing and may even be off key. The purpose is not to be pitch perfect but to trust that the perfect healing will take place.

1. Place your hands approximately 3 inches (6cm) to 2 feet (50cm) from the body of the client with your palms facing them.
2. First mentally begin toning the names of the symbols. You can create patterns by mixing the symbols together using your intuition.
3. Take a deep breath and begin the toning out loud. Allow the vowels to resonate.
4. Focus on the part of the body where you wish to direct the energy to.
5. Continue for as long as you feel necessary.

Violet Breath

Non-traditional breath technique used with attunement process

- Level 3 technique
- Introduced to the system of Reiki in Raku Kei Reiki and practiced in Tera Mai Reiki, Usui/Tibetan Reiki, Ichi Sekai Reiki, Johrei Reiki, Karuna Reiki, Karuna Ki, Seichim, Reiki Jin Kei Do and practiced by various Independent Reiki Masters

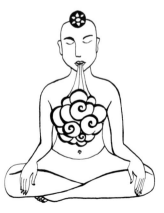

A variation of this technique is *breath of the fire dragon.

1. Visualize a white mist around you.
2. Contract the *hui yin point and place your tongue behind the upper teeth.
3. Visualize a white light coming down through the crown chakra, through the tongue and down the front of the body. It then moves through the *hui yin point and up the spine to the center of the head.
4. Visualize white mist filling the head.
5. Visualize the white mist turning blue, then indigo blue and then rotating clockwise. Now it begins to turn violet.
6. In the violet mist visualize a golden Dumo symbol.
7. In an attunement blow this breath out onto the student's crown chakra visualizing the symbol going into the head as you say the mantra three times.

Water Ritual

Changing water into energized healing water

- Level 3 technique
- Introduced to the system of Reiki by the West and taught in Tera Mai Reiki

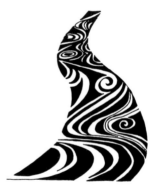

This is often used as a preparation for an attunement.

1. Students sit in chairs back to back with about 4 feet (1 ¼ metres) between them or in a circle.
2. The teacher uses Symbol 3 over cups of water.
3. Each student holds the cup of water at the solar plexus.
4. Students take a deep breath, hold it and close their eyes, exhaling forcibly a blue mist into the water.
5. After each breath the students pass the cup to the person on their right.
6. Throughout the technique the teacher will place the left hand on the crown saying Symbol 2 while using the *hui yin breath.
7. Students hold the cup in their left hand and then with their right hand draw Symbol 1 over the cup (horizontally) saying: I exorcise thee O SUI CHING (spirit of the water) to receive the Divine Benediction of Fire. That as I partake of this water, so shall I receive the Divine Benediction of Fire. I declare this to be True,

and so in the name of the Holy of Holies – So Be It.

8. Students draw Symbol 1 over the top of the cup again (vertically) and drink the water.

9. Students are now ready for the attunement.

Part IV

Directory

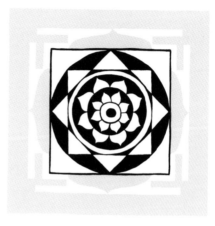

Reiki Branches

Under the heading of Reiki Branches[1] all forms of teaching that have at one time or another been based on Mikao Usui's teachings are included. There are so many branches it has been impossible to include each of them here in one directory. New branches of the system of Reiki are continually being developed. An overview of popular and less popular branches has been chosen to give a sense of what has evolved from Mikao Usui's teachings since the early 1900s.

The Reiki Sourcebook has included the claims that have been made by the branches but this in no way means that these branches are legitimate or that what is claimed is true. There are many varied 'original' histories and lots of individual creativity as far as branches of Mikao Usui's teachings are concerned. When reading through the branch information it is likely that you will feel confused. Don't lose sight of the fact that Mikao Usui's teachings are Japanese in origin. If you become overwhelmed by all the inter-galactic activity take a deep breath and head back to Part II – Reiki History.

It is good to remember that nothing can (as of yet) be proven to be of a 'higher vibration', 'stronger than' or be 'more penetrating' as far as energy is concerned. This is truly subjective, and these statements will only colour your personal experience of the energy.

In spite of extensive checking it is impossible to be 100 per cent correct about some of the information contained in the following pages. This is, of course, because of the changeable nature of life, Reiki practices and histories told (and not told). The authors are more than happy to update any information and offer their apologies here for any mistakes that may have slipped through.

---

[1] For the characteristics of what constitutes a Reiki Branch see page 171.

Alchemia Reiki

Founder: Reiki Master Kamala Renner.

Branch claims: Alchemia Reiki utilizes transformational and transmutational energy. It activates the Universal Fifth dimension Energy that involves being in the moment and accepting responsibility for your own reality.

Contact details:

> Dove Star
> 50 Whitehall Rd, Hooksett, NH, 03106-2104, UK
> Phone: 669 9497 or 669 5104
> Fax: 625 1919
> E-mail: nhdove@dovestar.edu
> Website: www.dovestar.edu

Amanohuna Reiki

Founder: Channeled by Arthur Cataldo in Hawaii.

Levels: Ten levels called degrees.

Branch claims: Amanohuna means the 'Abundance of the Right Way of Life'.

Contact details:

> Arthur Cataldo
> PO Box 1491, Sanibel, FL 33957, USA

Angelic RayKey

Lineage: Said to be channeled teachings from Archangel St Michael.

Founder: Reiki Master Sananda.

Levels: Three levels with approximately three days teaching for each level. The third level is the Reiki Master/Teacher level.

Mantras/Symbols: Uses traditional symbols/mantras and brings in other non-traditional symbols as needed.

Branch claims: Angelic RayKey teaches how to direct energy with prayer and intention, *distant healing, colour healing and also the importance of ceremony. It includes additional body/mind/spirit healing such as physical body energy systems and mental body creative powers. The focus is on healing and uplifting all aspects of body, mind, and spirit.

Ascension Reiki

Lineage: Said to be channeled from the Ascended Masters.

Founder: Channeled by Karuna Reiki Master Alan Harris with extra information from Robert Nutt.

Levels: Three levels.

Mantras/Symbols: Nine non-traditional symbols. These include seven symbols for seven chakras and two symbols for male and female energy.

Branch claims: Ascension Reiki is a powerful tool for healing but its main purpose is for expansion of consciousness and to accelerate the spiritual growth of mankind.

Comments: The Ascension Reiki system claims to be an entirely separate system from Mikao Usui's teachings and in the future will be entitled Ascension Chakra Therapy instead of Ascension Reiki. There is another Ascension Reiki taught in the USA. This is a completely different system.

Contact details:
3 Wood Green Road, Wednesbury, West Midlands WS10 9AX, UK
Phone: (0121) 502 4831

Blue Star Reiki

Lineage: Said to be channeled from Makuan.

Founder: Reiki Master John Williams channeled Blue Star Celestial Energy from his guide, Makuan, in January 1995. In April 1995 John initiated Gary Jirauch into this system. Gary then went on to modify it into Blue Star Reiki.

Levels: Available for Reiki Masters and Karuna Reiki Masters.

Branch claims: Also known as Blue Star Celestial Energy. John's guide Makuan received the knowledge of the Blue Star Celestial Energy System from Os-Mo-Ro-Pup. Os–Mo-Ro-Pup is from an Ancient Egyptian Mystery School. Blue Star Celestial Energy is a vehicle for bringing peace and planetary healing. It is not primarily concerned with immediate benefits or things pertaining to the needs of everyday life. Rather, it is aimed towards spiritual growth. It protects against the psychological fragmentation that could threaten the psyche during its exposure to multi-dimensional experiences of inter-time travel.

Brahma Satya Reiki

Lineage: Said to be channeled from a Master.

Founder: Reiki Master Deepak Hardikar.

Levels: Three levels plus extra levels called Healings Through Balance (HTB) and the Astral Travel levels.

Mantras/Symbols: Non-traditional symbols are used as needed.

Branch claims: In 1997 Deepak Hardikar heard a voice explaining revolutionary concepts about the universe and the system of Reiki. From this point on he began to intuit new symbols for his students. Deepak Hardikar then met a being – his Swami, the Master. He does not wish to disclose the identity of his Master, as he believes it may be controversial. At a later date he heard the voice say, 'This from now would be the Brahma Satya Reiki.' One other experience was when he felt his crown chakra being forced open and milk being poured into it from two great kalashes.

Contact details:
Based in India
E-mail: shardikar@satyam.net.in
Website: http://education.vsnl.com/brahmasatya

Dorje Reiki

Lineage: Mikao Usui – Chûjirô Hayashi – Hawayo Takata – Phyllis Lei Furumoto – Phillip Morgan – Robert Vaughan – Linda Nickel – Lawton R. Smith.

Founder: Lawton R. Smith.

Levels: Available for Reiki Masters. Non-traditional attunements are performed focusing on all chakras.

Mantras/Symbols: Non-traditional symbols are added as needed.

Branch claims: Dorje is a Tibetan word meaning 'diamond-like' or 'lightning' and stands for the divine universal diamond-like light, which permeates all of existence and energizes all living things. It also represents the understanding of which can arrive to an individual in a flash of light. It is energetically a synthesis of all dualities such as Kundalini and Tumo practice in the sense of the merging of spiritual energy with the physical for the purpose of healing and enlightenment. It is similar to the energy of Vajra Reiki merged with Karuna Ki. It can be used as both a healing system and a system of personal development. As only a healing system it is taught without the elements of meditation, and the attunement is simpler. Lawton R. Smith claims to have created Dorje Reiki from a combination of elements of Traditional Usui Reiki, Karuna Ki, Prema Reiki, Usui/Tibetan Reiki, Non-Traditional Reiki, and Seichim Reiki. It also has elements of Tibetan Tantric Buddhism and shamanism plus Lawton's own experiences and insights.

Contact details:
  Based in USA
  E-mail: lrsmith@sover.net
  Website: www.sover.net/~lrsmith

EnerSense-Buddho (see Reiki Jin Kei Do)

Gendai Reiki Hô

Lineage: Mikao Usui – Kanichi Taketomi – Kimiko Koyama – Hiroshi Doi (also trained with Mieko Mitsui, Hiroshi Ohta, Manaso, Chiyoko Yamaguchi).

Founder: Hiroshi Doi.

Levels: Four levels being *shoden, okuden, shinpiden* and *gokui kaiden. Gokui kaiden* has one integrated attunement. *Reiju* is also performed at each level.

Mantras/Symbols: Four traditional Japanese mantras/symbols are taught.

Branch claims: Gendai Reiki Hô is set up to respect Mikao Usui's system while blending Western and Japanese methods. His techniques are 'simplified and standardized' and structured in such a way that they are easily practiced in daily life. Some of the Westernized techniques taught are: *chakra kassei kokyû hô*, *communicating with your higher self, *deprogramming technique, *reiki box, *making contact with higher beings, *reiki meditation, *reiki shower and *solar image training. Gendai Reiki Hô teaches many traditional Japanese techniques too and these are listed under Part III – Reiki Techniques, Japanese Reiki Techniques.

Comments: Hiroshi Doi is a member of the Usui Reiki Ryôhô Gakkai. He has also been trained in western styles of Reiki. He does not speak English but offers English manuals.
Contact details:
> Based in Japan
> E-mail: g_reiki@yahoo.co.jp
> Website: www.geocities.jp/g_reiki

Ichi Sekai Reiki

Founder: Andrea Mikana-Pinkham.
Levels: Four levels with a non-traditional heart attunement.
Mantras/Symbols: Non-traditional Johre White Light Symbol is added, as is the *antakharana (male/female master symbol). No Symbol 4 is taught.
Branch claims: Ichi Sekai Reiki teaches the *breath of the fire dragon technique which originated from Raku Kei Reiki.
Comments: Said to be similar to Johrei Reiki.
Contact details:
> Website: www.SerpentsofWisdom.com

Imara Reiki

Founder: Channeled information by Reiki Master Barton Wendell.
Level: One level available to Reiki Masters with a 'new and easy' attunement.
Mantras/Symbols: None.
Branch claims: Imara means 'more'. It is a higher vibrational energy than most common forms of the system of Reiki because of its focused intentions. This course consists of the Imara Reiki Master handbook, a distant attunement to the Master Level of Imara Reiki, and a certificate for US$35.
Contact Details:
> Reiki Blessings
> PO Box 2000, Byron, GA, 31008, USA
> Fax or Voice Mail: (801) 7051802 – 24 hours
> E-mail: reikiblessings@earthlink.net
> Website: www.reikiblessings.homestead.com

Independent Reiki Master

Comments: This is a generic term for a branch that doesn't actually exist, as there is no underlying foundation. Independent Reiki Masters can come in two categories:
1. Those who teach from a number of different lineages and offer these to their students. These teachers show clearly which branches they practice.
2. Then there are those who claim to teach 'Usui Reiki', 'Traditional Usui Reiki' or something that sounds vaguely familiar to another branch of Reiki. They do not align themselves with a definitive branch of Reiki but instead teach bits and pieces from various branches. Independent Reiki Masters often teach some of these

non-traditional techniques: *antakharana, *breath of the fire dragon, *chakra balancing, *crystal healing (crystal grid), *group distant healing, *healing the past and the future, *hui yin breath, *manifesting grid, *open heart exercise, *power sandwich, *reiki aura cleansing, *reiki boost, *reiki box, *reiki guide meditation, *scanning, *symbol meditation, *smudging and *talismans.

Jikiden Reiki

Lineage: Mikao Usui – Chûjirô Hayashi – Chiyoko Yamaguchi – Tadao Yamaguchi.

Founders: Chiyoko Yamaguchi and Tadao Yamaguchi.

Levels: Four levels. Shoden and *okuden* are taught over five days with five attunements in total. Level 3 is the Assistant Teacher Level and lasts from six to 12 months. Level 4 is the Teacher Level.

Mantras/Symbols: Chiyoko Yamaguchi initially taught three mantras/ symbols before the system became known as Jikiden Reiki. Symbol 4 was not taught and the mantras and symbols were slightly different.

Branch claims: Jikiden Reiki means 'Reiki as taught or initiated directly' by Chûjirô Hayashi. This is a purely Japanese form of Reiki without Western influence. Copies of original photos of Mikao Usui and Chûjirô Hayashi are available to students only and cost a large additional sum of money. Covered under that cost is a copy of a work of calligraphy of the five precepts as written by Chûjirô Hayashi called the *gokai no sho*. Techniques taught are *distant reiki with one hand on the thighs, *nentatsu hô and *ketsueki kôkan hô.

Comments: Tadao Yamaguchi has published a book on the life of Chûjirô Hayashi. Tadao and Chikoyo Yamaguchi teach the courses together. Chiyoko studied *shoden* and *okuden* with Chûjirô Hayashi in a five-day course in 1938. Many of her family members were practitioners trained by Chûjirô Hayashi. One of them taught her the attunement so that she could help out at a course that the relative was hosting for Chûjirô Hayashi. Therefore, she has only learnt a part of *shinpiden* (not fully or formally).[2] Neither Chiyoko nor Tadao Yamaguchi speaks English but English manuals and translators are available.

Contact details:

Jikiden Reiki Association
Ayakouji Aburakoji Nishiiru, Shimogyouku, Kyôto City, Japan
Phone: (075) 343 0101
Fax: (075) 343 0064
E-mail: fwiv8655@mb.infoweb.ne.jp
Website: homepage2.nifty.com/reiki

---

[2] Information supplied by Hyakuten Inamoto who trained with Chiyoko Yamaguchi before her system was officially called Jikiden Reiki. Chiyoko Yamaguchi passed away in August, 2003.

Jinlap Maitri Reiki Branch (see also Tibetan Reiki)

Founder: Reiki Master Gary Jirauch.

Levels: Five levels available for Karuna Reiki Masters only. Non-traditional attunements are based on Medicine Buddha Initiations.

Mantras/Symbols: 25 non-traditional symbols.

Branch claims: Jinlap Maitri Reiki is Tibetan Reiki in the Medicine Buddha Tradition. It teaches the Tibetan concept of the five elements in relation to initiation, purification and healing; meridian therapy, information on the energetic body including eight wondrous channels, *violet breath, psychic pathways and etheric template expansion; *distant healing, psychic surgery, trauma release, self-empowerment, and clearing the emotional body.

Johrei Reiki or Jo Reiki

Lineage: Offshoot from Raku Kei Reiki.

Levels: One level that covers Level 1 to 3 in two days.

Mantras/Symbols: Four non-traditional symbols. The master symbol is very different from the traditional Symbol 4.

Branch claims: Teaches specific hand positions and uses the raku breath also called *breath of the fire dragon.

Comments: Johrei Reiki is a combination of Raku Kei Reiki and the Religion of Johrei. The Johrei Fellowship does not recognize it as part of what they do and have since trademarked the name Johrei so that any unauthorized usage is forbidden. Johrei Reiki is no longer practiced under this name. Vajra Reiki is an adaptation of Johrei Reiki.

Karuna Reiki

Founder: Reiki Master William Lee Rand.

Levels: Four levels with an attunement for each or just two levels (taught over three days) for established Reiki Masters.

Mantras/Symbols: 12 non-traditional symbols. Various Reiki Masters not including William Lee Rand channeled the symbols.

Branch claims: Some of the symbols used are the same as other schools but the attunements and the intention are different creating a unique system. The *violet breath, *chanting and *toning, *scanning and *Reiki meditation are all taught in Karuna Reiki.

Comments: In the early 1990s William Lee Rand created Sai Baba Reiki, which was influenced by Usui Shiki Ryôhô and Tera Mai Reiki. When the Sai Baba foundation found out that Sai Baba's name was being utilized in conjunction with profit making they asked that the system change its name. The name then changed to Karuna Reiki meaning 'compassion Reiki'.[3] Kathleen Milner, the founder of Tera Mai Reiki and William Lee Rand have been to court concerning the origins of their Reiki branches. Today neither branch mentions the other. Tera Mai Reiki and Karuna Reiki have both become trademarked names.

[3] *Reiki News*, Center for Reiki Training, Spring 1995.

Contact details:
The International Center for Reiki Training
21421 Hilltop St., Unit 28, Southfield, Michigan 48034, USA
Toll Free phone: (800) 332 8112
Phone: (248) 948 8112
Fax: (248) 948 9534
E-mail: center@Reiki.org
Website: www.Reiki.org

Karuna Ki

Founder: Reiki Master Vincent P. Amador.
Levels: Three levels or just one Master level (with one non-traditional attunement) for Reiki Masters.
Mantras/Symbols: Non-traditional symbols are used. These are the same as those used in Karuna Reiki but with different purposes.
Branch claims: Karuna Ki is the Way of Compassionate Energy. It shares early development with Karuna Reiki and Tera Mai Reiki. Techniques used are *violet breath, *chanting and *toning, *scanning and special *karuna ki do meditations.
Comments: Karuna Ki as a separate branch appears to initially have been a reaction to the trademarking of Karuna Reiki by its founder William Lee Rand.
Contact details:
E-mail: ShanTao@aol.com
Website: angelreiki.nu/karunaki

Komyo Reiki Kai

Lineage: Mikao Usui – Chûjirô Hayashi – Chiyoko Yamaguchi – Hyakuten Inamoto.
Founder: Hyakuten Inamoto.
Levels: Four levels. *Shoden, chuden, okuden* and *shinpiden*.
Mantras/Symbols: Traditional Japanese mantras and symbols, slightly different than are taught in the West.
Branch claims: Komyo Reiki was developed by Hyakuten Inamoto and is based on Chûjirô Hayashi's teachings. Komyo Reiki puts an emphasis on spiritual personal transformation or *satori* (enlightenment) through Reiki practice.
Comments: Hyakuten Inamoto has been the translator for a number of traditional Japanese teachers in Japan including Chiyoko Yamaguchi and Hiroshi Doi. He is a Pure Land monk and this added knowledge and experience makes him popular with his students. Some even say he looks like Mikao Usui!
Hyakuten Inamoto teaches for the URRI projects that have been organized worldwide. Hyakuten Inamoto completed the translation of Mikao Usui's Memorial Stone and the Meiji Emperor's waka used in this book.
Contact details:
Based in Kyôto, Japan and teaches internationally.

Cell Phone: 90 1910 5015
Phone: (75) 551 9666
E-mail: komyo100@yahoo.co.jp
Website: www.h4.dion.ne.jp/~reiki

Lightarian Reiki

Founder: Reiki and Karuna Reiki Master Jeanine Marie Jelm is said to have channeled information from Ascended Master Buddha.

Levels: Six Energetic levels have been adapted into four training levels (each with own non-traditional attunement and certificate). Prerequisite – Usui Reiki Master and Karuna Reiki Master. In lieu of Karuna Mastership, a Lightarian Buddhic Boost attunement can be received.

Mantras/Symbols: None.

Branch claims: Lightarian Reiki awakens humanity to six higher vibrational bands of Reiki energies. Ascended Master Buddha requested that Jeannine bring forth new levels of information about Reiki in order to clarify, demystify and expand the system of Reiki for humanity at this time. Created in 1997.

Contact Details:

Lightarian Institute for Global Human Transformation
PO Box 396, Pleasant View, TN 37146, USA
Toll Free phone: 1888 596 1071
E-mail: info@lightarian.com
Website: www.lightarian.com

Mahatma Reiki

Founder: Reiki Master Leonie Owen-Rosenberg.

Levels: Four levels.

Mantras/Symbols: Nine non-traditional symbols (three taught in each of the first three levels) with one attunement in each of the first three levels.

Branch claims: Mahatma Reiki is a mixture of the system of Reiki and the Mahatma 'I AM' presence. It is empowering and helps students to remember who they are. For more information about the Mahatma energy read Brian Grattan's book: *Mahatma 1 & 2*.

Contact details:

Leonie Owen-Rosenberg
8620 E. San Miguel Ave, Scottsdale, AZ 85250, USA
Phone: (480) 675 8675
E-mail: Leonie@Mahatmareiki.com
Website: www.mahatmareiki.com

Mari-EL

Lineage: Mikao Usui – Chûjirô Hayashi – Hawayo Takata – Ethel Lombardi.

Founder: Reiki Master Ethel Lombardi.

Levels: One level with one attunement (additional advanced classes available).

Mantras/Symbols: Three non-traditional symbols are taught in the first level.

Branch claims: Mari El teaches set hand positions; a *distant healing method and meridians are traced on the body after a treatment. The name is a combination of Mary (Mother of Jesus) and El (a name for God).

Comments: This was the first breakaway from what people thought of as the traditional system of Reiki in the West after Hawayo Takata's death (apart from The Radiance Technique). Ethel Lombardi created it in 1983 at a time when students of Hawayo Takata were deciding how they would organize the future of the system of Reiki. Ethel Lombardi only taught one teacher.

Contact details:
  Joan Baggett
  Phone in Portland USA: (503) 417 8092
  Phone in Vancouver Canada: (360) 690 1180
  E-mail: joan@joanbaggett.com
  Website: www.joanbaggett.com

Men Chhos Reiki (or Medicine Dharma Reiki or Universal Healing Reiki)

The claims to authenticity by the founder of this lineage, Richard Blackwell aka Lama Yeshe, are controversial.

Medicine Dharma Reiki (see also Men Chhos Reiki or Universal Healing Reiki)

The claims to authenticity by the founder of this lineage, Richard Blackwell aka Lama Yeshe, are controversial.

Method To Achieve Personal Perfection

Lineage: Mikao Usui – Suzuki san
Founder: Mikao Usui.
Levels: Three levels. The next sentence should begin *shoden, okuden,* and *shinpiden*. These levels are also divided up into sub levels. *Reiju* is received at meetings between student and teacher.
Mantras/Symbols: Depending on the student's abilities a meditation or a mantra or a symbol in conjunction with a mantra are practiced.
Branch claims: Suzuki san is a family member of Mikao Usui who was born in 1895 and is still alive today. She is passing on Mikao Usui's notes and teachings to Chris Marsh. The teachings are solely about the healing of self. This information was first called Usui teate when it came to the West – this reflects what Mikao Usui did, not what he was teaching. Some Japanese techniques taught are *kenyoku hô and *jôshin kokyû hô.
Comments: Mikao Usui is said to have spoken of his teachings as Method to Achieve Personal Perfection therefore that is the name that the authors have chosen to use in *The Reiki Sourcebook* to describe the teachings.

New Life Reiki

Founder: Reiki Master Dr V. Sukumaran.
Levels: Four levels (divides the third level into 3a and 3b)
Mantras/Symbols: 20 non-traditional symbols at level 2 and up to 150 non-traditional symbols in total.
Contact details:
  Indian Reiki Foundation
  23/5 A Govindan Street, Ayyavu colony, Aminjikarai,
    Chennai 600 029, India
  Phone: (44) 3740 085
  Website: www.newlifereiki.com

Newlife Reiki Seichim (see also Sekhem, Seichem, Seichim and SKHM)

Lineage: Mikâo Usui – Chûjirô Hayashi – Hawayo Takata – Barbara Weber Ray – Patrick Zeigler – Phoenix Summerfield – Marsha Burack – Margot Deepa Slater.
Founder: Reiki Master and Seichim Master Margot Deepa Slater.
Levels: Seven levels (approximately 740 hours of training in total) with non-traditional attunements
Mantras/Symbols: 36 non-traditional symbols from origins such as Tibetan, Chinese, Japanese and Egyptian. About a dozen mantras are used over the seven levels.
Branch claims: Margot Deepa Slater studied with Marsha Jean Burack in 1991 as a Reiki and Seichim Master. She found links between the ancient traditions of the Mystery Schools, Enochian Magic, Tantra, Taoism and Tibetan mysticism. She has therefore included traditional Western Reiki/Seichim/ Seventh Facet Seichim/Sekhem/SKHM into one course. The primary thrust of the Newlife Reiki Seichim lineage is one of a spiritual nature. The lineage aims to create understanding and awareness through the mystical secrets of body, mind and speech encouraging students on a path to self-discovery, understanding and self-mastery.
Contact details:
  PO Box 148, Pambula, NSW, 2549, Australia
  E-mail: newlife@asitis.net.au
  Website: www.newlifereikiseichim.com.au

Rainbow Reiki

Founder: Reiki Master Walter Lubeck.
Levels: Level 1 has four attunements and one Rainbow Reiki initiation and is taught over one evening and two full days. Level 2 has three attunements and is one evening and two days long. Level 3 is three days long and has one attunement.
Mantras/Symbols: One symbol is used in Level 1 plus three Rainbow Reiki mantras. Three traditional symbols are used in Level 2 and one traditional symbol in Level 3.

Branch claims: Rainbow Reiki is a spiritual way based on Usui Shiki Ryôhô and includes some Japanese Reiki techniques as well as *Reiki guide meditations, shamanism, feng shui, meditation, spiritual psychology/ psychotherapy, karma clearing, astral traveling, *crystal healing, inner child techniques, NLP, aura/chakra reading and channeling.

Contact details:
Reiki-Do Institute International Reinerstr. 10A, D-31855 Aerzen, Germany
Phone: (51) 54 97 00 40
Fax: (51) 54 97 00 42
E-mail: rainbowreikiwl@compuserve.de
Website: www.rainbowreiki.net

Raku Kei Reiki

Lineage: Mikao Usui – Chûjirô Hayashi – Hawayo Takata – Iris Ishikuro and Arthur Robertson (both deceased).

Founder: Reiki Master Arthur Robertson.

Levels: Four levels with Level 1 and 2 taught in one class with two non-traditional attunements. Third level has one non-traditional attunement plus an 'initiation'.

Mantras/Symbols: Johre Symbol.

Branch claims: Arthur Robertson first studied with Hawayo Takata's student, Virginia Samdahl in 1975. He then went on to study and work with another of Hawayo Takata's students, Iris Ishikuro in the early 1980s. Together they created Raku Kei Reiki. Iris Ishikuro was a member of the Johrei Fellowship[4] and this would account for the introduction of the Johre symbol or 'white light symbol' in these teachings. In a 1983 Raku Kei Reiki manual the non-traditional techniques taught included the *breath of the fire dragon, the *hui yin breath and the *kanji* hand mudras. (This was probably the first time they had been used in connection with the system of Reiki.) The *water ceremony and the chakra system are also practiced in Raku Kei Reiki. The seven major chakras are linked with the seven colours of the rainbow, seven musical notes and seven atomic seals to create healing and balance. Master Frequency Plates with an *antakharana inside must be bought and used by students of Raku Kei Reiki. The history for Raku Kei Reiki is said to be Tibetan in origin as researched by Rolf Jensen. He lived in Japan during Mikao Usui's lifetime as a medical doctor in the US Army (this has not been verified).

Comments: This was one of the first branches to break away from the Western Usui Shiki Ryôhô teachings and introduced the concept of a Tibetan history to the system. Raku Kei Reiki methods are practiced in many branches of Reiki and by Independent Reiki Masters.

Contact details:
American Reiki Master Association

---

[4] Information supplied to the authors by Light and Adonea's website: www.reiho.org

Omega Dawn Sanctuary of the Healing Arts
Cheri L. Robertson, PO Box 130, Lake City, FL 32056 0130, USA
Phone/Fax: (904) 755 9638
E-mail: arma@atlantic.net
Website: www.atlantic.net/~arma

Reido Reiki

Founder: Reiki Master Fuminori Aoki.

Levels: Seven levels.

Mantras/Symbols: The four traditional symbols are used and they have
one extra symbol called 'Koriki' which is the Force of Happiness and
brings inner peace.

Branch claims: Reido Reiki means 'to start again or be reborn'. It stresses
the importance of both spiritual emotional aspects of our being. Reido
Reiki teaches to clear or clean oneself at all the levels and to know what
is preventing us from happiness and how we can attain it. The focus is
on self-growth.

Comments: This is a fusion between Japanese and Western styles of the
system of Reiki.

Contact details:
  Based in Japan

Reiki Jin Kei Do

Lineage: Mikao Usui – Chûjirô Hayashi – Takeuchi – Seiji Takamori
– Ranga J. Premaratna.

Founder: Reiki Master Ranga Premaratna

Levels: Three levels followed up by four levels of a practice called Buddho-
EnerSense.

Mantras/Symbols: Traditional Reiki symbols are used except that the
Symbol 2 is slightly altered.

Branch claims: Reiki Jin Kei Do teaches from an Indian and Tibetan
Buddhist background. Seiji Takemori traveled through Tibet and India
developing this system. The chakra system and the nadis are taught as
well as techniques such as the *metta meditation, *Reiki boost, *breath
of the fire dragon, *Reiki shower, *seated chakra treatment and *six
point meditation for energy awareness.

Comments: There is no verification that Takeuchi or Seiji Takamori ever
existed. This teaching appears to be based on the chakra system while
Chûjirô Hayashi never taught it. There are many similarities with early
Kathleen Milner teachings. Ranga Premaratna studied the Levels 1 and 2
with a student of Kathleen Milner, Beth Sanders.

Contact details:
  Ranga Premaratna
  40 Killarney St, Mosman, Sydney, NSW, 2088, Australia

Reiki Plus

Lineage: Mikao Usui – Chûjirô Hayashi – Hawayo Takata – Phyllis
Furumoto – David Jarrell (deceased). David Jarrell also trained with

Virginia Samdahl and Barbara McCullough. He believed his true initiation was through the spirit of a Tibetan Master in 1981.

Founder: Reiki Master David Jarrell.

Levels: Four Practitioner levels plus Master level.

Branch claims: The Reiki Plus Institute teaches Usui Shiki Ryôhô with additional information such as the knowledge and understanding of etheric bodies, divine metaphysics, the Masters of the Rays and creative healing meditations. It offers 310 hours of formal training. The Practitioner's Certification requires 155 hours of hands on training plus an exam. Students are offered the opportunity of becoming ministers in the Pyramids of the Light Church.

Contact details:
> Reiki Plus Institute
> Richelle Jarrell
> 707 Barcelona Road, Key Largo, FL 33037, USA
> Phone: (305) 451 9881
> E-mail: reikiplus@terranova.net
> Website: www.reikiplus.com

Reiki Tummo

Founder: Reiki Master Irmansyah Effendi. (He has learnt both Usui Reiki and Tibetan Reiki and calls himself a Grandmaster.)

Levels: Three levels.

Branch claims: Reiki Tummo claims to have been taught by Buddha himself as the way to achieve enlightenment within one lifetime. It is said to be a more ancient and complete system than Reiki, Tibetan Reiki, Tibetan/Usui or gTummo Reiki.

Contact details:
> Irmansyah Effendi, 3/276 McDonald St, Yokine, WA, 6060,
> Australia
> Phone: (402) 235 942
> E-mail: ieffendi@hotmail.com
> Website: www.padmajaya.com

Sacred Path Reiki

Lineage: Mikao Usui – Chûjirô Hayashi – Hawayo Takata – Iris Ishikuro – Arthur Robertson – Rick and Emma Ferguson – Margarette L. Shelton – Gail Tola – Alice 'Leigha Dreamweaver' Wildman – Paula and John Steele.

Founders: Reiki Masters John and Paula Steele.

Branch claims: Sacred Path Reiki is a mixture of Raku Kei Reiki, Tibetan Reiki and Traditional Usui Reiki plus the teachers' own ideas for their students' development. Paula and John Steele were considering calling it 'Traditional/Additional Tibetan Raku Kei Reiki' but decided 'Sacred Path Reiki' sounded better.

Contact details:
> 3431 LaSalle Drive, Ann Arbor, Michigan, 48108-2900, USA
> E-mail: sacredpath@sacredpath.org
> Website: www.sacredpath.org/index.htm

Saku Reiki

Lineage: Mikao Usui – Chûjirô Hayashi – Hawayo Takata – Iris Ishikuro – Arthur Robertson – Rick and Emma Ferguson – Margarette L. Shelton – Kathleen Ann Milner-Derrick – William Lee Rand – Frank A. Petter – Hunan and Lino Alelyunas – Eric Bott – Bill Pentz.

Founder: Reiki Master Eric Bott.

Levels: Six levels in total. Level 1 and 2 are traditional Western levels with additions. A series of initiations from Tera Mai Reiki and Karuna Reiki are taught in Level 3. Those wishing to go on from there take the fourth and fifth levels that focus on additional energy and vibrational healing techniques. Level 6 imparts energizing techniques and starts the student on the Saku Ascension Program and the Saku Teaching Master Apprenticeship Program. Both take a number of years to complete.

Mantras/Symbols: Traditional and non-traditional symbols (some from Tera Mai Reiki and Karuna Reiki) are taught. The non-traditional Tibetan Saku master symbols are taught in Level 6.

Branch claims: Saku Reiki uses vibrational healing, nutrition, exercise, herbs, *crystal healing and other natural remedies to help heal.

Comments: This branch is also a combination of Tera Mai, Karuna Reiki, Usui Shiki Ryôhô and the founder's own personal practices.

Satya Reiki

Lineage: Mikao Usui – Toshihiro Eguchi – Goro Miyazaki – Mieko Mitsui – Takahashi – Toshitaka Mochizuki – Shingo Sakuma.

Founder: Reiki Master Shingo Sakuma.

Levels: Three levels called degrees with three or four attunements in the first level, three attunements in the second level and one attunement in the third level. Uses the traditional Mochizuki attunement.

Mantras/Symbols: Three traditional symbols for the second level and one for the third level.

Branch claims: Satya Reiki teaches the chakra system from an Indian viewpoint, set hand positions and *anti-clockwise energy spirals, *the morning prayer, *chakra balancing and the *symbol meditations.

Comments: This is said to be a Japanese lineage (as it is not from Hayashi/ Takata) but Mieko Mitsui has also studied and taught The Radiance Technique. This has been a definite influence on Satya Reiki. The Usui Reiki Ryôhô Gakkai's spokesman, Hiroshi Doi, wrote that Toshihiro Eguchi was a friend of Mikao Usui and a well-known healer but that he had never studied to become a Reiki teacher. If this were true, it would mean that what Goro Miyazaki taught was not the system of Reiki but a system devised by Toshihiro Eguchi. Shingo Sakuma has been teaching from India, where it is popular, since 1996.

Contact details:

Satya Reiki Communion Training Center: Pyramids Survey no. 81-82 Pingle Estate, North Koregaon Park Rd, Pune 411001, India
Phone: (212) 62 59 13
Fax: (212) 63 98 82

Seichem

Lineage: Mikao Usui – Chûjirô Hayashi – Hawayo Takata – Barbara Weber Ray – Patrick Zeigler – T'om Seaman – Phoenix Summerfield – August Star[5] – Kathleen Milner.

Founder: Reiki and Seichim Master Kathleen Milner.

Comments: See Kathleen Milner's Tera Mai Reiki for more information.

Contact details:

    Tera-Mai Healing
    PMB 102-125, 9393 North 90th Street, Scottsdale, Arizona 85258, USA
    Phone: (480) 314 5722
    Fax: 1-(480) 314 9905
    E-mail: kathleenmilner@earthlink.net
    Website: www.kathleenmilner.com

Seichim (see also Sekhem, Seichem, SKHM and Newlife Reiki Seichim)

Lineage: Mikao Usui – Chûjirô Hayashi – Hawayo Takata – Barbara Weber Ray – Patrick Zeigler.

Founder: Reiki Master Patrick Zeigler.

Levels: Five levels called facets. Four attunements in Level 1; two attunements in Level 2; one attunement in Level 3; one attunement in Level 4 plus separate attunements for animals and inanimate objects; one attunement in Level 5 and a personal empowerment attunement.

Mantras/Symbols: Three traditional symbols and several variations on Symbol 4. Additional symbols are added in the fourth and fifth level. Some of the symbols used under variations of Seichim are: Chokuret; Blue DKM; Pink DKM; Mai Yur Ma/Shining Everlasting Flower of Enlightenment (three versions); Tan Ku Rei; Ta Ku Rei; Shining Everlasting Living Waters of Ra; Shining Everlasting Living Facets of Eternal Compassionate Wisdom; Divine Balance; Eternal Pearl of Wisdom and Love/Blue Pearl of Wisdom; Healing Triangle; Symbol of Divinity; Heart of the Christos; Heart of Gaia; Align with God; Eeftchay; Angel Wings; Merge Consciousness; as well as the Infinity symbol.

Branch claims: This was the original Seichim system. Patrick Zeigler first tapped into the Egyptian feel of Seichim in 1980 when he spent a night in the King's chamber in the Great Pyramid in Egypt. He considers this to be his first initiation. After this he spent time with a group of Sufis who provided the teachings that went with his experience. Some of the techniques which have been taught under this name are the *power sandwich, *de-programming technique and *breath of the fire dragon or *violet breath, *distant healing and mental/emotional balancing.

Comments: Some Seichim systems have different spellings to enunciate their different approaches on the same theme. Seichim may not have the word 'Reiki' in its name but the system of Reiki is often considered

---

[5] Information supplied by Vincent Amador's website: angelreiki.nu/karunaki/karuna.html.

to be the foundation from where it began. In 1983/84 Patrick Zeigler studied the system of Reiki. In 1984 he taught Seichim for the first time. Two Seichim teachers, T'om Seaman and Phoenix Summerfield, turned Seichim into a popular form of healing. Many Independent Reiki Masters have taught versions of Seichim all around the world. In 1991, Kathleen Milner began teaching Tera Mai Seichem while Helen Belot created Sekhem. Patrick Zeigler had remained in the background until 1998 when he began teaching an updated version of Seichim called SKHM. Some Independent Reiki Master's teach the Seichim Master Level and the Reiki Master level together.

Contact details: Patrick Zeigler no longer teaches this particular system though there are many independent Reiki Masters who do teach their own system under the name Seichim. Apart from the versions of Seichim mentioned in *The Reiki Sourcebook* there is also Isis Sekhem, Renegade Seichim, Seichim-Sekhem-Reiki (SSR), Seven Facet Seichim, etc ...

Sekhem

Lineage: Mikao Usui – Chûjirô Hayashi – Hawayo Takata – Barbara Weber Ray – Patrick Zeigler – T'om Seaman – Phoenix Summerfield – Helen Belot.

Founder: Reiki and Seichim Master Helen Belot.

Levels: Four levels.

Mantras/Symbols: Traditional symbols are taught plus many more non-traditional symbols.

Branch claims: Helen Belot has 're-introduced' and adapted these teachings and is the custodian to this ancient Egyptian Energy System of Sekhem. She remembers a number of lifetimes as a high priest in early Egypt. This is not just healing energy but a complete energetic system. Though Helen is a Reiki Master she says that Sekhem is totally different to the system of Reiki.

Comments: A further variation on Seichim. Helen Belot has trademarked Sekhem in Australia, America, Hong Kong, China and possibly the EU.

Contact details:
> The International Sekhem Association Inc
> PO Box 98, Kangaroo Ground, Victoria 3097, Australia
> Phone: (07) 5545 3850
> Fax: (07) 5545 3870
> E-mail: hbelot@austarnet.com.au
> Website: www.sekhem.org

Seven Level System

Lineage: Mikao Usui – Chûjirô Hayashi – Hawayo Takata – Barbara Weber Ray – Gary Samer (Independent Reiki Master who resigned from The Radiance Technique in 1990).

Founder: Reiki Master Gary Samer.

Levels: Seven levels based on the Indian chakra system.

Mantras/Symbols: Traditional symbols are taught plus non-traditional symbols. These are often the Serpent Fire, Gateway, Daiki Ro Se (wisdom symbol), Cho Ka Ku (third eye symbol), Chi Ka So (throat chakra symbol), and the Shi Ka Sei Ki (heart chakra symbol). The well-known infinity symbol (a sideways 8) is used in the seventh level. Generally the infinity symbol is used in Seichim only.

Branch claims: Various *seventh level techniques are taught. Some of its teachers claim to teach the 'original' system of Reiki.

Comments: The Seven Level system is a generic term used to cover teachers who have broken away from The Radiance Technique (which is a breakaway from Usui Shiki Ryôhô). One of these is Gary Samer. This is a non-traditional system of Reiki. As there is no set system or foundation for this branch there are a multitude of teachings under its banner. Some Seven Level teachers claim to be able to re-attune the student (this means to take away the current attunement and replace it with a 'better' one – something that is inherent in existence cannot be taken away!). Also offered by some of these teachers is an attunement that lasts only a few days. Energy cannot be timed and this is a misrepresentation of the system of Reiki. Attunements are not 'given' by a teacher – students draw as much energy as they need at that particular moment in time (each individual is unique). This concept is about power – not about healing. The seven levels correlate with the Indian chakra system, which was introduced after Hawayo Takata's death in 1980.

Shamballa Multi-Dimensional Healing/Reiki

Lineage: Said to be channeled teachings from St Germain.

Founder: Reiki Master John Armitage.

Levels: Three levels.

Mantras/Symbol: 352 symbols one for each level between here and the Source.

Branch claims: Shamballa Reiki teaches the student to work with *crystals; the *antakharana; *how to connect people to their higher selves; the Mahatma energy; how to cleanse the 50 chakras and activate the 36-strand DNA; meet one's *Reiki guides, and the Ascended and Galactic Masters.

Comments: Includes a mixture of information from branches such as Usui Shiki Ryôhô, Raku Kei Reiki and Usui/Tibetan Reiki. John Armitage claims to have received these complete teachings direct from St Germain (bypassing Mikao Usui, the founder of Reiki, and any other teachers in his lineage). It is interesting to note that his information about the system of Reiki bases its history on that told by Hawayo Takata.

Contact details:

139 Kenn Rd, Clevedon, North Somerset, UK, BS21 6JY

E-mail: drdas@globalnet.co.uk

Website: www.mahatma.co.uk/p2.htm

SKHM (see also Sekhem, Seichem, Seichim and Newlife Reiki Seichim)

Lineage: Mikao Usui – Chûjirô Hayashi – Hawayo Takata – Barbara Weber Ray – Patrick Zeigler.

Founder: Reiki Master Patrick Zeigler.
Levels: No attunements.
Mantras/Symbols: No symbols.
Comments: This is the latest version of Seichim that is taught by Seichim's founder Patrick Zeigler.
Contact details:
E-mail: info@SKHM.org
Website: www.SKHM.org

Sun Li Chung Reiki

Lineage: Said to be channeled information from Mikao Usui; the Council of Nine; the Brotherhood of Light; the Peladian Council and the Crystal Council.
Founder: Yosef Sharon (calls himself a Grandmaster).
Levels: Five levels called degrees. The fifth level is the Grandmaster level and will only be taught to one person who will then take over from Yosef Sharon.
Mantras/Symbols: Thousands of symbols, which are never actually given to the student but are instead put into the aura.
Comments: Yosef Sharon claims not to have been attuned to the system of Reiki at all but says he received the whole Sun Li Ching system through channeling.

Tara Reiki

Founder: Reiki Master Richard Morningstar.
Levels: Five levels. The first level is the '$99 Usui Reiki Master Teacher On-line Course' where the student is initiated into all three traditional levels in one go (all students must complete this level even if they are already Reiki Masters). The other four levels are additions to the system of Reiki called Tara Reiki. Tara Reiki claims that the traditional attunement process is dangerous as it is not complete.
Contact details:
World Center for Tara Reiki
PO Box 7300, Ann Arbor, MI 48107, USA
Fax: (309) 416 6778
Website: www.tara-reiki.org

Tera Mai Reiki and Tera Mai Seichem

Lineage: Mikao Usui – Chûjirô Hayashi – Hawayo Takata – Iris Ishikuro – Arthur Robertson – Rick and Emma Ferguson – Margarette L. Shelton – Kathleen Ann Milner.
Founder: Reiki Master Kathleen Ann Milner.
Levels: Tera Mai Reiki I, II and Mastership and Tera Mai Seichem I, II and Mastership with non-traditional Egyptian attunements. The YOD initiation performed is said to connect the student with the energies of the Arc of the Covenant. Tera Mai Seichem has two more symbols than Tera Mai Reiki.

Mantras/Symbols: Some of the symbols are Harth, Zonar, two Double CKRs, Halu, Iava, Shanti, Sati.

Branch claims: The Tera Mai Reiki system is followed up by the Tera Mai Seichem system. They teach *breath of the fire dragon technique, *deprogramming techniques, the *Reiki boost and the *water ceremony amongst other techniques. Kathleen Milner claims that Hawayo Takata had left out a symbol and half of the attunement process. New symbols continued to be added to the system continuously raising the system of Reiki's energetic level.[6]

Comments: Tera Mai appears to be drawn from Seichim (through the lineage of Patrick Zeigler) and Raku Kei Reiki (created by Arthur Robertson) with altered information and added symbols. Kathleen Milner first taught what she called 'Reiki' after contacting a 'highly evolved being' with 'brown skin, orange clothes and an Afro hairstyle.'[7] The branch name later changed to Tera Mai Reiki and Tera Mai Seichem. Kathleen Milner trademarked Tera Mai Reiki and Tera Mai Seichem in 1995.

Contact details:

> Tera-Mai Healing
> PMB 102-125, 9393 North 90th Street, Scottsdale, Arizona 85258, USA
> Phone: (480) 314 5722
> Fax: 1-(480) 314 9905
> E-mail: kathleenmilner@earthlink.net
> Website: www.kathleenmilner.com

The Radiance Technique (or Authentic Reiki or Real Reiki)

Lineage: Mikao Usui – Chûjirô Hayashi – Hawayo Takata – Barbara Weber Ray.

Founder: Reiki Master Barbara Weber Ray.

Levels: Initially three levels are described in her book, The Reiki Factor (1983), but this changed in later editions to seven levels. Level 1 has four non-traditional attunements and level 2 has one non-traditional attunement. The system works like this: From Level 3 a student can teach the levels beneath them. This same system continues through to Level 7 from where the student can teach all levels.

Mantras/Symbols: The traditional symbols are taught plus non-traditional symbols. The names for the traditional symbols are different though. They are Cosmic Pattern 1 (Symbol 1), Cosmic Pattern 4 (Symbol 2) and Cosmic Pattern 22 (Symbol 3). After completing Level 2 these are replaced with the traditional Japanese mantras.

Branch claims: Hawayo Takata taught Barbara Weber Ray in 1979 as a Reiki Master. After Hawayo Takata's death in 1980 she claimed to have been the only Master student to receive her true teachings. The Radiance Technique website asserts that any other form of the system of Reiki is 'an imitation, a copy, a part and a fabrication'. The nature of these

---

[6] *Reiki and Other Rays of Touch Healing*, Kathleen Milner, 1995.
[7] *Reiki and Other Rays of Touch Healing*, Kathleen Milner, 1995.

teachings appears to have changed or developed over a period of time and includes a Tibetan history with New Age leanings. The Radiance Technique uses the *de-programming technique.

Comments: It has been suggested that the seven levels were introduced to The Radiance Technique after a student, Mieko Mitsui, traveled to Japan in 1985 and met a member of the Usui Reiki Ryôhô Gakkai. The Usui Reiki Ryôhô Gakkai teaches three major levels with a number of sub-levels of proficiency. It does not teach that Mikao Usui's teachings are from Tibet or have any other link to The Radiance Technique.

Contact details:
The Radiance Technique International Association, Inc. (TRTIA)
PO Box 40570, St. Petersburg, FL 33743 0570, USA
Phone/Fax: (727) 347 2106
E-mail: TRTIA@aol.com
Website: www.trtia.org

Tibetan Reiki

Comments: Generic term which covers Usui/Tibetan Reiki, Tibetan/Usui Reiki or Wei Chi Tibetan Reiki. Many Independent Reiki Masters teach variations of these systems (often without being aware of their origins).

Traditional Japanese Reiki (see Usui Dô)

Universal Healing Reiki (see also Men Chhos Reiki or Medicine Dharma Reiki)

The claims to authenticity by the founder of this lineage, Richard Blackwell aka Lama Yeshe, are controversial.

Usui Dô

Lineage 1: Mikao Usui – Toshihiro Eguchi – Yûji Onuki – Dave King.
Lineage 2: Mikao Usui – Chûjirô Hayashi – Tatsumi – Dave King.
Founders: Dave King and Melissa Riggall.
Levels: 13 levels from *Rokkyû* to *Shichidan*. Jigorô Kanô initially developed these levels for the practice of jûdô. Eight transformations (or attunements) over eight levels are given. These eight levels correlate to the teacher level. The eighth to the thirteenth level are by invitation only.
Mantras/Symbols: Four symbols of Chinese Taoist/Buddhist origin used in the Chinese manner. These are the traditional Japanese symbols but with a different context.
Branch claims: Usui Dô is said to be a close reconstruction of what was taught by Tatsumi (a student of Chûjirô Hayashi from 1927 to 1931) and by Yûji Onuki (a student of Toshihiro Eguchi). There is also additional information from a living nun who is said to have studied with Mikao Usui called Mariko Obaasan. It is a meditative, spiritual system.
Comments: Dave King claims that Mariko Obaasan is providing him with information from Mikao Usui's teachings and life from 1920 to 1926. There is no verification of this material at present. In a group

photo including Mikao Usui (from Toshitaka Mochizuki's book) Dave King claims that Mariko Obaasan has said that Jigorô Kanô, founder of jûdô, is standing on the far right hand side at the front. Major jûdô associations including the Kodokan Jûdô Institute in Japan have denied this claim.

Dave King also founded Traditional Japanese Reiki. It is based on information taught in the Vortex School in Japan by Toshitaka Mochizuki. The Usui Reiki Ryôhô Gakkai's spokesman, Hiroshi Doi, wrote that Toshihiro Eguchi was a friend of Mikao Usui and a well-known healer but that he had never became a teacher in Mikao Usui's method. If this were true, it would mean that what Yûji Onuki taught was not Mikao Usui's teachings but a system devised by Toshihiro Eguchi.

Contact details:
>The Usui-Do Foundation
>Toronto, Canada
>Phone: (403) 437 5481
>E-mail: askme@usui-do.org
>Website: www.usui-do.org

Usui Reiki

Comments: Generic term that is used by Reiki Masters who are unsure as to what lineage they belong to. All Reiki stems back to Mikao Usui therefore all Reiki is Usui Reiki. This name does not indicate what the teacher teaches. Many Independent Reiki Masters will use the term 'Usui Reiki' or 'Traditional Usui Reiki' on their certificates.

Usui Reiki Ryôhô

Lineage: Mikao Usui – Kanichi Taketomi – Kimiko Koyama – Hiroshi Doi.

Founder: Hiroshi Doi (also trained with Mieko Mitsui, Hiroshi Ohta, Manaso, Chiyoko Yamaguchi).

Levels: Three levels with four traditional Japanese attunements in the first level, three in the second level and one in the shinpiden or teacher level. The Tatsumi attunement is used as well as a reiju.[8] The reiju is a creation by Hiroshi Doi in which he has replicated the reiju used by Kimiko Koyama (former president of the Usui Reiki Ryôhô Gakkai).

Mantras/Symbols: Four traditional symbols/mantras that are hand drawn copies from traditional Japanese teachers.

Branch claims: Usui Reiki Ryôhô uses techniques which are/were once used by the Usui Reiki Ryôhô Gakkai. Other traditional Japanese methods may be included in these teachings depending on the teacher. Techniques included are *hatsurei hô, *byôsen reikan hô and *reiji hô.

Contact details 1:
>International House of Reiki
>Frans and Bronwen Stiene

---

[8] *Reiju* is a Japanese name for attunement and is performed without mantras and symbols. For more information about *reiju* see page 97.

PO Box 9, Glebe, Sydney, NSW, 2037, Australia
Freecall: 1800 000 992
E-mail: info@reiki.net.au
Website: www.reiki.net.au
Contact details 2:
Southwestern Usui Reiki Ryôhô Association
Adonea
PO Box 5162, Lake Montezuma, Arizona 86342 5162, USA
Phone: (520) 567 0559
E-mail: adonea@msn.com
Website: www.reiho.org

Usui Reiki Ryôhô Gakkai

Lineage: (list of Presidents) Mikao Usui – Jûzaburô Ushida – Kanichi Taketomi – Yoshiharu Watanabe – Hôichi Wanami – Kimiko Koyama – Masaki Kondô.

Founder: Mikao Usui.

Levels: Three major levels with sub-levels of proficiency. Reiju[9] is performed at each meeting by the shihan (Masters).

Branch claims: The Usui Reiki Ryôhô Gakkai only accepts members by invitation and it is closed to foreigners. The focus is very much on self-development. Meetings are held three times a month. This is a society that supports its members rather than a branch or school. The Usui Reiki Ryôhô Gakkai teaches *hatsurei hô, *byôsen reikan hô and *reiji hô.

Comments: The Usui Reiki Ryôhô Gakkai has changed over the years as each shihan introduces or takes away material but the Usui Reiki Ryôhô Gakkai does try to preserve the essence of the teachings. Mikao Usui either started the Usui Reiki Ryôhô Gakkai in 1922 or his students created it shortly after his death.

Usui Shiki Ryôhô

Lineage: Mikao Usui – Chûjirô Hayashi – Hawayo Takata.

Founder: Hawayo Takata.

Levels: Three levels or degrees. The first has four attunements, the second has one or two attunements and the third level is the Reiki Master level, which has one attunement.

Mantras/Symbols: Four traditional symbols and mantras. Three are taught in the second level and one is taught in the third level.

Branch claims: Hawayo Takata taught 22 Reiki Masters. Hawayo Takata's granddaughter, Phyllis Lei Furumoto, has continued on with what is said to be Hawayo Takata's teachings. In 1983 she was joined by a number of the other Reiki Masters who together created an association called The Reiki Alliance.

Comments: Phyllis Lei Furumoto was dubbed the Grandmaster and

---

[9] *Reiju* is a Japanese name for attunement and is performed without mantras and symbols. For more information see page 97.

lineage bearer of Usui Shiki Ryôhô by The Reiki Alliance. Some of the techniques taught are *distant reiki, *de-programming techniques and * the finishing treatment or *nerve stroke (*ketsueki kôkan hô). Since 1995 Phyllis Furumoto is no longer a member of the Alliance though she still retains her position as Grandmaster and lineage bearer. Usui Shiki Ryôhô is just one of the names that Hawayo Takata gave this system. She is also known to have called it Usui Reiki Ryôhô.[10] The techniques practiced are *distant healing, *the finishing stroke or nerve stroke, *the deprogramming technique, *scanning and *group Reiki.

Contact details:

> The Reiki Alliance
> PO Box 41, Cataldo, ID 83810, USA
> Phone: (208) 783 3535
> Fax (208) 783 4848.
> E-mail: info@reikialliance.com
> Website: www.reikialliance.com
> Postbus 75523, 1070 AM Amsterdam, The Netherlands
> Phone: (020) 6719276
> Fax: (020) 6711736
> E-mail: europeoffice@reikialliance.com

Usui Teate (see Method to Achieve Personal Perfection)

Usui/Tibetan Reiki

Lineage: Mikao Usui – Chûjirô Hayashi – Hawayo Takata – Phyllis Lei Furumoto – Carrell Ann Farmer – Leah Smith – William Lee Rand (William Lee Rand has also studied with Diane McCumber, Marlene Schilke, Beth Gray, Harry Kuboi, Bethel Phaigh, Phyllis Lei Furumoto, Hyakuten Inamoto and Chiyoko Yamaguchi).

Founder: William Lee Rand.

Levels: Four levels called degrees. Levels 1 and 2 are taught in one class with two attunements in total. ART or (Advanced Reiki Training) has one attunement. The fourth level or Master Level has a non-traditional Usui/Tibetan Reiki Master attunement.

Mantras/Symbols: Three traditional symbols and two non-traditional 'Tibetan' initiatory symbols. One of these is Dumo (claimed by some to be a modern Symbol 4 – there is no relationship between the two symbols).

Branch Claims: The first two levels include most of the traditional Usui Shiki Ryôhô information. Level 3a or ART and Level 3b or 4 is where most of the non-traditional techniques have been added. Usui/Tibetan Reiki teaches *Reiki meditation; psychic surgery; healing attunement; distance and self-attunement; *violet breath; *manifesting; four variations of the *antakharana symbol with description and usage.

---

[10] Transcript of a tape of Mrs Takata talking about Dr Usui, 1979.

Comments: Usui/Tibetan Reiki is a mix of Raku Kei Reiki (through Diane McCumber), Usui Shiki Ryôhô (through Phyllis Lei Furumoto), and most recently, Japanese techniques (through Frank Arjava Petter). The center no longer advertises the classes as Usui/Tibetan Reiki but instead have returned to naming them as 'Reiki I, II, ART and IIIM/T'. Individual teachers have previously called these teachings Tibetan Reiki or Tibetan/Usui. There are many Independent Reiki Masters who teach this system or parts thereof.

Contact details:

> The International Center for Reiki Training
> 21421 Hilltop St., 28, Southfield, MI 48034 1023, USA
> Phone: (248) 948-8112
> Fax: (248)-948-9534
> E-mail: center@reiki.org
> Website: www.reiki.org

Vajra Reiki

Founder: Wade Ryan.

Levels: Three levels with the first level, Shokuden, having three attunements and four symbols. The second level is *shinpiden* with one attunement where the student learns to teach Shokuden. The third level is the Vajra Raku Kei Reiki Master Level where another attunement is received.

Mantras/Symbols: Four symbols and one Om-Ah-Hum Mantra all influenced by Raku Kei Reiki and Johrei.

Branch claims: Vajra Reiki is a mixture of Raku Kei Reiki and Johrei Reiki with Usui Shiki Ryôhô. Claims to be excellent for working on the damaging bacteria and viruses that are appearing on our planet at this time.

Wei Chi Tibetan Reiki

Lineage: Said to be the channeled teachings of Wei Chi.

Founders: Reiki Masters Thomas A. Hensel and Kevin Rodd Emery.

Levels: Three Practitioner levels and three teacher levels. The teacher levels comprise 1135 contact hours plus 200 documented and reviewed practice hours.

Branch claims: Wei Chi Reiki stems from Tibet 5000 years ago. Wei Chi said that he and his brothers had created the original system that is the basis of the system of Reiki today. He claims that when the system was rediscovered in the nineteenth century, only a small portion of the original was actually found as much had been lost through the centuries.

Contact details:

> LightLines
> PO Box 5067, Portsmouth, NH, 03802 5067, UK
> Phone: (603) 433-5784
> E-mail: weichireiki@aol.com
> Website: www.weichireiki.com

Reiki Schools

This directory lists Reiki schools throughout the world. They are from an array of branches with some schools teaching more than one branch of Reiki. When looking for contact details of the original branches of Reiki please see the previous section. These schools are not personal recommendations simply a list compiled for the reader's interest and convenience.

Argentina:

Sólo Reiki
Claudio Márquez
Aguilar 2612
Buenos Aires
Phone: 4787 6414
E-mail: reiki@reikihoy.com.ar

Australia:

International House of Reiki
Frans and Bronwen Stiene
PO Box 9, Glebe, Sydney, NSW 2037, Australia
Freecall: 1800 000 992 within Australia
E-mail: info@reiki.net.au
Website: www.reiki.net.au
Frans and Bronwen Stiene teach Usui Reiki Ryôhô.

Austria:

Akasha – Zentrum für neue Erfahrungen
Mooswiesengasse 1/6, A-1140 Wien, Austria
Phone: 015771053
Cell Phone: 0676-7253886
E-mail: 41antakarana8@aon.at
Website: www.Akasha-Zentrum.at.tf

Belgium:

Anne Fredholm
Belgium
E-mail: ann.reiki@pandora.be
Website: www.users.pandora.be/annreiki/index.htm
Anne Fredholm has monthly Reiki gatherings and organizes Reiki
workshops for international teachers.

Canada:

Soul Connection
12 Oakridge Crescent
Guelph, Ontario, Canada
Phone: (519) 823 2162
Website: www.soulconnection.ca

Chile:

International Reiki Center Armonia Natural
Viviana Puebla
Escuela Mount Vernon, Quebec 560, Santiago, Chile
Phone: (56) 2 2749111
E-mail: armonianatural@yahoo.es
Website: www.geocities.com/armonianatural/reiki.html
Viviana Puebla teaches Gendai Reiki Hô.

Czech Republic:

International Association of Reiki
Mari Hall
Czech Republic
E-mail: reikimari@hotmail.com
Website: www.wisechoices.com
Mari Hall teaches internationally and organizes International Reiki
Conferences.

Finland:

Reiki TMI
Attila Kupi
Finland
E-mail: attila@reiki.fi
Website: www.reiki.fi
Attila Kupi teaches Gendai Reiki Hô.

Germany:

Brigitte Müller
Auf der Schanz 1, D-65936 Frankfurt, Germany
Phone: (69) 34 826 338
Fax: (69) 34 826 339
E-mail: brigitte_mueller@breathenet.de
Website: brigitte-mueller.de
Brigitte Müller is a member of The Reiki Alliance.

Carola Zedzianowski
Dominicusstr. 46, D-10827 Berlin, Germany
Phone: (030) 7844594
E-mail: zedzis@t-online.de
Internet: www.reiki-tiefenentspannung.de

Christoph Graf von Keyserlingk, Reiki Zentrum Dresden
Böhmische Strasse 19, D-01099 Dresden, Germany
Phone: (0351) 8015554
E-mail: ckeyserlingk@gmx.net
Internet: www.reiki-zentrum-dresden.de

Frank Arjava Petter
Am Seestern 12
40547 Duesseldorf, Germany
Phone: (211) 50 73 810
E-mail: arjava@reikidharma.com
Website: www.reikidharma.com
Frank Arjava Petter is one of the founding researchers of the system
of Reiki in Japan.

Stefanie Krupp
Hamburg, Germany
E-mail: stefanie.krupp@web.de
Stefanie Krupp teaches Usui Reiki Ryôhô.

Italy:

Associazione Culturale 'Reiki On'
Casella postale 250, Via Pellicceria 3, 50100 Firenze, Italy
E-mail: cristian@harno.it, lucia.damerino@tin.it, sara@harno.it
Website: www.usuireiki.it

Gabriella Campioni
Via dei Tigli, 2/F. 20090 Rodano, Milan, Italy
E-mail: amitiel@libero.it
Gabriella Campioni teaches Usui Shiki Ryôhô, Karuna Reiki and
Japanese Reiki techniques.

Hong Kong:

Angeline Pui-Yee Yeung
Shop 111, 1/f, Allied Plaza, 760 Nathan Rd, Kowloon, Hong Kong
Phone: (852) 2399 7390
E-mail: angeline@crystalage.com.hk
Angeline Pui-Yee Yeung teaches Usui Reiki Ryôhô.

Japan:

Joynus Healing Center
Dr Koki Matsuoka
2093 Nakabata, Gotemba-Shi, Shizuoka-Ken, Japan
Phone/Fax: (81) 55089 8125
E-mail: wbs22867@mail.wbs.ne.jp
Dr Koki Matsuoka speaks English and teaches Reiki throughout Japan.

Komyo Reiki Kai
Rev. Hyakuten Inamoto
182-26 4-chome, Higashiyama-ku, Kyôto, Japan
Phone/Fax: (075) 551 9666
E-mail: komyo100@yahoo.co.jp
Website: www.h4.dion.ne.jp/~reiki
Reverend Hyakuten Inamoto speaks fluent English and teaches a
  system based on traditional Japanese Reiki including the non-
  Western, Chûjirô Hayashi system.

Reiki Center for Healing Arts
Rev. Fran Brown
Tôkyô, Japan
E-mail: joshua22@cg.mbn.or.jp
Website: plaza3.mbn.or.jp/~franbrown
Reverend Fran Brown teaches Usui Shiki Ryôhô and is a native
  English speaker.

SP Net Co., Ltd. Healing Academy
Yashuhide Tanaka
194-1 Naruto Narutomachi Chiba, Tôkyô, Japan
Tel: (03) 3371 1611
Fax: (03) 3371 1640
E-mail: co-spi@ss.iij4u.or.jp
Website: www.reikijapan.com
Yashuhide Tanaka speaks English and English manuals are available.

Y&Y Healing Center
Kyôto, Japan
Phone/Fax: (077) 533 3078
E-mail: tcey@mb.infoweb.ne.jp
Website: www.yandyhc.com
Yukio and Yuko teach Gendai Reiki Hô and Karuna Reiki, have
  English manuals available and speak English fluently.

New Zealand:

Anka & Ljubomir Bosanac
Mt Eden, Auckland, N.Z.
Phone: (09) 623 2620
E-mail: lj.bosanac@xtra.co.nz

Rod Gordon
2 Kea St, Burkes Bay, Dunedin, N.Z.
Phone: (03) 4710970
Cell Phone: (021) 322 088

Russia:

Usui Reiki Ryôhô – Traditional Japanese School
Moscow, Russia
Phone: (095) 120 23 31, 344 74 72, 344 84 48,
E-mail: reiki@reiki.ru
Website: www.reiki.ru
This school teaches Usui Reiki Ryôhô.

South Africa:

Beverley Marsden
42 Tugela Crescent, Gallo Manor, Sandton, Gauteng 2052, South Africa
Phone: 011 656 5401
E-mail: maniacs@iafrica.com
Website: www.reikihealing.co.za

Switzerland:

Claudine Chiquet
Oeschenweg 1,CH-3047 Bremgarten b. Bern, Switzerland
Phone: (031) 301 50 87 or 078 632 82 54
E-mail: chiquet.im@bluewin.ch

Gabriella Keller
Bändlistrasse 31, CH-8064 Zürich, Switzerland
Phone: (0) 14327282
Website: www.reiki-kurse.com

Lichtinsel
St. Urbangasse 25, CH-4500 Solothurn, Switzerland
Phone: (78) 751 42 19
E-mail: info@lichtinsel.ch
Website: www.lichtinsel.ch

The Netherlands:

Healing Energy Focusing
Ing. Carl W. Berlage
Camera Obscuralaan 260, 1183 KE Amstelveen, The Netherlands
Phone/Fax: (020) 643 8542
E-mail: carlberlage@zonnet.nl
Carl Berlage teaches Gendai Reiki Hô, Karuna Reiki and Sekhem-Seichem.

Praktijk Parcival
Monique Hendriks
Groenendijk 74, 4587 CX Kloosterzande, The Netherlands
Phone: 065 3216824
E-mail: praktijkparcival@wanadoo.nl
Website: home.wanadoo.nl/praktijkparcival
Monique Hendriks teaches the system of Reiki and practices on animals.

UK:

Christine Johnston
Hall Cottage, Sandy Lane, Sternfield, Suffolk, IP17 1RT, UK
Phone: (44) 0 1728 605 888
E-mail: cjele@easynet.co.uk

Dave Hedger
'Conifers', 27 The Street, Rockland All Saints, Attleborough, Norfolk, UK
Phone: (44) 0 1953 483 385
E-mail: dave.hedger@btinternet.com

Doreen Sawyer
Weyhill, Andover, Hampshire, SP11 0PZ, UK
Phone: (44) 0 1264 771163
E-mail: doreen.therapy@tesco.net
Doreen Sawyer teaches Usui Shiki Ryôhô.

Kay Zega
Worcester, U.K.
Phone: (44) 0 1905 26002
E-mail: kayzega@telco4u.net
Kay Zega teaches Usui Shiki Ryôhô.

USA:

Reiki Center for Healing Arts
Rev. Fran Brown
1764 Hamlet St., San Mateo, CA 94403, USA
Phone: (413) 345 7666
Reverend Fran Brown teaches Usui Shiki Ryôhô.

Reiki Healing Institute
Marsha Burack
449 Sante Fe Dr 303, Encinitas, CA 92024, USA
Phone: (619) 436 6875

Reiki Outreach International
Mary Alexandra McFadyen
PO Box 191156, San Diego, CA 92159-1156, USA
Website: www.annieo.com/reikioutreach

Southwestern Usui Reiki Ryôhô Association
Adonea
PO Box 5162, Lake Montezuma, Arizona 86342-5162, USA
Phone: (520) 567 0559
E-mail: adonea@msn.com
Website: www.reiho.org
Adonea teaches Usui Reiki Ryôhô and has trained in many Reiki branches.

The International Center for Reiki Training
William Lee Rand
21421 Hilltop St., 28, Southfield, Michigan 48034, USA
Toll Free phone: (800) 332 8112
Phone: (248) 948 8112
Fax (248) 948 9534
E-mail: center@reiki.org
Website: www.reiki.org
William Lee Rand teaches Karuna Reiki and Usui/Tibetan Reiki.

The Reiki System
Robert Fueston
Saluda, Northern Carolina, USA
E-mail: fueston@reikisystem.com
Website: www.reikisystem.com
Robert Fueston teaches Usui Reiki Ryôhô.

Reiki Associations

Associations have been set up throughout the world to provide a place of community for Reiki Practitioners. They are also there to set and keep standards. Each association has its own views as to what these standards are and how they should be implemented.

Some associations are created for specific branches of Reiki while others have an open membership for all Reiki practitioners. There is even an association for registered nurses.

It is important that an association is there for its members rather than for those who direct it. For associations to be successful they must meet the needs of their members and, at the same time, the needs of the general public.

Argentina:

Asociación Argentina de Reiki
en Av. Los Incas 4112 C.P. (1427), Argentina
Phone: 4787 6414
E-mail: info@reikihoy.com.ar
Website: www.reikihoy.com.ar

Australia:

Australian Reiki Connection
WendyJoy Smith, President
40 Jarvis Crescent, North Dandenong, Vic 3175, Australia
Phone: (03) 9791 2564
Fax: (03) 9793 4515
E-mail: help@australianreikiconnection.com.au
Website: www.australianreikiconnection.com.au

Canada:

Atlantic Usui Reiki Association
Judith Settle, Secretary
RR#2 Stewiacke, Nova Scotia, B0N 2J0, Canada
E-mail: jsettle@atcon.com

Canadian Reiki Association
PO Box 74072, Hillcrest RPO, Vancouver, BC, V5V 5C8, Canada
Phone: 1800 835 7525
E-mail: reiki@reiki.ca
Website: www.reiki.ca

Croatia:

Croatian Reiki Society
Vera Alexander
Centar za poboljšanje kvalitete života
Veslaèka 27, Zagreb, Croatia
Phone: (385) 1619 00 99 or 619 22 99
E-mail: verica.aleksander@zg.tel.hr

Italy:

European Reiki Association
Prof. Dr Stefano Maria Rattazzi, Founder
Dr Giacomo Motta, Manager
Viale S. Antonio 59, 21100 Varese VA, Italy
Phone: (0332) 966064
Fax: (0347) 4180414
E-mail: caocis@tin.it

New Zealand:

Reiki New Zealand Inc.
PO Box 60-226, Titirangi, Auckland, NZ
E-mail: reiki@ihug.co.nz
Website: www.reiki.org.nz

South Africa:

The Reiki Association of Southern Africa
PO Box 1344, Pinegowrie, 2123, Gauteng, South Africa
Phone: (2782) 857 5999
E-mail: karen@reikiassociation.co.za
Website: www.reikiassociation.co.za

The Netherlands:

Reiki Alliance - Europe
Honthorstraat 40, 1071 DG, Amsterdam, Netherlands
Phone: (020) 671 9276
Fax: (020) 671 1736
E-mail: europeoffice@reikialliance.com

UK:

UK Reiki Federation
Doreen Sawyer, Secretary
PO Box 1785, Andover SP11 OWB, UK
Phone: (01264) 773774
E-mail: enquiries@reikifed.co.uk
Website: www.reikifed.co.uk

USA:

International Association of Reiki Professionals (IARP)
PO Box 104, Harrisville, NH 03450, USA
Phone: (603) 827 3290
E-mail: info@iarp.org
Website: www.iarp.org

The Reiki Nurse Network
Marion Yaglinski
1248 Hunt Club Lane, Media, PA 19063, USA
Phone: (610) 566 5669
E-mail: karunarn@aol.com
Website: members.aol.com/KarunaRN

Reiki Newsletters

Hand To Hand

The John Harvey Gray Center for Reiki Healing
PO Box 696, Rindge, NH 03461-0696, USA
E-mail: lgray@reiki.mv.com
Website: www.mv.com/ipusers/reiki/index.html
This is a quarterly publication.

Reiki Federation Magazine and Newsletter

resonance@reikifed.co.uk
Kay Zega
Worcester, U.K.
Phone: (44) 0 1905 26002

Reiki Magazin

Jürgen Kindler Verlag
Gaudystr. 12, D-10437 Berlin, Germany
Phone: (0700) 2332 3323
Fax: (0700) 2332 3324
E-mail: verlag@reiki-magazin.de or verwaltung@reiki-magazin.de
Website: www.reiki-magazin.de
This is a quarterly publication.

Reiki Magazine International

Rolf and Li-Li Holm
Sumatrakade 747, 1019 PX Amsterdam, The Netherlands
Phone: (020) 419 3755
Fax: (020) 419 4144
E-mail: publishers@reikimagazine.com
Website: www.reikimagazine.com
This is a 48-page, full colour magazine published six times a year.

Reiki Magazine Italia

redazione@reikimagazine.it or abbonamenti@reikimagazine.it

Reiki News Magazine

The International Center for Reiki Training
21421 Hilltop St., 28, Southfield, Michigan 48034, USA
Toll Free phone: (800) 332 8112
Phone: (248) 948 8112
Fax: (248) 948 9534
E-mail: center@reiki.org
Website: www.reiki.org
This is a quarterly publication.

Reiki One Newsletter

E-mail: teri@reikione.com
Website: www.reikione.com
This is a free weekly 'e-zine' newsletter containing regular columns,
advice, stories, discussions, and more.

The Reiki Newsletter

International House of Reiki
Frans and Bronwen Stiene
PO Box 9, Glebe, Sydney, NSW 2037, Australia
Freecall: 1800 000 992 within Australia
E-mail: info@reiki.net.au
Website: www.reiki.net.au
This is a bi-monthly e-mail newsletter from the authors of *The Reiki
Sourcebook*.

Reiki Internet Resources

One of the greatest inventions of the last century (apart from the computer) must be the Internet. The World Wide Web has laid the globe at our feet. Billions of pages of information are accessible with just a tap of the fingers and a 'click' of a mouse.

The Internet is a weird and wonderful place. Listed below are sites for chatting, joining forums, registering for free distant Reiki and sites to help practitioners become pro-active and heal the earth. Hopefully none of these sites will have been hacked into and turned into sex sites by the time they are logged onto.

An added element of caution has also entered our lives with the advent of the Internet. In the writing of this book many wonderful sites have been accessed and some strange ones too. It is true that all that is read cannot be believed. This must be held in one's thoughts as the Reiki roller web is ridden. Reiki pages have taken to the Internet like a duck to water and there is no shortage of viewpoints out there. Their validity is another point entirely. Once again the chats, forums and distant healing groups are not here through special recommendation – their existence is simply noted.

Life on the Internet can be short lived for many sites so if any alterations are found please contact the authors and they will be updated.

Reiki Chat/Forum

Practitioners from all levels can come together and chat over the Internet to ask questions, provide information and make friends.

Animal Reiki
Website: groups.yahoo.com/group/animal_reiki
Reiki on animals based forum.

Australian Reiki Connection
Website: www.australianreikiconnection.com.au
Australian forum.

Reiki Centrum
Website: www.reikicentrum.nl
Dutch forum and chat site.

Reiki Chat
Website: www.reikichat.net
German chat site.

Reiki-Chat
Website: www.lehrpraxis.de
German forum and chat site.

Reiki Forums
Website: www.groups.yahoo.com/search?query=reiki&submit=Search
Almost 1000 Reiki forums listed under Yahoo Groups.

ReiKi News
Website: www.imparare-reiki.it/reikinews.htm
Italian forum and chat site.

Reiki On
Website: www.groups.yahoo.com/group/reiki_on

Reiki-Teachings from the Heart
Website: www.reikifire.ca/school/chatroom.html
German/French/English chat site.

The Reiki Cafe
Website: www.nexuscafe.com
This site has around the 4000 members.

Usui Reiki Ryôhô International – English
Website: www.groups.yahoo.com/group/urri
Canadian forum.

Usui Reiki Ryôhô International – Japanese
Website: www.egroups.co.jp/group/urriJP
Japanese forum.

Distant Healing

These sites provide distant healing for the general public and are also open for practitioners to join as members.

Distance Healing Request Center
Website: www.sacredpath.org/hrb/index.htm

The Circle of Light
Website: www.yourangels.com

The Distant Healing Network
Website: www.the-dhn.com

Reiki Earth Healing

This site provides the opportunity for Level 2 and 3 practitioners to send healing to the earth.

Global Reiki Network – Earthsend
E-mail: InnateFoundation@aol.com
Website: www.innatefoundation.com/earthsend.html

Reiki Research

This site is dedicated to collecting data from Reiki practitioners about their treatments. Interesting to either take part in or, at least, to read the results.

The Rose Carr Reiki Center
Website: www.reiki-research.co.uk/home.html

Appendices

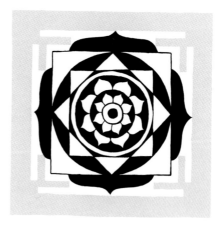

Appendix A
Reiki Glossary

 A

Advanced Reiki Training
– Sometimes called ART, 3a or Reiki Master/Practitioner. It is a Western addition to the system of Reiki often practiced in Usui /Tibetan Reiki but has also been adopted by many Independent Reiki Masters. Some techniques taught at this level are *crystal grid work, a healing attunement, *Reiki guide meditation, psychic surgery, *Reiki symbol meditation and the *antakharana symbol. Students are taught 'the master symbol' (Symbol 4 and/or Dumo) but not how to perform the attunement.

Alchemia Reiki – Complete details listed in Part IV of *The Reiki Sourcebook* under Reiki Branches.

Amanohuna Reiki – Complete details listed in Part IV of *The Reiki Sourcebook* under Reiki Branches.

Amida Nyorai – This deity is taught as the connection to Symbol 2. Amida Nyorai is the main deity of the Pure Land School. Amida in Sanskrit is 'Infinite Light'. Amida's compassion is therefore also infinite. The main practice of the Pure Land School is to recite *Namu-*

Amida-Butsu, which is an expression of Oneness. *Namu-Amida-Butsu* literally translates to, 'I take refuge in Amida Buddha.'

Angelic RayKey – Complete details listed in Part IV of *The Reiki Sourcebook* under Reiki Branches.

*Antakharana Symbol – Non-traditional Reiki healing symbol. This symbol has been added to the system of Reiki by some Western Reiki teachers such as Arthur Robertson and is used in Usui/Tibetan Reiki as a meditation method. The antakharana is a two dimensional cube with three 7s on its face. Myth has it that this symbol comes from Tibet and China. It is said if you meditate on the antakharana you will connect the physical brain with the Higher Self.

*Anti-Clockwise Energy Spirals – Non-traditional technique used to ease the client into a change that is about to happen.

Araki, George – He became a Reiki Master in 1979. One of Hawayo Takata's 22 Reiki Master students. According to Robert Fueston, George initially became a Reiki Master when he was head of the Department of Natural Healing at San Francisco State University and was interested in completing a study about it. He did not teach many people preferring to refer them to either Fran Brown or Shinobu Saito.

Ascension Reiki – Complete details listed in Part IV of *The Reiki Sourcebook* under Reiki Branches.

Attunements – An attunement is the Western method of initiating students into the system of Reiki. Attunements are integral to the system of Reiki. There are many different attunement methods as teachers have added to or taken away from the traditional process. It is believed that Chûjirô Hayashi may have created the attunement process that is used in the West. Attunements were initially called *reiju* in Japan but when the system moved to the West this changed and they became known as initiations, empowerments, attunements or transformations. Something as profound as an attunement cannot be analyzed on the human level – merely experienced. As an attunement is a powerful clearing of the body's meridians it is impossible to be able to undo this or 'wipe-it-out'. Each attunement you receive takes you a step further to re-aligning yourself with the natural function of your body – mentally, physically, emotionally or spiritually. For these reasons it is also impossible to 'make' an attunement last for a limited period of time.

 B

Baba, Dorothy – One of Hawayo Takata's 22 Reiki Master students who has since passed away.

Baylow, Ursula – One of Hawayo Takata's 22 Reiki Master students. She is no longer teaching the system of Reiki. She became a Master in 1976.

Beaming – Non-traditional technique in which Reiki is directed to a person/place or thing by turning the palms toward them/it. This technique does not include touch. It is taught in the Usui/Tibetan branch of Reiki and is practiced by Independent Reiki Masters.

Beggar Story – Most Western practitioners know the beggar story as a parable told by Hawayo Takata. It teaches practitioners that Reiki must be paid for or it will not be respected. Many teachers dispute this concept today and there exist groups of teachers and practitioners who offer Reiki for free – for more information see Internet Yahoo Group, Grass Roots Reiki. There is an account of the 'beggar story' in *Living Reiki, Takata's Teachings* by Fran Brown

Blue Book, The – Paul Mitchell and Phyllis Lei Furumoto wrote *The Blue Book – Reiki* in 1985. It includes historical information as taught by Hawayo Takata, a photo of Mikao Usui, Chûjirô Hayashi, Hawayo Takata and Phyllis Lei Furumoto and some information about The Reiki Alliance.

Blue Star Reiki – Complete details listed in Part IV of *The Reiki Sourcebook* under Reiki Branches.

Bockner, Rick – One of Hawayo Takata's 22 Reiki Masters. He became a Reiki Master on 12 October 1980 at Bethal Phaigh's house in Slocan Valley. He had received his first degree on 10 October 1979 and his second degree on 20 October 1979. He is currently a member of The Reiki Alliance.

Bowling, Andrew – He is the Western researcher who first made contact with Hiroshi Doi, member of the Usui Reiki Ryôhô Gakkai. Today he practices Usui Teate, otherwise listed as Method to Achieve Personal Perfection in *The Reiki Sourcebook*. These teachings are from Suzuki san who is said to be the 108-year-old cousin of Mikao Usui.

Brahma Satya Reiki – Complete details listed in Part IV of *The Reiki Sourcebook* under Reiki Branches.

*Breath of the Fire Dragon – Non-traditional breath technique used with attunement process. Variations of this are the *blue kidney breath, *Reiki breathing and *violet breath.

Brown, Barbara – One of Hawayo Takata's 22 Reiki Masters. She became a Reiki Master in October 1979 in Cherryville, BC, Canada. The inaugural Reiki Alliance meeting was held at Barbara Brown's house in British Columbia in 1983. She passed away on Easter Sunday, 2000 and was in her mid-80s.

Brown, Fran – One of Hawayo Takata's 22 Reiki Masters. She was the seventh Reiki Master trained by Hawayo Takata. She completed her First Degree on 3 June 1973 with Hawayo Takata. She then took her Second Degree training from John Gray in 1976. She became a Reiki Master on 15 January 1979 in Keosauqua, Iowa. She has been a member of The Reiki Alliance. Though she is in her late 70s she continues to teach all over the world, including Japan.

Buddho Symbol – Non-traditional symbol utilized in Enersense/Reiki Jin Kei do. Claimed to be a 'Tibetan' symbol and is used with meditation.

Budô – *Budô* refers to the traditional art of self-defence in Japan. Some different kinds of *budô* are: *jûdô*, karate, aikidô, kendô and iaidô.

*Byôsen Reikan Hô 病腺霊感法 – (lit. Japanese) sense imbalances in the body. Traditional Japanese technique similar to the Western technique of *scanning.

C

Certificate – Certification is often given to students on completion of a course or level. There is no one true form of Reiki certification. In the West a certificate signifies that a student has simply completed whatever it is that the Reiki Master teaches. There are no across the board standards. It is possible to finish Levels 1, 2 or even 3 in a weekend. This leaves the student feeling temporarily powerful without actually becoming empowered. When an individual receives attunements over a couple of days the body's energy cannot differentiate between having received a Level 1, 2 or 3 certificate. Reiki is not about certification it is about personal practice. In traditional Japanese teachings a certificate is given to indicate that certain levels of proficiency have been reached and that the student is just beginning that actual level.

Chakra – Chakra is a Sanskrit word often translated as 'wheel of energy'. Chakras, though Indian in origin, are popularly used in many forms of energetic work today including the system of Reiki. It does not seem that Mikao Usui or Hawayo Takata used the chakra system and yet both the Western and some Japanese methods today have adapted to using them. Chakras have been taught in the system of Reiki by a number of Hawayo Takata's students including John Gray and Iris Ishikuro. Barbara Weber Ray also bases The Radiance Technique on the chakra system. Hawayo Takata spoke of the 'true energy' in the body that 'lies in the bottom of the stomach about 2 inches below the naval' in notes which are included in *The*

Gray Book. Here she is writing about the *hara* method that is used in Japan.

*Chakra Balancing – Non-traditional Western technique to balance the chakras with one another.

*Chakra Kassei Kokyû Hô – Non-traditional Western breathing method to activate the chakras.

*Chanting – Non-traditional technique that enhances the qualities of symbols with the sound of mantras.

Chiba 千葉 – The name of Mikao Usui's ancestors. The Chiba clan was one of the most famous and influential *samurai* families in all of Japan according to the Chiba family records. The Usui family crest, otherwise known as the Chiba *mon*, is a design comprising the moon and a star. The memorial stones states that the famous *samurai*, Tsunetane Chiba (1118–1201) was Mikao Usui's ancestor.

Chiryô Hô 治療法 – (lit. Japanese) treatment. This term is used in the description of a number of Japanese Reiki techniques.

Cho Ku Ret Symbol – A non-traditional symbol taught in Seichim. Channeled by students of Patrick Ziegler.

Cleansing Process – With any form of natural healing method there exists a cleansing. This may happen immediately after a treatment or within a few days. The client's body draws in energy and allows it to wash through, clearing the body out on a physical, mental, emotional or spiritual level. Also called a 'clearing' or a 'healing crisis'. See also Three-Week Cleansing Process.

Clearing – see Cleansing Process.

*Communicating with Your Higher Self – A Western technique used to re-connect one's self with the Higher Self.

Connection – This is the name most Japanese schools call Symbol 3. The word 'connection' is used to describe the action of the symbol. Symbol 3 helps practitioners to remember that everything is connected. Therefore it is not possible to 'send' Reiki to someone, instead one becomes One with the person.

*Crystal Healing – Crystals are renowned as excellent healers. There are now many versions of crystal healing being used in the Western system of Reiki. This includes *crystal chakra healing and the *crystal grid.

 D

Dainichi Nyorai – This deity is sometimes taught as the connection to Symbol 4. Dainichi Nyorai is the Great Shining Buddha because this Buddha is the life force of the Buddhas that illuminate everything. Dainichi dispels the darkness of the world by casting light everywhere, giving life to and nurturing all living things.

Daiseishi Bosatsu – This deity is sometimes taught as the connection to Symbol 1. The name means 'He Who Proceeds With Great Vigour'.

Dan 段 – (lit. Japanese) level or degree. In some Japanese branches of Reiki the name of the levels end with *dan*. This is taken from martial arts levels in Japan.

Den 伝 – (lit. Japanese) legend, tradition and teachings. In some Japanese branches of Reiki the name of the levels end with *den*. This is taken from martial arts levels in Japan.

*De-programming Techniques – There are two traditional Japanese techniques that work on releasing set mental patterns. One is *nentatsu hô* and the other is *seiheki chiryô hô*. In the West, a number of variations of these techniques are practiced.

Distance Symbol – This symbol is also known as Symbol 3 in traditional Japanese systems and is taught in Level 2 or *okuden zenki*. It is the third of the four symbols and is commonly used for *distant healing. According to the Western system of Reiki it creates a bridge between the sender and receiver/place or thing. Most Japanese schools call it 'connection' as it helps one remember that the connection already exists. This stimulates Oneness by becoming One with the person that receives the Reiki. The symbol itself is Japanese *kanji* and can literally be translated. One meaning is 'my original nature is a correct thought' and another translation used by Hiroshi Doi is 'Right consciousness is the origin of everything'.

Distant Attunements – Attunements in the West were initially performed in person but in the event of globalization, attunements are now being sent by distance. This method is an extension of the concept of *distant healing, which has been used in both Western and Japanese systems of Reiki. See also attunements.

***Distant Healing** – Distant healing is used to send Reiki for the purpose of healing to someone who is not physically present. Symbol 3 is said to activate this method and it is taught in Level 2. In the West, the methods used are the photo technique, healing lists or the teddy bear technique. The similar Japanese technique is called *enkaku chiryô hô*.

Distant Reiki – Send Reiki to a person, place or thing in the past, present or future with *distant healing.

Dô 道 – (lit. Japanese) treatment, method or way. It is commonly used in Japan to describe a teacher's method. Like aikidô and jûdô. Mikao Usui's teachings (not his healings) were traditionally called Usui dô, the way of Usui.

Doi, Hiroshi – Teacher of Gendai Reiki Hô and one of the initiators of the URRI projects. Hiroshi Doi is also a member of the Usui Reiki Ryôhô Gakkai. He officially joined the society on 22 October 1993. Hiroshi Doi has studied many styles of Reiki, Western and Japanese, as well as numerous energetic and spiritual techniques. He was one of the first Japanese to study Levels 1 and 2 with Mieko Mitsui who was teaching Barbara Weber Ray's The Radiance Technique in Japan. He also studied all three levels of a system of Reiki called Neo Reiki and has trained with Chiyoko Yamaguchi.

Dôjô – (lit. Japanese) a place of the path. Generally speaking a place where we learn something and most often used in martial arts like jûdô, karate, kendo, etc. On Mikao Usui's memorial it says that he set up a *dôjô* at Nakano in Tôkyô.

Dorje Reiki – Complete details listed in Part IV of The Reiki Sourcebook under Reiki Branches.

Dumo – Dumo is a non-traditional symbol and was introduced to the system of Reiki in the West. It is sometimes called the Tibetan master symbol and is taught in the Usui/Tibetan Reiki branch as well as by various Independent Reiki Masters. It is claimed to be a 'Tibetan symbol' though this has not been verified. It is also claimed to be a 'modern-day Symbol 4'. Those who teach this believe that the energy today is different to that of Mikao Usui's time. Though this may be so, the traditional Symbol 4 has specific meanings, which have no correlation to the Dumo.

E

Eguchi, Toshihiro 江口俊博
– Friend and student of Mikao Usui. According to Hiroshi Doi, Toshihiro Eguchi did not study to the teacher level with Mikao Usui. Toshihiro Eguchi created the *Tenohira Ryôji Kenkyû Kai* (Hand Healing Research Center) in 1928 and wrote a number of books: *Te No Hira Ryôji Nyûmon (Introduction to healing with the palms)* in 1930 and *Te No Hira Ryôji Wo Kataru (A story of healing with the palms)* in 1954. Dave King states Toshihiro Eguchi worked with Mikao Usui for several months in 1921. In late 1923 he returned to teach Mikao Usui and his students. Hiroshi Doi states that he studied the teachings between 1925 and 1927. According to Chris Marsh, Toshihiro Eguchi played a large role in the formation of the teachings that became known as the system of Reiki in the West. In 1929 he taught members of the Ittoen commune his new system.

Empowerment – This word is often used to describe the Japanese *reiju* and/or the Western attunement process.

Energy Exchange – This term is a Western concept that ensures students take responsibility for their own health. It has also been used to justify Reiki practitioners charging for treatments. The client is asked to return the favour of a Reiki treatment by doing 'something' for the practitioner. In this way the client is more respectful of the Reiki treatment, leaving him/her with a sense of self-responsibility for his/her own health.

EnerSense-Buddho Reiki – Complete details listed in Part IV of *The Reiki Sourcebook* under Reiki Branches.

Enkaku Chiryô Hô 遠隔治療法 – (lit. Japanese) remote healing. This is the practice called *distant healing in the West.

Enryaku Ji – Main Tendai temple on *hiei zan*, near Kyôto, Japan. Mikao Usui is said to have trained and studied there. Copies of sutras with his Buddhist name on it are alleged to still exist there.

Enzui Bu 延髄部 – (lit. Japanese) medulla oblongata. This is the fourth head position as taught by Mikao Usui.

Ewing, Patricia – One of the 22 Reiki Master students trained by Hawayo Takata.

F

Facet – A variation of the word 'level' used by some branches of Reiki e.g. Facet 2 instead of Level 2.

***Finishing Treatment** –Blood cleansing method. Also called the *nerve stroke. In Japan traditional versions of this are *zenshin kôketsu hô, *hanshin kôketsu hô and *ketsueki kôkan hô. Hawayo Takata taught this technique in level 2.

Fire Serpent – A non-traditional symbol used in the 'Tibetan' branches of Reiki. Also called nin gizzida, Serpent Raku or Tibetan Fire Serpent. The Fire Serpent Symbol is drawn with a horizontal line across the top of the crown, snaking down the spine, and spiraling clockwise at the base of the spine thus grounding energy into the lower body. It can be practiced in healing, meditation or in an attunement for more balance and receptivity.

Five Head Positions – They are: *zentô bu* – forehead; *sokutô bu* – both temples; *kôtô bu* – back of your head and forehead; *enzui bu* – either side of neck; *tôchô bu* – crown on top of head. These head positions were taught to Mikao Usui's cousin Suzuki san and are included in the *Reiki Ryôhô Hikkei* and Chûjirô Hayashi's *Ryôhô Shishin*. Toshihiro Eguchi, a well-known healer around the time of Mikao Usui, is said to have used a similar set of hand positions in his manuals.

Five Precepts – For today only: Do not anger; Do not worry; Be humble; Be honest in your work; and Be compassionate to yourself and others.

These precepts are the cornerstone of Mikao Usui's teachings and are guidelines to aid students in their journey toward spiritual development. The Usui Reiki Ryôhô Gakkai perform *gokai sansho*, or the chanting of the five precepts, three times, at the end of their regular group meetings. The precepts are spiritual teachings rather than religious teachings and students were asked to practice them in their daily lives. Recently, it has been asserted that the origins of the five precepts actually date back to 9th century Japanese Buddhist precepts.

Fueston, Robert – Reiki researcher who focuses mainly on Hawayo Takata, her teachings and her students. Robert Fueston has trained with some of Hawayo Takata's Master students as well as more traditional teachers from Japan like Hiroshi Doi and Hyakuten Inamoto.

Funakoshi, Gichin – (1868–1957). Founder of modern karate. He is said to have known Mikao Usui.

Shinpei Goto knew both Gichin Funakoshi (he wrote a calligraphic work for Gichin Funakoshi's first book in 1922) and Mikao Usui. In 1922 Mikao Usui moved his seat of learning to Tôkyô where Gichin Funakoshi taught and Shinpei Goto lived.

Furumoto, Alice Takata – She was the daughter of Hawayo Takata and the mother of Phyllis Lei Furumoto. Alice Takata Furumoto compiled *The Gray Book* (called *Leiki*), which was handed out to some of Hawayo Takata's teacher students.

Furumoto, Phyllis Lei – Phyllis Lei Furumoto is the granddaughter of Hawayo Takata. She became a Reiki Master in April of 1979 in Keosauqua, Iowa. She is a founding member of The Reiki Alliance. The Reiki Alliance honoured her with their 'title of holder' of the 'Office of the Grandmaster' and also called her the lineage bearer of the system of Reiki. Phyllis Lei Furumoto is said to have apprenticed with her grandmother for the year and a half before she passed on. In the mid 1990s this headline headed an article in The Reiki Alliance 1996 newsletter, 'Does The Reiki Alliance want to follow the evolving teachings of the Office of the Grand Master?' After discussions, Phyllis Lei Furumoto resigned as a member though retained her official title.

Futomani Divination Chart – The Futomani Divination Chart stems from the *Hotsuma Tsutae*. Copies of the *Hotsuma Tsutae* have been stored in *iwamuro* (cave storage) in a Tendai temple at *enryaku ji* (*hiei zan*, Kyôto). These copies were given to Saichô (767–822), the founding priest of *enryaku ji*. The origin of this text is controversial. Tendai priests were believed to give lectures on the *Hotsuma Tsutae*. The divination chart has 48 syllables that are attributed to deities, forming the matrix of magic signs. One of the letterforms in the divination chart, the *wa*, resembles the essence of Symbol 1.

 G

Gasshô 合掌 – (lit. Japanese) to place the two palms together. This is a Japanese gesture of respect, gratitude, veneration and humility. This simple act balances both the mind and body. There are many varieties of *gasshô*.

*Gasshô Kokyû Hô 合掌呼吸法 – (lit. Japanese) *gasshô* breathing method. Also called **seishin toitsu* and is part of the technique **hatsurei hô*.

****Gasshô* Meditation** – A meditation method concentrating on the hands.

Gateway Symbol – A non-traditional symbol taught at the 7th level in the 7 Level System. Also known as the infinity symbol.

*Gedoku Hô – A similar technique to **tanden chiryô hô*. One hand is placed on the front of the *hara* and the other hand on the back of the *hara*. This technique is in the *shiori* for Usui Reiki Ryôhô Gakkai members.

Gendai Reiki Hô – Complete details listed in Part IV of *The Reiki Sourcebook* under Reiki Branches. This is a branch created by Hiroshi Doi and is a fusion between East and West.

Gnosa Symbol– A non-traditional symbol used in Karuna Reiki, Tera Mai, and Karuna Ki. It is said to connect the higher self with lower self, improve learning ability, communication and increase creativity.

Gokai 五戒 – (lit. Japanese) Five precepts.

Gokai No Sho – A copy of a work of calligraphy of the five precepts as brushstroked by Chûjirô Hayashi.

Gokai Sansho 五戒三唱 – (lit. Japanese) to sing the five precepts three times. This is a Buddhist term. It is still practiced by the Usui Reiki Ryôhô Gakkai at the end of their meetings.

Gokui Kaiden – Teacher level in Gendai Reiki Hô, Hiroshi Doi's branch of Reiki.

Golden Age Reiki – Complete details listed in Part IV of *The Reiki Sourcebook* under Reiki Branches.

Go Shimbô ご辛抱 – (lit. Japanese) patience, endurance or perseverance. The technique is also called 'Dharma for Protecting the Body'. This is a Tendai ritual that has similarities to the *reiju*.

Goto, Shinpei – (1857–1929). After studying at medical school he worked in various important Government positions. He became well known for advocating philanthropy and the principle of a 'Large Family' when he became Governor of the Standard of Railways. After the Kanto earthquake in September 1923, he played an active role in rebuilding Tôkyô. As a politician his nickname was 'Big Talker'. Shinpei Goto became the Mayor of Tôkyô in 1920 and it has been said that Mikao Usui had worked for him. Shinpei Goto wrote a calligraphic work in Gichin Funakoshi's first book in 1922 called *Ryukyu Kempo: Tode*. Gichin Funakoshi is also said to have been an acquaintance of Mikao Usui. In 1924, Citizen's forerunner, the Shokosha Watch Research Institute produced its first pocket watch. Shinpei Goto named the watch CITIZEN with the hope that the watch (a luxury item of those times) would become widely available to ordinary citizens and be sold throughout the world.

Grandmaster – The name Grandmaster in conjunction

with Reiki came into being with the advent of The Reiki Alliance. Phyllis Lei Furumoto, Hawayo Takata's granddaughter, received the title 'Office of the Grandmaster' from this association in 1983–4. This term was never used by Mikao Usui or Chûjirô Hayashi.

Gray, Reverend Beth – Beth Gray completed Levels 1 and 2 with Hawayo Takata. Her then husband, John Harvey Gray, became a Reiki Master with Hawayo Takata in 1976. He initiated Beth Gray as a Reiki Master while Hawayo Takata was alive even though it's believed she had asked that her students should not initiate any Reiki Masters until she died. In 1976, Beth Gray ordained Hawayo Takata as a minister on the basis of the spiritual nature of her teachings. Hawayo Takata eventually accepted her as a teacher and her name is included in the list of 22 Reiki Masters that Hawayo Takata had left with her sister. Beth Gray no longer practices after having a stroke in 1993.

Gray Book, The – Also called the *Leiki* booklet by some. Alice Takata Furumoto compiled this booklet in 1982. It includes notes and photographs of Hawayo Takata, a copy of Hawayo Takata's certificate signed by Chûjirô Hayashi, a list of Hawayo Takata's teacher students and the *Ryôhô Shishin – Healing Method's Guideline*. Chûjirô Hayashi wrote this guide especially for distribution in America. It shows hand positions for treating specific illnesses.

Gray, John Harvey – One of Hawayo Takata's 22 Reiki Master students. He was initiated on 6 October 1976 in Woodside, California. He was the third Reiki Master initiated by Hawayo Takata. He was once married to Beth Gray but has since remarried.

*Grounding – A method of connecting to the center of the earth energetically.

*Group Distant Healing – A method where a group of Reiki practitioners send Reiki.

*Group Reiki – Healing with Reiki in a group. Based on a traditional Japanese technique **shûchû Reiki*.

Gyoho (Gyotse) – Claimed to be Mikao Usui's Buddhist name by some. The name is written on the memorial stone. It has previously been translated as a 'pen name' or 'extra name'. According to Chris Marsh, a Tendai practitioner, there are still copies of old sutras with Mikao Usui's Buddhist name on it at *hiei zan*.

Gyosei 御製 – *Gyosei* is used to denote *waka* (poetry) written by the Meiji Emperor. It is said that the Emperor had written over 100,000 *waka* and his Empress Shoken over 30,000. Mikao Usui had added over 100 *gyosei* to his *Reiki Ryôhô Hikkei* for students to recite for spiritual purposes. The Usui Reiki Ryôhô Gakkai recite *gyosei* at the beginning of each meeting.

*Gyôshi Hô 凝視法 – (lit. Japanese) healing by staring method.

Gyôsho – *Kanji* drawn in modern, semi cursive style. A simplification of the standard style of writing *kanji*, allowing it to be written in a more flowing and faster manner.

 # H

*Hadô Kokyû Hô 波動呼吸法 – (lit. Japanese) vibrational breathing method.

*Hadô Meiso Hô 波動瞑想法 – (lit. Japanese) vibrational meditation method.

Hall, Mari – She is an American Reiki Master living in Prague who organizes large Reiki conferences around the world. She has written numerous books about the system of Reiki and teaches internationally.

Halu Symbol – A non-traditional symbol used in Karuna Reiki, Tera Mai, and Karuna Ki. It is said to heal unconscious patterns, the shadow, sexual and physical abuse issues and works on psychic and psychological attack. This was the third symbol retrieved by a 'Very High Being' from the Inner Planes and given to Kathleen Milner and Marcy Miller from the USA.

Hand Positions – Hand positions refer to the specific hand positions used when performing a Reiki treatment. Practitioners place their hands on specific body regions with the intention of assisting the energy to move through the body. The purpose is to clear and strengthen the client's spiritual and energetic connection. A one-hour Reiki treatment is made up of a practitioner placing hands on (or just off) the body of the client.

It appears that in Mikao Usui's traditional method only five head positions were used. Similar head positions are written up in the *Reiki Ryôhô Hikkei* and the *Ryôhô Shishin*. Toshihiro Eguchi, a well-known healer around the time of Mikao Usui, is said to have used a similar set of hand positions in his manuals. It is claimed that Hawayo Takata taught 12 positions (including the head, front and back of torso). Other Reiki systems may use a different number of positions. In the Western system students practice hand positions on themselves.

Hanko – A *hanko* is also called an *inkan* and is a personal seal. This seal is used to sign formal and legal documents in conjunction with a signature. Without this seal business in Japan would stagnate.

The *hanko* is necessary for filling in application forms or banking slips, or for when you receive registered mail. There are different kinds of *hanko*: cheap ready made ones – *sanmon ban*; ones that are officially registered – *jitsu in*; and those that are for banking mainly – *ginkô in*. Mikao Usui would have used his *hanko* on his documents. The use of *hanko* will help modern researchers verify the authenticity of any documents that lay claim to Mikao Usui as their writer.

*Hanshin Kôketsu Hô 半身交血法 – (lit. Japanese) half body blood exchange. This is a part of the technique **ketsueki kôkan hô.*

Hara 腹 – (lit. Japanese) belly or abdomen. Though the abdomen is generally called the *hara* there are also two other energetic centers in the body. One is the head and the other is the heart. The *hara* is like a battery that can be recharged through physical and spiritual techniques. Energy is stored at this point of the body. From here it expands through the whole body. In Mikao Usui's and the Usui Reiki Ryôhô Gakkai's teachings many techniques are taught to stimulate the *hara* centers. This is not unique in itself as the *hara* is an innate element of Japanese philosophy and culture. Whether practicing *go* (a Japanese game), *sadô* (flower arrangement) or *budô* (martial arts) the focus is on the *hara*.

Harajuku – Harajuku, Aoyama, Tôkyô. The place where Mikao Usui started his first official seat of learning in 1922.

Harth Symbol – A non-traditional symbol used in Karuna Reiki, Tera Mai, and Karuna Ki. It is said to help heal relationships, develop good habits, heal addictions, develops compassionate action and to contact spiritual beings. This was the second symbol retrieved by a

'Very High Being' from the Inner Planes and given to Kathleen Milner and Marcy Miller from the USA.
Hatamoto 旗下 – The *hatamoto* were the shogun's personal guard. Mikao Usui's family was *hatamoto samurai* – a high level within the ranks of *samurai*.
*Hatsurei Hô 発霊法 – (lit. Japanese) to generate greater amounts of spiritual energy. This technique includes the techniques **kenyoku hô*, **jôshin kokyû hô* and **seishin toitsu*. Kaiji Tomita describes a version of this technique, using *waka*, in his book *Reiki To Jinjutsu – Tomita Ryû Teate Ryôhô* that was published in 1933. Hiroshi Doi claims that the Usui Reiki Ryôhô Gakkai also practiced this technique.
Hayashi, Chie – The wife of Chûjirô Hayashi. She continued on at her husband's clinic after his death, becoming the second President of the *Hayashi Reiki Kenkyû Kai*.
Hayashi, Chûjirô 林忠次郎 – (1880–1940). One of the 21 teacher students of Mikao Usui. He was a Sôtô Zen practitioner who naturally included Shintô into his personal practices. In May 1925, Chûjirô Hayashi became a student of Mikao Usui's school in Tôkyô. He was a retired naval officer (still in the reserves) and surgeon and was about 45 years old when he met Mikao Usui. The length of his study with Mikao Usui was relatively short as he only studied the teachings for 10 months before Mikao Usui's death in March 1926.

It is interesting to note that Chûjirô Hayashi didn't teach the *reiju* but instead taught an attunement, which includes the mantras and symbols. Some researchers today question whether Chûjirô Hayashi actually was one of the 21 teacher students trained by Mikao Usui. Chûjirô Hayashi was known to have a healing guide

called the *Ryôhô Shishin*. It appears to be an almost exact copy of the *Reiki Ryôhô Hikkei*'s own healing guide. Today people believe that Chûjirô Hayashi may well have written the *Ryôhô Shishin* at Mikao Usui's request. Chûjirô Hayashi is thought to have been a member of the Usui Reiki Ryôhô Gakkai at first but broke away in 1931 developing his own branch called *Hayashi Reiki Kenkyû Kai*.

He wrote in 1938 that he had trained 13 Reiki Masters. Some of his students were Tatsumi, Shûô Matsui (not a teacher), Hawayo Takata, Chie Hayashi, and Chiyoko Yamaguchi.

He passed away on 10 May 1940. Hawayo Takata reported that he died ceremoniously of a self-induced stroke, Chiyoko Yamaguchi recounts that he had killed himself by 'breaking an artery' while others say that as he was a military man the honourable method of death would certainly have been *seppuku*.
*Hayashi Reiki Kenkyû Kai 林霊気研究会 – (lit. Japanese) Hayashi Spiritual Energy Research Society. Chûjirô Hayashi started this society in 1931. After his death his wife, Chie Hayashi, became known as the second president.
Head Positions – see Five Head Positions.
Healing Attunements – William Lee Rand developed this non-initiatory attunement with the intent that it increases healing. Some Masters are concerned that it gives the recipients the ability to practice Reiki yet they don't have the knowledge to work with the energy.
Healing Crisis – see Cleansing Process.
*Healing the Past and the Future – Send Reiki to yourself to heal your past, present and future.
*Heso Chiryô Ho 臍治療法 – (lit.

Japanese) healing at the navel method.

Hibiki 響き – (lit. Japanese) sound, echo, vibration. *Hibiki* is sensed when the body is being scanned or treated. It may feel like heat/cold/ tingling/pain/itchiness/pulsating, etc … in the palm of the hand.

Hiei Zan 比叡山 – A mountain near Kyôto where there is a main Tendai temple complex, *enryaku ji*. Mikao Usui is said to have studied Tendai Buddhism here. It has been suggested that old sutra copies on *hiei zan* have Mikao Usui's Buddhist name on them of Gyoho or Gyotse.

*Hikari No Kokyû Hô 光の呼吸法 – (lit. Japanese) breathing in the light method. Also called **jôshin kokyû hô* and is part of the technique **hatsurei hô*.

Hikkei 必携 – (lit. Japanese) companion, often called manual in the West.

Hiragana ひらがな – *Hiragana* is used to write the inflectional endings of the conceptual words that are written in *kanji*. It also is used for all types of native words not written in *kanji*. This was an attempt to cut down on the amount of *kanji* needed to express a multi-syllabic Japanese word.

Hô 法 – (lit. Japanese) method. This word is used in the description of a number of Japanese Reiki techniques.

Hosanna Symbol – A non-traditional symbol used in Tera Mai for clearing. Originally channeled by Eileen Gurhy from the USA.

Hotsuma Tsutae – Its first parts, 'Book of Heaven' and 'Book of Earth', were recorded and edited around 660 BC (according to the Nihonshoki calendar) by Kushimikatama-Wanihiko. His descendant, Ootataneko, recorded the third part, 'Book of Man', which contains the stories after Emperor Jinmu (660 BC), and offered the complete *Hotsuma Tsutae* to Emperor Keiko (the twelfth emperor) in AD 126. The origin of the *Hotsuma Tsutae* is controversial. It is guessed to be very old while some researchers challenge the dates written above.

Copies of *Hotsuma Tsutae* have been stored in *iwamuro* (cave storage) in a Tendai temple at *enryaku ji* (*hiei zan*, Kyôto). These copies may have been given to Saichô (767–822), the founding priest of *enryaku ji*. Tendai priests were also known to give lectures on the *Hotsuma Tsutae*.

*Hui Yin Breath – Non-traditional breath technique used with the attunement process.

I

Iava Symbol – A non-traditional symbol used in Karuna Reiki, Tera Mai, and Karuna Ki. It is said to heal co-dependence, empower goals and heal the earth. Catherine Mills Bellamont from Ireland channeled this symbol.

Ichi Sekai Reiki – Complete details listed in Part IV of *The Reiki Sourcebook* under Reiki Branches.

Imara Reiki – Complete details listed in Part IV of *The Reiki Sourcebook* under Reiki Branches.

Imperial Rescript on Education – The Imperial Rescript was written by the Meiji Emperor in 1890 and is an edict that became a fundamental Japanese moral code until the end of World War II. Jigorô Kanô, an acquaintance of Mikao Usui, also used this text as a moral code in his teachings and according to Frank Arjava Petter the five precepts are based on the rescript. The full rescript can be found in Appendix D.

In and *Yô* 陰陽 – Japanese word for yin and yang. These are the cosmic dual forces of heaven and earth. The *samurai* of the seventeenth century used the principles along with Chinese Confucianism. The first two mantras and Symbol 1 and 2 used in Mikao Usui's teachings are said to help the student become One with the *in* and *yô*.

Inamoto, Reverend Hyakuten – Teacher of Komyo Reiki Kai. He has studied the system of Reiki under different teachers such as Chiyoko Yamaguchi and is one of the guest teachers at the URRI (Usui Reiki Ryôhô International). He is also a translator for Hiroshi Doi and a Pure Land Buddhist monk. Hyakuten Inamoto's excellent translation of the memorial stone and the Meiji Emperor's *waka*, poetry, is included in *The Reiki Sourcebook*.

Independent Reiki Master – Independent Reiki Master is a term used to describe people who are Reiki Masters but are not aligned with a particular branch of Reiki. They might use an eclectic approach drawing on techniques from many schools. The vast majority of Reiki Masters in the West are Independent Reiki Masters. For complete details see Part IV of *The Reiki Sourcebook* under Reiki Branches.

Individual Attunement – An attunement is a ritual performed on students (often on their back and front while they are seated) by Reiki teachers. This ritual is generally performed as an individual attunement meaning that the teacher completes the attunement on each student individually before moving to the next student. With the advent of large courses some teachers began to line students up and walk down the front of the line – performing the first part of the attunement and then walking down the back of the line – completing the back.

Some teachers have expressed concern that the individual energetic link between teacher and student is broken or weakened by this 'group' method.

Initiation – This word is often used to describe the Japanese *reiju* and/or the Western attunement process.

Integrated Attunement – Attunement created and taught by Hiroshi Doi in the *gokui kaiden* level of Gendai Reiki Hô. It integrates all mantras and symbols into one attunement.

Intent – Reiki is an intent driven system. Intent is the key to working with Reiki in healing and attunements. Intent ensures the outcome. If one's intent is to be unhappy in life be assured that this will be the outcome. If one's intent is to be compassionate in life, well the choice is there. Intent rules every aspect of life and yet there is often obliviousness to this strength that humans possess and use.

The practitioner does not need to work hard to make Reiki work. The intent is there once the thought to place the hands on the body takes place. It is this intent which sparks the movement of energy. *Ki*, or energy, follows the mind. As far as Reiki is concerned, if the practitioner intends to use Reiki in the manner they were taught, then that is what will happen. If a practitioner intends to treat a client with Reiki then that person will receive a Reiki treatment.

Ishikuro, Iris – One of Hawayo Takata's 22 Reiki Master students. She was the tenth Master to be trained by Hawayo Takata. She was told to only train three people to the Master level. Iris Ishikuro only trained two people to this level, her daughter and Arthur

Robertson. Arthur Robertson worked with Iris Ishikuro and together they had an immense impact on the future of the system of Reiki with their system Raku Kei Reiki. They introduced a great deal of the 'Tibetan' information into the system. This included the 'Tibetan' symbols, the Johre symbol and 'Tibetan' techniques such as *breath of the fire dragon and the *hui yin technique. Iris Ishikuro died in 1984.

 J

Jakikiri Jôka Hô 邪気きり浄化法 – (lit. Japanese) energetically cleansing and enhancing inanimate objects.

Jikiden Reiki – Complete details listed in Part IV of *The Reiki Sourcebook* under Reiki Branches.

Jiko Joka Hô 自己浄化法 – (lit. Japanese) self-purification method.

Jinlap Maitri Reiki – Complete details listed in Part IV of *The Reiki Sourcebook* under Reiki Branches.

Jisshû Kai 実習会 – (lit. Japanese) practice or training meetings. The Usui Reiki Ryôhô Gakkai held these meetings after the *shûyô kai*.

Jôdo Shû 浄土宗 – (lit. Japanese) School of the Pure Land. The goal of this Buddhist school is to be reborn in the pure land of Amida Buddha. The main practice of the Pure Land school is to recite *Namu-Amida-Butsu*, which is an expression of Oneness. *Namu-Amida-Butsu* literally translates as 'I take refuge in Amida Buddha.'

Mikao Usui is buried in a Pure Land temple in Tôkyô. Hyakuten Inamoto believes that Mikao Usui

belonged to this sect. According to some traditional Japanese branches, Symbol 2 is connected to Amida Buddha.

Johrei – Johrei began in 1935 in Japan as a spiritual healing activity by Mokichi Okada and also uses a form of *reiju*. A 'Johrei Reiki' was developed from Raku Kei Reiki using the Johre symbol as part of its practices and attunements. Once the Johrei fellowship discovered this illegal use of their name the system became known as Vajra Reiki.

Johrei Reiki or Jo Reiki – Complete details listed in Part IV of *The Reiki Sourcebook* under Reiki Branches.

Johre Symbol – A non-traditional symbol used in 'Tibetan' branches of the system of Reiki. Said to have been added by Iris Ishikuro who created Raku Kei Reiki with Arthur Robertson. It is said to release blockages. This symbol has been taken from the religion, Johrei and is known as White Light.

Jôshin Kokyû Hô 浄心呼吸法 – (lit. Japanese) focusing the mind with the breath. Also called *hikari no kokyû hô* and is a part of *hatsurei hô*.

Jûdô – Modernized, sport oriented form of jujutsu. Founded by Jigorô Kanô (1860–1938) who is said to have been an acquaintance of Mikao Usui.

Jumon 呪文 – (lit. Japanese) spell, incantation. This is the Japanese word used for mantra, a sound that invokes a specific energetic vibration. Some Japanese teachers use the mantras taught by Mikao Usui in this way. For more information about Reiki *jumon* see page 82.

---

[1] Pictographs are pictures that represent ideas.
[2] Ideographs are symbols (*kanji*) that represent the sounds that form its name.

K

Kaisho – *Kanji* in modern, standard style. This style is similar to the printed style of *kanji*, and is taught in schools.

Kanji 漢字 – *Kanji* are Japanese written characters that are both pictographs[1] and ideographs.[2] In China, *kanji* originated in the Yellow River area about 2000 BC. During the third and fourth centuries AD it was brought across from China and Korea to Japan. Until this time Japan had only ever used the spoken language. The Chinese characters were used phonetically to represent similar sounding Japanese syllables, the actual meaning of the characters were ignored.

Kanji **Hand Mudras** – Mudras are hand gestures that stimulate specific energy. Introduced to the system of Reiki in an Omega Dawn Sanctuary of Healing Arts manual in 1983 from the branch Raku Kei Reiki. This was created by Arthur Robertson in conjunction with Iris Ishikuro.

Kannon – This deity is sometimes taught as the connection to Symbol 3. Kannon is the 'Bodhisattva Who Perceives the Sounds of the World'.

Kanô, Jigorô – (1860–1938). The founder of jûdô. According to Chris Marsh he knew Mikao Usui. Dave King believes that Mikao Usui started to use jûdô levels in his teachings in 1923: *rokkyû, gokyû, yonkyû, sankyû, nikyû, ikkyû, shodan, nidan, sandan, yondan, godan, rokudan* and *shichidan*. He states that the first four levels correspond to *shoden* and the next three to four levels correspond to *okuden zenki* and *kôki* in Mikao Usui's teachings.

The last five levels he asserts are not taught today. Jigorô Kanô is not in the photo with Mikao Usui that is found in Toshitaka Mochizuki's book about the system of Reiki.

Karuna Ki – Complete details listed in Part IV of *The Reiki Sourcebook* under Reiki Branches.

Karuna Reiki – Complete details listed in Part IV of *The Reiki Sourcebook* under Reiki Branches.

Katakana カタカナ – *Katakana* became phonetic shorthand based on Chinese characters. It was used by students who, while listening to classic Buddhist lectures, would make notations on the pronunciations or meanings of unfamiliar characters, and sometimes wrote commentaries between the lines of certain passages.

Katsu – This is a method of infusing life into a person and is mentioned on page 35 of the Chûjirô Hayashi *Ryôhô Shishin*[3] as a method to aid resuscitation.

Kenkyû Kai 研究会 – (lit. Japanese) Research or Study Society. This is the name that the Usui Reiki Ryôhô Gakkai use for their regular meetings today.

*Kenyoku Hô 乾浴法 – (lit. Japanese) dry bathing or brushing off method. This is similar to purification methods practiced in Shintôism. Purification rites are a vital part of Shintôism. A personal purification rite is the purification by water; this may involve standing under a waterfall, also known as *misogi*.

*Ketsueki Kôkan Hô 血液交換法 – (lit. Japanese) blood exchange method. Variations are **hanshin kôketsu hô* – half body blood exchange, **zenshin kôketsu hô* – whole body blood exchange, **finishing treatment* or **nerve stroke*. Sometimes also called **kôketsu hô*.

[3] This is the *Healing Method's Guideline* created by *Chûjirô* Hayashi.

Ki 気 – (lit. Japanese) Universal energy. *Ki* is considered to be an integral element to everyday Japanese life. Many Japanese traditions are based on a strong connection to *ki* apart from the martial arts and religious training. The success of the world renowned tea ceremony, the ancient game of *go* and the art of calligraphy are all based on the practitioner's ability to channel free-flowing *ki*.

Ki Ko – Qi Gong. Physical and meditative exercises, which are practiced in China and help to regulate the body, mind and breath. These exercises are both Taoist and Buddhist in origin.

King, Dave – Teacher in Canada who met a student of Toshihiro Eguchi called Yûji Onuki, in Morocco in the 1970s. In 1995, he met Tatsumi, a teacher student of Chûjirô Hayashi, in an out of the way village in Japan. He was allowed to make copies of Tatsumi's notes and symbols and was also taught Tatsumi's attunement. Dave King taught this attunement to Rick Rivard who in turn taught it to students at the URRI in Vancouver, 1999. This attunement has become popular amongst practitioners wishing to practice in a more traditional Japanese manner. Today, Dave King denies having passed on the full information relating to the attunement (or transformation as he calls it) to Rick Rivard. In his most recent research Dave King states that he is in contact with a Tendai nun called Mariko Obaasan who was a student of Mikao Usui.

Kiriku – This is the name for a seed syllable. A seed syllable is a letterform used solely for meditation and is a part of esoteric Buddhism practiced in China and Japan. The *kiriku* calls upon the energy of Amida Nyorai. Amida Nyorai is the main deity in Pure Land Buddhism. Symbol 2 is derived from the *kiriku*.

Kokoro – (lit. Japanese) heart, mind or core.

*Kôketsu Hô 交血法 – Also called **ketsueki kôkan hô*. **Kôketsu hô* is an abbreviation of **ketsueki kôkan hô*.

Kôki 後期 – (lit. Japanese) second half. This is the term used to describe the second level of *Okuden* (Level 2).

*Koki Hô 呼気法 – (lit. Japanese) sending *ki* with the breath method.

Komyo Reiki Kai – Complete details listed in Part IV of *The Reiki Sourcebook* under Reiki Branches.

Kondô, Masaki – Seventh President of the Usui Reiki Ryôhô Gakkai. He is also a University Professor.

Koriki Symbol – A non-traditional mantra/symbol taught in Reido Reiki. Also called the force of happiness.

Kôtô Bu 後頭部 - (lit. Japanese) back of the head. This is the third head position as taught by Mikao Usui.

Kotodama 言霊 – (lit. Japanese) words carrying spirit. Words have a particular power. Hiroshi Doi uses the word *kotodama* to address the mantra. Morihei Ueshiba an acquaintance of Mikao Usui and founder of aikidô also used the word *kotodama* in his teachings. He belonged to the Oomoto sect who had formulated effective meditation techniques and powerful chants based on *kotodama*. *Kotodama* in Shintôism invoke specific energies/deities. For more information about Reiki Kotodama see page 82.

Koyama, Kimiko – (1906–99). Sixth President of the Usui Reiki Ryôhô Gakkai.

Kriya Symbol – A non-traditional mantra/symbol used in Karuna Reiki, Tera Mai, and Karuna Ki. It is said to ground, manifest goals, create priorities and heal the human race.

Kuboi, Harry M. – The sixth of Hawayo Takata's 22 Reiki Master students. He believes that 99 per cent of people who learn the system of Reiki have 'negative' Reiki and therefore doesn't teach it anymore. Instead he does exorcisms where people's 'negative' Reiki becomes 'positive'. He told Robert Fueston that Barbara Weber Ray had sent him a letter stating that if he wanted to become a certified Reiki Master he would have to re-train with her and pay several thousand dollars. He also said that he had channeled Mikao Usui who gave him the title of 'Reiki Master of Masters'. Robert Fueston was further told that he could be trained to the Master Level for US$10,000 but he would have to receive a Reiki exorcism first. He would not be allowed to train others as a Reiki Master after this either.

Kun Yomi 訓読み – Here Chinese *kanji* are used to express Japanese words that have a similar meaning to the original Chinese word. When a Japanese word's sound uses *kanji* this is then called a *kun yomi* reading.

Kurama Yama 鞍馬山 – Mount Kurama near Kyôto, Japan. It is states on the memorial stone of Mikao Usui that he became enlightened while performing a meditation on *kurama yama*. According to the Kurama Temple Mikao Usui has no specific connection to them.

Kushu Shinren – (lit. Japanese) Painful and difficult training. A form of *shûgyô*. *Kushu shinren* was the word used for Mikao Usui's practice on *kurama yama* on his memorial stone.

 L

Leiki – Hawayo Takata sometimes wrote 'Leiki' instead of Reiki. This seems to be a translation mistake. To pronounce the word, Reiki, in Japanese it is necessary to forego any preconceptions about language that you may have. The first sound in *'rei'* is neither an 'R' nor an 'L', as some Westerners believe. In Japanese the sound is in fact somewhere in between the two letters. The Japanese language has no correlation with English or its pronunciations. The *kanji* for *'rei'* is officially spelt with an 'R' when translating into English and is therefore pronounced with an 'R' (even though the Japanese pronunciation might sound similar to what is understood as an 'L' in English).

Light and Adonea – Teachers of the Usui Reiki Ryôhô Tradition and founders of the Southwestern Usui Reiki Ryôhô Association. They are also Gendai Reiki Hô *gokui kaiden* (Teachers), Traditional and Contemporary Reiki Master/ Teachers. In addition to being Reiki Teachers, Light and Adonea are also Ordained Ministers and Spiritual Counsellors. Light passed away in 2003.

Lightarian Reiki – Complete details listed in Part IV of *The Reiki Sourcebook* under Reiki Branches.

Ling Chi – This is the pronunciation of the two *kanji* that represent the word 'Reiki' in Chinese. Ling Chi has a similar context to the word Reiki.

Lombardi, Ethel – She was the second of Hawayo Takata's 22 Reiki Master students. In 1976 she became a Reiki Master and in 1983 she created the system Mari-EL. Though this is based on the system of Reiki it was filled out with her own interpretations. She did not wish to be a member of either of the post- Hawayo Takata organizations.

Love and Light – The salutation 'Love and Light' is used by some Reiki practitioners in the West.

Lubeck, Walter – German author of many Reiki books and founder of a branch of Reiki called Rainbow Reiki. Has also written a book in conjunction with Frank Arjava Petter and William Lee Rand called *The Spirit of Reiki*.

 M

Mahatma Reiki – Complete details listed in Part IV of *The Reiki Sourcebook* under Reiki Branches.

*****Making Contact with Higher Beings** – Non-traditional technique of connecting and asking for guidance from higher beings.

*****Manifesting** – Non-traditional technique to manifest what you need or want.

Mantra – It is a power-laden syllable or series of syllables that manifest certain cosmic forces. Traditionally there are only four mantras in Mikao Usui's teachings. For more information about the traditional mantras see page 82. The mantras were given to students as a device for tapping into specific elements of energy. The Japanese words to describe the word mantra are either *kotodama* or *jumon*.

Mari-EL – Complete details listed in Part IV of *The Reiki Sourcebook* under Reiki Branches.

Mariko Obaasan – (1897–). Also known by her Buddhist name Tenon in. She is a Buddhist nun who was taught by Mikao Usui from 1920- 1926.

Marsh, Chris – A student of Suzuki san (Mikao Usui's cousin). He is a Tendai practitioner, iaidô practitioner and professional musician.

Matsui, Shûô – He studied with Chûjirô Hayashi in 1928. His first level was completed in five lots of one and a half hour sessions. Shûô Matsui wrote in an article called 'A Treatment to Heal Diseases, Hand Healing' in the magazine *Sunday Mainichi*, 4 March 1928, about the levels *shoden* and *okuden* and mentions that there were further unknown levels.

McCullough, Barbara Lincoln – One of Hawayo Takata's 22 Reiki Master students.

McFadyen, Mary Alexandra – One of Hawayo Takata's 22 Reiki Master students. She took her second level training with John Harvey Gray and her Master Level with Hawayo Takata. She teaches in California, USA.

Meiji 明治 – (lit. Japanese) name of an era.

Meiji Emperor – (1852–1912). The Meiji Emperor ruled Japan from 1867–1912. Mikao Usui used *waka*, poetry, written by the Meiji Emperor in his teachings.

Memorial Stone – This is the engraved memorial stone of Mikao Usui's life at his gravesite at the Pure Land Buddhist Saihôji Temple in Tôkyô. It was placed there by a number of his students, just one year after his death in 1927. The memorial stone is one aspect of Mikao Usui's life as seen through the eyes of his students from the Usui Reiki Ryôhô Gakkai. Unfortunately, the students who wrote this information up are said to not have consulted Mikao Usui's family and therefore may have left out information that was relevant in a memorial about him.

Men Chhos Reiki (or Medicine Dharma Reiki or Universal Healing

Reiki) – Complete details listed in Part IV of *The Reiki Sourcebook* under Reiki Branches.

Menkyo Kaiden – (lit. Japanese) Licence of complete and total transmission. It is a certificate given in traditional arts to show full proficiency for a lineage or style. It normally denotes a licence indicating a very high level of skill. For some lineages, it might be given to the headmaster. It is said that Mikao' Usui received *menkyo kaiden* in a specific branch of martial arts.

Meridian – These are interconnected energy lines in the body. The system originates from traditional Chinese medicine.

Method To Achieve Personal Perfection – Complete details listed in Part IV of *The Reiki Sourcebook* under Reiki Branches.

*Metta Meditation – Non-traditional meditation focusing on goodwill and sending love and compassion to all beings.

Mikkyô 密教 – (lit. Japanese) the secret teaching, esoteric Buddhism. There are five general areas taught in Tendai Buddhism. They are the teachings of the Lotus Sutra; esoteric Mikkyô practices; meditation practices; precepts; and Pure Land teachings. This form of Buddhism reached Japan at the beginning of the ninth century. There is a clear connection between Mikao Usui's teachings and Mikkyô. As Mikao Usui is believed to have been a Tendai lay priest he must have studied Mikkyô as it is an integral part of Tendai.

Misogi 禊 – (lit. Japanese) purification. Purification rites are a vital part of Shintôism. A personal purification rite is the purification by water; this may involve standing under a waterfall, which is known as *misogi*. In Mikao Usui's traditional teachings there is a technique called **kenyoku*

hô – a method of dry bathing or brushing off, which is a form of *misogi*. Shintô priests practice **kenyoku hô* according to some Usui Reiki Ryôhô teachers. One Shintô practitioner said that he performed a similar ritual with a group of men from his village where they wore only a red loincloth at the *hekogaki* festival (putting on the loincloth festival).

Mitchell, Paul – One of Hawayo Takata's 22 Reiki Master students. He studied Level 1 in 1978 and later became a Reiki Master in November of 1979 in San Francisco, California. He is a founding member of The Reiki Alliance though he resigned in 1995. Robert Fueston states that according to Rick Bockner, Paul Mitchell was initiated into the Master level around the same time as Rick Bockner, which was October 1980.

Mitsui, Mieko – A Japanese Reiki practitioner living in New York, who visited her native country in 1985. She began a revival of the system of Reiki in Japan by teaching the first two levels of The Radiance Technique. Here, she met Fumio Ogawa, a member of the Usui Reiki Ryôhô Gakkai. In 1986 there was an article in a Japanese magazine called *Twilight Zone* with a photo of her practicing the system of Reiki and of Fumio Ogawa reading a book written by the founder of a Western style of Reiki called The Radiance Technique. Hiroshi Doi was also one of the first Japanese to study Levels 1 and 2 with Mieko Mitsui.

Mochizuki, Toshitaka – Writer of two Japanese Reiki books and founder of the Vortex school in Japan. In his 2001 book, *Chô Kantan Iyashi No Te*, there is a photo of Mikao Usui and 19 of his students as well as family and friends in 1926. In the first edition of this book *Iyashi No Te (Healing Hands)*, he claims to have healed 3000 people. In his 2001 condensed version with pictures he claims to have healed up to 5200 people. *Reiki To Jinjutsu – Tomita Ryû Teate Ryôhô (Reiki and Humanitarian Work – Tomita Ryû Hands Healing)*, a book written by Tomita Kaiji in 1933 was re-published in 1999 with the help of Toshitaka Mochizuki. Included in this book are many anecdotes about healing, hand positions for specific diseases and some techniques like *hatsurei hô*.

Mon, or **Kamon** – (lit. Japanese) family crest. It originated in the eleventh century when court nobles and warriors used emblems as symbols of their families. The designs were drawn from a variety of objects like the sun, moon, stars, animals, geometrical patterns and letters. Families marked their clothing, banners and many other things with their crest. The most famous crest is the 16-petalled chrysanthemum possessed by the Imperial family. Mikao Usui's Chiba crest is a circle with a dot at the top. The circle represents the universe, and the dot or Japanese star represents the North Star. The North Star never moves while the universe circumambulates it.

*Morning Prayer – Non-traditional prayer to be practiced each morning. This is a prayer that is practiced in Satya Reiki by, mainly, the Pune, India branch.

 N

*Nadete Chiryô Hô 撫手治療法 – (lit. Japanese) stroking with the hands method.

Nagao, Tatseyi – He completed Levels 1 and 2 with Hawayo Takata in Hawaii and while in Japan in

1950 received *shinpiden* (Master or teacher level) from Chie Hayashi (Chûjirô Hayashi's wife). He returned to Hawaii to teach the system of Reiki to students and died in 1980.

Nakano – A suburb of Tôkyô where Mikao Usui moved his *dôjô* to in February 1925.

*Nentatsu Hô 念達法 – (lit. Japanese) sending thoughts method. Also called **seiheki chiryô hô*.

*Nerve Stroke – Also called **finishing stroke*, **zenshin kôketsu hô* or **ketsueki kôkan hô*. Hawayo Takata taught this technique in Level 2.

New Life Reiki – Complete details listed in Part IV of *The Reiki Sourcebook* under Reiki Branches.

Newlife Reiki Seichim – Complete details listed in Part IV of *The Reiki Sourcebook* under Reiki Branches.

 O

Ogawa, Fumio – Member of the Usui Reiki Ryôhô Gakkai in 1942 who completed six levels of proficiency in 14 months. His certificates were displayed in a Japanese magazine called *Twilight Zone* in 1986. In the same magazine was a photo of him reading a book written by the founder of a Western style of Reiki called The Radiance Technique. He met with Mieko Mitsui and with Frank Arjava Petter. Fumio Ogawa's stepfather, Kôzô Ogawa, ran a healing center in Shizuoka during Mikao Usui's lifetime. Fumio Ogawa's certificates read *rokkyû*, *gokyû*, *yonkyû*, *sankyû*, *okuden zenki* and *okuden kôki*. These dated from 1942 to 1943.

Ogawa, Kôzô – The stepfather of Fumio Ogawa who ran a healing center in Shizuoka during Mikao Usui's lifetime. A student of Kôzô

Ogawa was the mother of Tsutomu Oishi, an acquaintance of Frank Arjava Petter.

Okada, Masayuki – He composed the text of Mikao Usui's memorial stone at the Saihôji Temple in Tôkyô in 1927 one year after the death of Mikao Usui.

Okudan 奥段 – (lit. Japanese) innermost level.

Okuden 奥伝 – (lit. Japanese) second stage (hidden). This term actually signifies that you have only begun to work at this level – it does do not signify that you have completed this level.

Oneness – A concept where you become One with the universe. No separation, you are the Universe and the Universe is you. Oneness is absolute truth. To face Oneness means to face everything – yourself, the world, every being, and everything – in its absolute truth.

Onuki, Yûji 小貫祐仁 – A student of Toshihiro Eguchi. Dave King met and studied with him in the 1970s in Morocco.

On Yomi 音読み – There are two methods of pronouncing Japanese *kanji*. One is *on yomi* where the Chinese reading and meaning are attached to the *kanji*. The other is *kun yomi*.

***Open Heart Exercise** – Non-traditional technique used to create a trusting and open relationship with others.

***Oshite Chiryô Hô** 押手治療法 – (lit. Japanese) a hand pressure method.

 P

Petter, Frank Arjava – In 1991, Frank Arjava Petter moved to Japan with his Japanese wife, Chetna, to live. Briefly returning to Germany, his homeland, he studied all three

levels of the system of Reiki. He claims that before long he became the first teacher to teach all three levels openly in Japan. In 1993, they began researching the system of Reiki's traditional roots. He also made contact with Fumio Ogawa, a Usui Reiki Ryôhô Gakkai member. In 1997, Tsutomu Oishi provided Frank Arjava Petter with a photo of Mikao Usui with the five precepts in the left hand corner and a manual. Frank Arjava Petter has written three books about his research in Japan. Now living back in Dusseldorf, Germany he has recently co-written a book with · Tadao Yamaguchi about Chûjirô Hayashi.

Phaigh, Bethel – One of the 22 Reiki Master students of Hawayo Takata. She wrote two books, one called *Gestalt and the Wisdom of the Kahunas* and the other, *Journey into Consciousness* (unpublished). According to Robert Fueston she studied over a short period of time with Hawayo Takata and wrote in *Journey into Consciousness*, 'The lessons (in life that I needed to learn) may have been particularly painful because my initiations had been timed so closely together. I had left Hawaii that spring not knowing of Reiki. I return this winter as a Reiki Master, a very green one.' Bethel studied to become a Reiki Master after meeting Barbara Brown who told her all about Hawayo Takata. She died on 3 January 1986.

Photo Technique – This is a technique used to send *distant healing and is based on the Japanese technique *enkaku chiryô hô*. A simple version of this is where a photo is held in the hands with the intent that Reiki be sent to who or whatever is in the photo.

***Power Sandwich** – A non-traditional technique said to

increase effectiveness of hands-on or distant treatments.

Precepts – see Five Precepts

Proxy Methods – Proxy methods are Western techniques used to send *distant healing and are based on the Japanese technique *enkaku chiryô hô*. There is the Knee method, Pillow method or Teddy Bear method. These items or parts of the body are used as a proxy for the individual to send Reiki to. This concept is to help those who have difficulty setting clear intent when performing *distant healing.

Pure Land Buddhism – Also called Jôdo shû. Hônen brought Pure Land to Japan. The goal of this school is to be reborn in the Pure Land of Amida Buddha. The main practice of the Pure Land school is to recite *Namu-Amida-Butsu*, which is an expression of Oneness. *Namu-Amida-Butsu* literally translates as I take refuge in Amida Buddha.

Mikao Usui is buried in a Pure Land temple in Tôkyô. Hyakuten Inamoto believes that Mikao Usui belonged to this sect. According to some Japanese schools of the system of Reiki Symbol 2 is connected to Amida Buddha.

 Q

Qi Gong – This means 'energy cultivation' and refers to exercises that improve health and longevity as well as increase the sense of harmony within oneself and in the world. Japanese *ki ko* techniques are based on Qi Gong.

 R

Rainbow Reiki – Complete details listed in Part IV of *The Reiki Sourcebook* under Reiki Branches.

Raku – A lightening-like non-traditional symbol that is practiced in 'Tibetan' branches of Reiki. It is used at the end of attunements and is said to separate the energies of the teacher and student.

Raku Kei Reiki – Complete details listed in Part IV of *The Reiki Sourcebook* under Reiki Branches.

Rama Symbol – A non-traditional symbol used in Karuna Reiki, Tera Mai, and Karuna Ki. It is said to clear the mind, clear the room of negative energies, harmonize upper chakras with lower chakras and create determination and completion. The non-traditional symbol Mara emerged from this. Originally channeled by Kellie-Ray Marine from the USA who called the symbol Rama.

Rand, William Lee – Founder of Karuna Reiki and Usui/Tibetan Reiki. William Lee Rand runs the International Center for Reiki Training in Michigan, USA. He has trained with numerous teachers and has written *Reiki The Healing Touch* and co-written *Reiki News Magazine* with Walter Lubeck and Frank Arjava Petter.

Ray, Barbara Weber – She became a Reiki Master with Hawayo Takata on 1 September 1979. She received Level 1 in August 1978 and Level 2 in October 1978. Barbara Weber Ray claims that she is the only student to have received the seven level system of Reiki from Hawayo Takata. Harry Kuboi said she had sent him a letter stating that if he wanted to become a certified Reiki Master he would have to re-train with her and pay several thousand dollars. She founded the American Reiki Association in 1980 (now called the American-International Reiki Association). She wrote a book in 1983 called *The Reiki Factor* that later changed its name to *The Reiki Factor in The Radiance Technique*. It is only in the later editions of this book that she states there are seven levels in the system of Reiki. The first edition notes that there are just three levels (the same as Hawayo Takata's other Reiki Master students).

Re-Attune – Some teachers claim to be able to re-attune you. As an attunement is a clearing of the body's meridians it is impossible to be able to undo this or 'wipe-it-out'. Each attunement received takes the student a step further to re-aligning oneself with the natural function of the body – either mentally, physically, emotionally or spiritually.

Reido Reiki – Complete details listed in Part IV of *The Reiki Sourcebook* under Reiki Branches.

Reiha 霊波 – (lit. Japanese) wave of *rei*. It describes the tingling sensation that is comparable to an electrical current. The heat created and the wave of *rei* are what constitute spiritual energy. This is according to the 1933 book written by Kaiji Tomita a student of Mikao Usui.

Reiho 霊法 – (lit. Japanese) spiritual energy method. This is the name that is used for the system of Reiki in Japan. It includes the techniques, meditations, chanting, use of Reiki and *reiju*.

*Reiji hô 霊示法 – (lit. Japanese) being guided by spirit method.

Reiju 霊授 – (lit. Japanese) offering of spiritual energy. This is the Japanese name for attunement/ initiations/transformations, etc … *Reiju* is integral to Mikao Usui's teachings. To practice the system of Reiki a *reiju* must first be received. It helps to strengthen the student's connection with spiritual energy and raises their personal energy levels. This in turn gives a sense of reconnection to one's true self. It also helps to clear the meridians allowing the student to conduct more energy through the body. *Reiju* is just the first step. Students are also asked to practice with the mind and the body using the five precepts and *waka* and the physical techniques respectively.

Reiju is the same for each level – there are no differences as it is the student's ability to draw on more energy that creates the differences not the *reiju* itself. No symbols or mantras are used in the *reiju*. The *reiju* does not 'attune' the student to the symbols as is believed in the West.

The *reiju* appears to have links ˙ to practices from within the more esoteric elements of Tendai called Mikkyô. It mirrors a Tendai ritual called *go shimbô* also known as Dharma for Protecting the Body.

Reiki 霊気 – (lit. Japanese) spiritual energy. 霊 is *rei* – (lit. Japanese) spiritual. 気 is *ki* – (lit. Japanese) energy.

Mikao Usui did not call his teachings by this name. The word Reiki appeared often in conjunction with his teachings but this was merely to point out that the teachings worked with spiritual energy.

Once his teachings came to the West in 1938 they became known as Reiki, the system.

*Reiki Aura Cleansing – A non-traditional technique for clearing the aura of heavy energy.

*Reiki Boost – A non-traditional technique that balances and harmonizes the chakras allowing a greater flow of Reiki in the body. Also called the **quick treatment*, harmonizing Reiki with another prior to a session, *preparative mini Reiki session.

*Reiki Box** – A non-traditional technique to send Reiki to a person, place or event in the past, present or future.

Reiki Circle** – A coming together of Reiki practitioners where *group Reiki is practiced.

*Reiki Guide Meditation** – A non-traditional technique to meet your Reiki guide.

Reiki Guides** – The concept of guides is an add-on to the system of Reiki. It might stem from shamanism yet witches were also known to have familiars. Mystics, too, have been guided throughout the centuries by angelic beings – so the concept of spiritual guidance is quite broad based. Diane Stein and William Lee Rand have both popularized this element in the modern Reiki system.

Reiki Jin Kei Do** – Complete details listed in Part IV of *The Reiki Sourcebook* under Reiki Branches.

Reiki Levels** – Levels to be attained in the system of Reiki. When Mikao Usui first started teaching he had no need for recognized levels – it was just the teaching and you would be given further teachings after you had progressed on your spiritual path. There are generally three levels taught today though these have also been broken up into sub levels. In Japan the three major levels are *shoden, okuden* and *shinpiden*. In the West the levels have varying names including degree or facet.

Reiki Master** – Someone who completed Level 3 or *shinpiden* and is allowed to teach other people the system of Reiki. The title might not necessarily mean that this individual can guide

you on your spiritual path or even understands the concept of Reiki. Some branches may only teach the attunement to their teacher students while others may offer an extensive training. The minimal requirement to become a 'Reiki Master' in the West is that you know how to perform the attunement.

Reiki Master/Practitioner** – A title used in the West for someone who has completed only half of the third level. This is a new innovation. It means that the student has not learnt the attunement only the fourth mantra and symbol. Commonly used in the 'Tibetan' branches of Reiki.

Reiki Master/Teacher** – A title used in the West for two different purposes. One is to signify that the student has completed both levels of a form of Reiki where the third level is split in two. The second purpose is that many Reiki 'Masters' today do not believe that the term 'Master' is relevant as a description of what they do. There is the suggestion that it is arrogant to call yourself a 'Master' after a 'weekend' course. The title Master/Teacher is meant to suggest that the person is in fact a teacher rather than a guru of some sort.

*Reiki Mawashi** 霊気回し – (lit. Japanese) a current of spiritual energy.

*Reiki Meditation** – A non-traditional meditation using Reiki to increase sensitivity and connection to the source.

Reiki Plus** – Complete details listed in Part IV of *The Reiki Sourcebook* under Reiki Branches.

*Reiki Ryôhô Hikkei** 霊気療法必携 – (lit. Japanese) *Spiritual Energy Method Manual*. The *Reiki Ryôhô Hikkei* is a 68-page document

---

⁴ Virginia Samdahl was Hawayo Takata's first trained Reiki Master in 1976.

divided up into four sections. It was given to *shoden* (Level 1) students of the Usui Reiki Ryôhô Gakkai. There is the introduction or explanation by Mikao Usui; a question and answer section with Mikao Usui; the *Ryôhô Shishin* or healing guide with specific hand positions and the *gyosei* (*waka*, poetry, of the Meiji Emperor). General thought today has it that Chûjirô Hayashi largely created the healing guide.

Frank Arjava Petter named one of his books, *The Original Reiki Handbook of Dr. Mikao Usui* after this manual. Kimiko Koyama compiled the *Reiki Ryôhô Hikkei* or manual for the Usui Reiki Ryôhô Gakkai's fiftieth anniversary and therefore it is not directly from Mikao Usui.

Reiki Salad – Hawayo Takata was renowned for her 'Reiki Salad' as she called it. Some of her recommended recipes for better health included sunflower seeds, red beet, grape juice and almonds. Two students of Virginia Samdahl's[4] wrote a book in 1984 called *The Reiki Handbook*, which includes Reiki recipes.

*Reiki Shower – A non-traditional cleansing technique that also increases energy flow in the body.

Reiki Stacks – Non-traditional Western technique used for sending distant Reiki. This is similar to the technique *Reiki box where lists are written up and Reiki is sent to them.

Reiki Teacher – A Reiki Master that does not wish to use the word Reiki 'Master' due to its implications.

Reiki Treatment – Reiki treatments come in all shapes and sizes. The client lies or sits and the practitioner's hands are placed on or just above the body. It is unnecessary for the client to remove one's clothes and no private parts of the body need be touched. There is no place for sexual contact or inference within the system of Reiki. The treatment may take from about five minutes to an hour.

Reiki Tummo – Complete details listed in Part IV of *The Reiki Sourcebook* under Reiki Branches.

*Reiki Undô 霊気運動 – (lit. Japanese) movement of spiritual energy.

Robertson, Arthur – He first studied with Hawayo Takata's student, Virginia Samdahl in 1975. He then went on to study and work with another of Hawayo Takata's students, Iris Ishikuro in the early 1980s. Together they created Raku Kei Reiki. In a 1983 Raku Kei Reiki manual the non-traditional techniques taught included the *breath of the fire dragon, the *hui yin breath and the *kanji* hand mudras. This appears to be the first time that they had been used in connection with the system of Reiki. Arthur Robertson also worked with Master Frequency Plates with an *antakharana inside. These additions to the system of Reiki have made a profound impact on how it is taught today. Most of the 'Tibetan' systems have stemmed from Arthur Robertson's teachings.

Ryôhô – (lit. Japanese) healing method.

Ryôhô Shishin 療法指針 – (lit. Japanese) *Healing Method's Guideline.* A guide that was written by Chûjirô Hayashi for his students. It contains almost identical hand positions for treating specific illnesses as the guide in the *Reiki Ryôhô Hikkei*. It is uncertain when Chûjirô Hayashi first used a healing guide. Its front cover reads *Healing Method's Guidelines* and explains that it had been set up for American distribution. The branch name on the cover was the *Hayashi Reiki Kenkyû Kai* or Hayashi Spiritual Energy Research Society. It also stated that it was not for sale and was a printed copy of the original.

Written in Japanese, Hawayo Takata is known to have handed it to a number of her students including Harue Kanemitsu. John Harvey Gray also received a copy from Alice Takata, Hawayo Takata's daughter.

 S

Sacred Path Reiki – Complete details listed in Part IV of *The Reiki Sourcebook* under Reiki Branches.

Saibo Kassei Kokyû Hô 細胞活性呼吸法 – (lit. Japanese) vitalizing the cells through the breath method.

Saihôji Temple 西方寺 – Pure Land Buddhist Temple in Tôkyô. The exact address is Toyotama district, 1-4-56 Umesato, Suginami Ku, Tôkyô. Here you can see the memorial stone that was engraved by Mikao Usui's students in 1927, one year after his death. Masayuki Okada composed it with brush strokes written by Juzaburo Ushida in 1927. The memorial stone is one aspect of Mikao Usui's life as seen through the eyes of his students from the Usui Reiki Ryôhô Gakkai.

Saito, Shinobu – One of Hawayo Takata's 22 Reiki Master students. She completed Level 1 in 1976 and Level 2 in 1978, and became a Reiki Master in May 1980 in Palo Alto, California with Hawayo Takata. Robert Fueston states that Hawayo Takata hoped she would help take the system of Reiki back to Japan.

Sakoku 鎖国 – (lit. Japanese) Japan's national isolation. From 1639–1854 Japan was shut under a policy called *sakoku* or 'national isolation' which had left it culturally prosperous though far behind the Western world technologically and militarily. Westerners were forbidden to enter Japan and trade.

Only the Dutch were excluded. Through the small port of Dejima in Nagasaki the traders became Japan's single link to the West for more than two centuries. This privilege was only extended to contact with Japanese merchants and prostitutes. Any Japanese who dared to venture abroad during this period were executed on their return to prevent any form of 'contamination'. Christianity was legalized in 1877.

The Meiji Emperor (1852–1912) introduced Japan to modernization and industrialization.

Saku Reiki – Complete details listed in Part IV of *The Reiki Sourcebook* under Reiki Branches.

Sama – This is a more polite version of *san* and is commonly used in formal situations or when writing letters. It may be too polite in a casual context.

Samdahl, Virginia – She was the first of Hawayo Takata's 22 Reiki Master students. She received Level 1 in 1974, Level 2 in 1975 and became a Reiki Master in 1976. Robert Fueston states that he was told that Virginia Samdahl introduced Barbara Weber Ray to Hawayo Takata. This may account for the fact that after Hawayo Takata's death Virginia Samdahl was a member of both of the groups that claimed to carry on Hawayo Takata's teachings, one was The Reiki Alliance and the other was Barbara Weber Ray's Radiance Technique. Virginia Samdahl retired from teaching Reiki in 1989 and died in 1994.

Samurai 侍 – (lit. Japanese) warrior. Mikao Usui's family was *hatamoto samurai* – a high level within the ranks of *samurai*.

San – This is a neutral title, and can be used in most situations. In formal situations it may not be polite enough.

Sati Symbol – A non-traditional symbol used in Tera Mai. It is said to open, integrate and balance. Originally channeled by Lawson Bracewall from New Zealand.

Satori – (lit. Japanese) spiritual enlightenment or awakening. The method of attaining spiritual enlightenment would differ depending on which Buddhist sect you belonged to. Zen emphasized meditation as a means of experiencing awakening while the Pure Land sect uses the chanting of a *nembutsu* (prayer to Amitabha).

Satya Reiki – Complete details listed in Part IV of *The Reiki Sourcebook* under Reiki Branches.

***Scanning** – A non-traditional technique sensing imbalances in the energy field.

***Seated Chakra Treatment** – A non-traditional technique stimulating the chakras.

Seichem – Complete details listed in Part IV of *The Reiki Sourcebook* under Reiki Branches.

Seichim – Complete details listed in Part IV of *The Reiki Sourcebook* under Reiki Branches.

***Seiheki Chiryô Hô** 性癖治療法 – (lit. Japanese) treatment of mental patterns. This is the same treatment as *nentatsu hô* but with the inclusion of mantra's and symbols.

***Seishin Toitsu** 精神統一 – (lit. Japanese) mental concentration. Also called *gasshô kokyu hô* and is a part of the technique *hatsurei hô*.

Seiza 正座 – (lit. Japanese) correct sitting. This is a traditional Japanese style of sitting on top of the ankles, with the legs folded underneath and the back erect. It is a formal way of sitting on a tatami. Sitting upright is *seiza*, sitting cross-legged is *agura*, informal or casual. *Seiza* is used when you attend a formal occasion while *agura* would be used for informal occasions.

Seiza 静座 – (lit. Japanese) sit still. This is a different reading of the word *seiza*. It is written in the 1933 book, *Reiki To Jinjutsu – Tomita Ryû Teate Ryôhô (Reiki and Humanitarian Work – Tomita Ryû Hands Healing)* by a student of Mikao Usui called Kaiji Tomita. It is used with this meaning in the first section of the technique *hatsurei hô*.

Sekhem – Complete details listed in Part IV of *The Reiki Sourcebook* under Reiki Branches.

***Sekizui Jôka Ibuki hô** 脊髄浄化息吹法 – (lit. Japanese) cleansing the spinal cord with breath method.

Self-Treatment – This is where students practice placing their hands on their bodies in a systemized fashion. Self-practice by placing hands on one's own body was not taught directly by Mikao Usui.

Sensei 先生 – (lit. Japanese) teacher, master. It is an honorific title, which people call their teachers or someone of a higher position. You must never call yourself a *sensei*.

Seppuku – Suicide by disembowelment. *Seppuku* was a death penalty to which high-ranking *samurai* warriors were condemned for crimes of great gravity. It was considered to be a less disgraceful punishment than beheading. It is seen as a solemn, almost ceremonial suicide achieved by a man thrusting a short sword into the side of the belly and then moving it across. Women would stab a dagger into their throat. By enduring the pain, the *samurai* was assumed to have made amends for his offense.

Seven Level System – Complete details listed in Part IV of *The Reiki Sourcebook* under Reiki Branches.

***Seventh Level Technique** – Non-traditional Western technique said to activate the gateway chakra.

Shamballa Multi-Dimensional

Healing/Reiki – Complete details listed in Part IV of *The Reiki Sourcebook* under Reiki Branches.

Shanti Symbol – A non-traditional symbol used in Karuna Reiki, Tera Mai, and Karuna Ki. It is said to create trust, heal insomnia, fear and panic and manifest the best results. Originally channeled by Pat Courtney from the USA.

Shihan 師範 – (lit. Japanese) instructor or teacher.

Shinpiden 神秘伝 – (lit. Japanese) mystery teachings. Japanese name for Level 3 or Master or Teacher level. These Japanese terms actually signify that you have only begun to work on that level – they do not signify that you have completed that level.

Shintô 神道 – (lit. Japanese) the way of the *kami* (gods). Shintô is the indigenous faith of the Japanese people, and it is as old as the culture itself. The *kami*, or gods, are the objects of worship in Shintô. It has no founder and no sacred scriptures like the sutras or the bible. Initially, it was so unself-conscious that it also had no name. The term, Shintô came into use after the sixth century when it was necessary to distinguish it from the recently imported Buddhism. It is not unusual for Japanese people to be followers of both Buddhism and Shintôism. Today many people visit Shintô shrines for self-purification services. Purification rites are a vital part of Shintôism. A personal purification rite is the purification by water; this may involve standing under a waterfall, which is known as *misogi*. In Mikao Usui's traditional teachings there is a technique called *kenyoku hô which is a kind of *misogi*.

The use of *kotodama/jumon* is an aspect of Shintôism that is also reflected in Mikao Usui's teachings.

Shiori 栞 – (lit. Japanese) guide, usually for beginners. This is a booklet exclusively for members of the Usui Reiki Ryôhô Gakkai and was written by Hôichi Wanami and Kimiko Koyama, both presidents of the Usui Reiki Ryôhô Gakkai. It consists of: the purpose, history and administrative system of the Usui Reiki Ryôhô Gakkai and includes the names of 11 of the 21 *shinpiden* students taught by Mikao Usui; how to strengthen Reiki and includes techniques such as *byôsen reikan hô, *gedoku hô, *kôketsu hô and *nentatsu hô; a teaching from Mikao Usui; a guide to treatment; characteristics of *Reiki Ryôhô*; remarks by medical doctors and explanation of the *Ryôhô Shishin* (healing guide).

Shirushi 印 – (lit. Japanese) symbol.

Shodan 初段 – (lit. Japanese) beginners level.

Shoden 初伝 – (lit. Japanese) first stage. This is the Japanese name for Level 1. This Japanese term actually signifies that you have only begun to work on this level – it does not signify that you have completed this level.

Shogun 将軍 – (lit. Japanese) a general.

***Shûchû Reiki** 集中霊気 – (lit. Japanese) concentrated spiritual energy. Also called *shûdan reiki*. This is what is called *group Reiki in the west.

***Shûdan Reiki** 集団霊気 – (lit. Japanese) group spiritual energy. Also called *shûchû reiki*.

Shûgyô 修行 – (lit. Japanese) Deep mind /body training. *Shûgyô* is a training performed in pursuit of deeper levels of consciousness. It is usually quite demanding, requiring unlimited amounts of effort, mindfulness and refinement. Mikao Usui performed a form of *shûgyô* on *kurama yama*.

Shûyô Kai 修養会 – (lit. Japanese) group meetings. *Shûyô* means to cultivate one's mind or improve

Oneself. This was the name of the group meetings of the Usui Reiki Ryôhô Gakkai. After the *shûyô kai* there was the *jisshû kai*, the practical gathering, where some techniques were performed. Today the meeting is called the *kenkyû kai*.

*Six Point Meditation for Energy Awareness – A non-traditional technique creating an even flow of energy in the body.

SKHM – Complete details listed in Part IV of *The Reiki Sourcebook* under Reiki Branches.

*Smudging – A non-traditional technique using the vibration of smell to affect energy.

*Sokutô Bu 側頭部 (lit. Japanese) both temples. This is the second head position as taught by Mikao Usui.

*Solar Image Training – A non-traditional technique to aid in letting go of dependency on symbols.

Sôsho – Kanji in modern, cursive style. This is a kind of simplified shorthand that is drawn according to esthetic standards.

Sôtô Zen – One of the two most important schools of Zen in Japan. *Zazan shikan taza* meditation is heavily stressed in this school.

Stein, Diane – Diane Stein's book, *Essential Reiki*, published in 1995 was a revolt against the 1980s system of Reiki and the elitism that was being practiced under its name. It also introduced many add-on elements to the system of Reiki and popularized the 'Tibetan' style.

Stiene, Bronwen and Frans – Authors of *The Reiki Sourcebook*. Bronwen and Frans ran a Reiki center in Darjeeling, India in 1998–9. They treated the local community and taught the system of Reiki to travelers passing through. Though Frans is from Holland, they moved to Australia (Bronwen's country of birth) in 1999. They now live in the Blue Mountains and run the International House of Reiki based in Sydney. Their passion is to study Mikao Usui's teachings and to research their origins. In 2001 they traveled to Japan to meet with Japanese Reiki teachers, visit *hiei zan* and *kurama yama* and pay their respects to Mikao Usui.

Sun Li Chung Reiki – Complete details listed in Part IV of *The Reiki Sourcebook* under Reiki Branches.

Suzuki, Bizan – Author of a book called *Kenzon No Genri*, written in 1914. It includes similar precepts to those taught by Mikao Usui. A translation of this similar section in Bizan Suzuki's book is: 'Today do not be angry, do not worry and be honest, work hard and be kind to people.' Another interesting fact is that the *kanji* for Bizan can be read as Miyama. Miyama cho is the modern name of the place where Mikao Usui was born.

Suzuki san – (1895–). A Tendai nun, cousin of Mikao Usui's wife and one of his students. She was born in 1895 and was aware of Mikao Usui her whole life. Her formal training with him began in 1915 when she was 20 years old and her relationship with him continued on a less formal basis until his death in 1926. It's believed that Suzuki san and 11 other living students of Mikao Usui have preserved a collection of his papers from 1920, which include the precepts, *waka*, meditations, and teachings.

Suzuki, Sadako – (?–1946). Mikao Usui's wife. She died on 17 October 1946. Sadako Suzuki's cousin is Suzuki san who is still alive today.

*Symbol Exercises – Non-traditional techniques to increase your connection to Reiki by meditating on the symbols.

Symbols – Traditionally there are only four symbols in Mikao Usui's teachings. It is believed that only later in Mikao Usui's life, around 1923 (once he began working with lay people who were not involved in spiritual practices), were symbols introduced. These symbols were extra tools that made it easier for students to practice Mikao Usui's spiritual teachings. The names of the traditional symbols are Symbol 1, 2, 3 and 4. See page 82 for more information.

 T

Takata, Hawayo – (1900–1980). One of the 13 teacher students of Chûjirô Hayashi. Hawayo Takata studied with Chûjirô Hayashi from 1936 to 1938 and was the first to bring Chûjirô Hayashi's teachings to the West. For 40 years she employed the method of storytelling to practice and eventually teach people about the system she called Reiki and its history. Before she died in 1980 she had taught 22 Reiki Masters to carry on her teachings.

Taketomi, Kanichi – (1878–1960). Third President of the Usui Reiki Ryôhô Gakkai. He was also a Rear Admiral. He became a member in 1925.

*Talismans – A non-traditional method of manifesting using an image as the focus.

Tamasura – A non-traditional symbol used in 'Tibetan' branches of Reiki. Said to be an antidote to fear.

Tanden 丹田 – (lit. Japanese) means the abdomen below the navel. It is used to mean the center of balance of the body. Also called *hara*.

*Tanden Chiryô Hô 丹田治療法 – (lit. Japanese) detoxifying and

purifying method.

Taniai 谷合 – Birthplace of Mikao Usui. He was born on 15 August 1865 in this village in the Yamagata county of the Gifu Prefecture, Japan. This village is now called Miyama cho.

Tara Reiki – Complete details listed in Part IV of *The Reiki Sourcebook* under Reiki Branches.

Tatsumi – (?–1996). One of the 13 teacher students of Chûjirô Hayashi. Tatsumi, trained in 1927 to become a teacher. Tatsumi did not appreciate the changes that Chûjirô Hayashi had made and finally left in 1931. Tatsumi said he was initially taught in a class with five other students. He learnt seven basic hand positions from Chûjirô Hayashi before 1931. These were formulated to cover specific acupuncture points on the body.

In 1995, Dave King met Tatsumi in an out of the way village in Japan. Though Tatsumi had never taught these teachings he still had the paperwork. These included hand written notes from Chûjirô Hayashi's teachings and copies of the four traditional symbols. Tatsumi died in 1996.

Teate 手当 – (lit. Japanese) hands-on healing. This was a very common practice during the time of Mikao Usui. Many individual groups were practicing *teate*, some of these teachings have spread worldwide. Usui teate would indicate what Mikao Usui did, not what he was teaching; this would have been called Usui dô.

Tendai 天台 – Buddhist sect in Japan. Mikao Usui is said to have been a Tendai lay priest and to have studied on *hiei zan* the main Tendai temple complex in Japan. Tendai was brought to Japan by Saichô in the early ninth century and names Nagarjuna as its patriarch. Their belief is that the Lotus Sutra is Buddha's complete and perfect teachings. There are five general areas taught in Tendai. They are the teachings of the Lotus Sutra; esoteric Mikkyô practices; meditation practices; precepts; and Pure Land teachings.

Tenohira Ryôji Kenkyû Kai 手のひら療治研究会 – (lit. Japanese) Hand Healing Research Center. Toshihiro Eguchi a student and friend of Mikao Usui created this society.

Tenon in – (1897–) The Buddhist name for Mariko Obaasan, who was a student of Mikao Usui.

Tera-Mai Reiki and Tera-Mai Seichem – Complete details listed in Part IV of *The Reiki Sourcebook* under Reiki Branches.

The Radiance Technique (or Authentic Reiki or Real Reiki) – Complete details listed in Part IV of *The Reiki Sourcebook* under Reiki Branches.

The Reiki Alliance – An organization formed by some of Hawayo Takata's Master students after her death in 1980. In 1982 they all came together, according to Carel Anne Farmer, and compared symbols and mantras (and attunements according to John Harvey Gray). They were surprised when they found that they differed. This group then standardized these elements of the system of Reiki. Hawayo Takata's granddaughter, Phyllis Lei Furumoto, was named as their Grandmaster and lineage bearer – the first time that these words had ever been used by anyone in conjunction with the system of Reiki. The Alliance maintains a requirement that the Master Level should cost US$10,000. An attempt was made by Phyllis Lei Furumoto in the 1990s to trademark words like 'Reiki', which failed in most countries except South America.

Three-Week Cleansing Process

– The cleansing process is also known as a healing crisis. It is a response to an attunement, *reiju* or Reiki treatment. The body is attempting to remove toxins and re-balance the body and this can often be felt physically, emotionally, mentally or spiritually. After an attunement it is often said that the student will undergo a 21-day cleansing process in which the student must practice Reiki to aid the process. Though this is a recent Western addition to Reiki it certainly has had its share of esoteric interpretations. Basically the popularity of the three-week cleansing process concept can be put down to the fact that it is successful – it achieves its aim. That aim is to get people practicing. Some smart individual knew that human nature technically takes 21 days to break a habit and therefore also takes 21 days to *make* a habit. After practicing Reiki for three weeks students don't want to stop practicing – it feels too good!

Tibetan Reiki – Complete details listed in Part IV of *The Reiki Sourcebook* under Reiki Branches.

Tôchô Bu 頭頂部 – (lit. Japanese) crown on top of head. This is the fifth head position as taught by Mikao Usui.

*Toning – A non-traditional method of using the voice as a healing tool.

Tomita, Kaiji – Said to be a student of Mikao Usui. He wrote a book called, *Reiki To Jinjutsu – Tomita Ryû Teate Ryôhô (Reiki and Humanitarian Work – Tomita Ryû Hands Healing)* in 1933. The book was re-published in 1999 with the help of Toshitaka Mochizuki. Included in his book are case studies, the technique **hatsurei hô* (which includes the use of *waka*), hand positions for specific illnesses. The name of his school was *Teate Ryôhô Kai* and it taught four levels *shoden, chuden,* *okuden* and *kaiden.*

Tomita Teate Ryôhô Kai – Name of the school created by Kaiji Tomita, a student of Mikao Usui. In his school he used four levels, which were called, *shoden, chuden, okuden* and *kaiden.*

Tôrô – (lit. Japanese) a lantern. These *tôrô* were first brought to Japan from China in the sixth century along with the introduction of Buddhism. Though they come in all shapes and sizes their one common factor is the hollow upper tier that is used for illumination purposes where a candle or oil lamp can be placed. A garden lantern is not so much an illumination as a sculptural ornament.

Toshitane, Chiba – A famous *samurai* warlord from the 1500s. In 1551 he conquered the city Usui and thereafter all family members acquired that name. The memorial stones states that the famous *samurai*, Tsunetane Chiba (1118–1201) was Mikao Usui's ancestor. Recently Hiroshi Doi notes that this was incorrect and that it was in fact Toshitane Chiba.

Traditional Japanese Reiki - Complete details listed in Part IV of *The Reiki Sourcebook* under Reiki Branches.

Transformation – This word is often used to describe the Japanese *reiju* and/or the Western attunement process.

Tsunetane, Chiba – (1118–1201). The memorial stones states that the famous *samurai*, Tsunetane Chiba was Mikao Usui's ancestor

Twan, Wanja – One of Hawayo Takata's 22 Reiki Master students.

 U

*Uchite Chiryô Hô 打手治療法 – (lit.

Japanese) patting with the hands method.

Ueshiba, Morihei – (1883-1969). Founder of aikidô. Morihei Ueshiba is claimed to be an acquaintance of Mikao Usui. Chris Marsh states that they had a teacher in common as well. Morihei Ueshiba used *kotodama* in his method, not unlike Mikao Usui.

Universal Healing Reiki (Men Chhos Reiki or Medicine Dharma Reiki) – Complete details listed in Part IV of *The Reiki Sourcebook* under Reiki Branches.

URRI – See Usui Reiki Ryôhô International.

Ushida, Jûzaburô – (1865-1935). Second President of the Usui Reiki Ryôhô Gakkai. He was also a Rear Admiral. He became a member of this society in 1925. Ushida Jûzaburô did the brush strokes on Mikao Usui's Memorial Stone in 1927.

Usui Dô 臼井道 – (lit. Japanese) the way of Usui. What Mikao Usui taught was called 'Usui dô' – 'the way of Usui', and what he practiced on people would have been called 'Usui teate' – meaning 'Usui hands-on healing'. Early students had never heard of the word Reiki in relation to the entirety of Mikao Usui's teachings.

There is also a branch of Reiki called Usui Dô, for more complete details of this branch see Part IV of *The Reiki Sourcebook* under Reiki Branches.

Usui, Fuji – (1908-1946). Mikao Usui's son. He was a teacher at the Tôkyô University.

Usui, Mikao 臼井甕男 – (1865-1926). Mikao Usui is the founder of the system of Reiki. Mikao Usui was born on 15 August 1865, in the village of Taniai mura in the Yamagata district of the Gifu Prefecture, in Japan. His father's name was Uzaemon and they were from the Chiba clan. Mikao Usui is understood to have been born a Tendai Buddhist and as a child studied in a Tendai monastery. He remained Tendai all his life and is believed to eventually have become a Tendai lay priest.

Mikao Usui married Sadako Suzuki and they had two children a boy and a girl, called Fuji and Toshiko respectively.

He is thought to have studied on *hiei zan* and practiced certain meditations on *kurama yama*. It has been suggested that old sutra copies on *hiei zan* have Mikao Usui's Buddhist name or extra name of Gyoho or Gyotse on them.

What Mikao Usui taught was called 'Usui dô' – 'the way of Usui'. His teachings included using *waka*, the five precepts, meditations and techniques, mantras and or symbols and *reiju*. What he practiced on people would have been called 'Usui teate' – 'Usui hands-on healing' and included hands on healing.

The names of 11 of the 21 Master students of Mikao Usui have been recorded in a booklet used by the Usui Reiki Ryôhô Gakkai.

Usui Reiki – Complete details listed in Part IV of *The Reiki Sourcebook* under Reiki Branches.

Usui Reiki Ryôhô 臼井霊気療法 – (lit. Japanese) Usui Spiritual Energy Healing Method. Hawayo Takata referred to the system of Reiki she learned from Chûjirô Hayashi as Usui Reiki Ryôhô in a recording of 1979 telling the story of the system of Reiki.

There is also a branch of Reiki called Usui Reiki Ryôhô, for more complete details of this branch see Part IV of *The Reiki Sourcebook* under Reiki Branches.

Usui Reiki Ryôhô Gakkai 臼井霊気療法学会 – (lit. Japanese) Society of the Usui Spiritual Energy

Healing Method. The Usui Reiki Ryôhô Gakkai claims to have been created by Mikao Usui in 1922. The society still exists today, and has its seventh president. It is closed to foreigners and members are asked not to discuss the details of the society with non-members. When this society was first started members of the Japanese navy largely attended it. They do not advertise and have not actively made contact with Westerners apart from Hiroshi Doi. Hiroshi Doi is a member of this society. There were once 80 divisions of the Usui Reiki Ryôhô Gakkai throughout Japan but today there are only five and all the teaching is now done in Tôkyô. There are three major levels in the Usui Reiki Ryôhô Gakkai. These are *shoden*, *okuden* and *shinpiden*, the teacher level. Within these levels there are six levels of proficiency. Each member is supplied with the *Reiki Ryôhô Hikkei* and *shiori*.

Here is a list of President's from Mikao Usui to modern day:

- Mikao Usui (1865–1926)
- Jûzaburô Ushida (Rear Admiral, 1865–1935)
- Kanichi Taketomi (Rear Admiral, 1878–1960)
- Yoshiharu Watanabe (Schoolteacher, ? –1960)
- Hôichi Wanami (Vice Admiral, 1883–1975)
- Kimiko Koyama (1906–1999)
- Masaki Kondô (University Professor)

Usui Reiki Ryôhô International (URRI) – A project, which began in 1999 in Vancouver. Since then it has been held in different countries each year. Teachers who have a strong Japanese influence in their teachings are generally invited to provide workshops. There has been discussion about setting up a formal URRI organization in the future.

Usui Shiki Ryôhô 臼井式療法 – (lit. Japanese) the Usui Way Healing Method. The Reiki Alliance and some Independent Reiki Masters teach under this title. Hawayo Takata used this name on the certificates she issued. It seems that she used two different names to indicate the system she taught, Usui Reiki Ryôhô and Usui Shiki Ryôhô. For more information about Usui Shiki Ryôhô see also Part IV of *The Reiki Sourcebook* under Reiki Branches.

Usui Teate 臼井手当 – (lit. Japanese) hands-on healing by Usui. Usui teate would indicate what Mikao Usui did, not what he was teaching; this would have been called Usui dô. According to the memorial stone Mikao Usui was a very well known healer. Even though his teachings were not about healing others rather about self-healing some of his students began to focus more on healing others e.g. Chûjirô Hayashi. It seems that this is what we practice in the West.

When the information first came to the West it was called 'Usui Teate'.

Usui/Tibetan Reiki – Complete details listed in Part IV of *The Reiki Sourcebook* under Reiki Branches.

Usui, Toshiko – (1913–1935). Mikao Usui's daughter.

V

Vajra Reiki – Complete details listed in Part IV of *The Reiki Sourcebook* under Reiki Branches.

*Violet Breath – Non-traditional breath technique used with attunement process. This is very similar to the *breath of the fire dragon.

W

Waka 和歌 – Classical Japanese poetry form. The word *waka* is made up of two parts: *wa* meaning 'Japanese' and *ka* meaning 'poem' or 'song'. *Waka* is a short form of poetry that contains 31 syllables. In English it is typically divided into five lines of 5,7,5,7 and 7 syllables. *Waka* as written by the Meiji Emperor is one of the components of Mikao Usui's teachings. All the *waka* Mikao Usui used in his teachings are written down in the *Reiki Ryôhô Hikkei*, a manual used by the Usui Reiki Ryôhô Gakkai. Kaiji Tomita, a student of Mikao Usui, wrote in his 1933 book that the technique *hatsurei hô included the student becoming One with the essence of the *waka*. Gichin Funakoshi, the founder of modern karate, also worked with *waka*. It was a popular cultural social interaction at the turn of the twentieth century and was very common amongst certain sections of the population.

Wanami, Hôichi – (1883–1975). Fifth President of the Usui Reiki Ryôhô Gakkai. He was also a Vice Admiral.

Watanabe, Yoshiharu – (? –1960). Fourth President of the Usui Reiki Ryôhô Gakkai. He was also a schoolteacher.

*Water Ritual – Non-traditional method of changing water into energized healing water.

Wei Chi Tibetan Reiki – Complete details listed in Part IV of *The Reiki Sourcebook* under Reiki Branches.

Y

Yamaguchi, Chiyoko – (1920/21 –2003). Chiyoko Yamaguchi was taught Levels 1 and 2 by Chûjirô Hayashi in 1938. She said that she learnt both *shoden* and *okuden* together over five consecutive days. Many of her family members were practitioners and from one of them she learnt to perform the attunement. Chiyoko Yamaguchi assisted her son, Tadao, teaching a style called Jikiden Reiki. Alive are some of their family members who are practitioners, but not teachers, in the system.

Yamaguchi, Tadao – Son of Chiyoko Yamaguchi and the founder of Jikiden Reiki. He has recently co-written a book about Chûjirô Hayashi with Frank Arjava Petter.

Yamashita, Kay – One of Hawayo Takata's sisters and trained by Hawayo Takata as a Reiki Master.

Yuri in – (1897–1997). According to Dave King, Yuri in studied Mikao Usui's teachings alongside Tenon in from 1920–1926.

 Z

Zaike 在家 – (lit. Japanese) lay priest. This priest has his own home and is not expected to reside in a monastery. Mikao Usui is said to have been a Tendai *zaike.*

Zazen Shikan Taza – A Tendai meditation practice that was supposedly practiced by Mikao Usui on *kurama yama.*

Zenki 前期 – (lit. Japanese) first stage. Used in conjunction with *okuden.*

***Zenshin Kôketsu hô** 全身交血法 – (lit. Japanese) whole body blood exchange. Also called *ketsueki kôkan hô.*

Hawayo Takata taught this as the *finishing treatment or *nerve stroke in her Level 2 classes. Here it is apparent that she knew some of the more traditional Japanese techniques.

Zentô Bu 前頭部 – (lit. Japanese) the front of the head. This is the first head position as taught by Mikao Usui.

Zeigler, Patrick – Founder of Seichim. Patrick Zeigler became initiated to an energy in a pyramid in Egypt. He was also influenced by Sufi teachings and eventually the system of Reiki.

Zonar Symbol – A non-traditional mantra/symbol used in Karuna Reiki, Tera Mai, and Karuna Ki. It is said to heal past life issues, child abuse and connect to Archangel Gabriel. This was the first symbol channeled by Kathleen Milner and Marcy Miller.

.

Appendix B

Mikao Usui's Memorial Stone

Reiho Choso Usui Sensei Kudoku No Hi
(Memorial of the merits of Usui Sensei, the founder of Reiho (Reiki Ryoho))

That which is attained within oneself after having accumulated the fruits of disciplined study and training is called 'Toku' and that which can be offered to others after having spread a path of teaching and salvation is called 'Koh'. Only with high merits and great virtues can one be a great founding teacher. Sagacious and brilliant men of the olden time or the founders of new teachings and religious sects were all like that. Someone like Usui Sensei can be counted among them. Sensei newly founded the method based on Reiki of the universe to improve the mind and body. Having heard of his reputation all over, people crowded around to seek his teachings and treatments. Ah, how popular it is!

Sensei, commonly known by the name 'Mikao', with an extra name 'Gyohan' is from Taniai-mura (village), Yamagata-gun (county), Gifu-ken (prefecture). He is descended from Chiba Tsunetane. His father's name was Taneuji, and was commonly called Uzaemon. His mother was from the Kawai family.

Sensei was born on 15 August of the first year of *Keio* (ad 1865). From his youth he surpassed his fellows in hard work and endeavour. When he grew up he visited Europe and America, and studied in China. Despite his will to succeed in life, he was stalemated and fell into great difficulties. However, in the face of adversity he strove to train himself even more with the courage never to yield.

One day, he climbed *Kurama-yama* and after 21 days of a severe discipline without eating, he suddenly felt One Great Reiki over his head and attained enlightenment and he obtained Reiki Ryoho. Then, he tried it on himself and experimented on his family members. The efficacy was immediate. Sensei thought that it would be far better to offer it widely to the general public and share its benefits than just to improve the well-being of his own family members. In April of the eleventh year of *Taisho* (AD 1922) he settled in Harajuku, Aoyama, Tokyo and set up the Gakkai to teach Reiki Ryoho and give treatments. Even outside of the building it was full of pairs of shoes of the visitors who had come from far and near.

In September of the twelfth year (AD 1923) there was a great earthquake and a conflagration broke out. Everywhere there were groans of pain from the wounded. Sensei, feeling pity for them, went out every morning to go around the town, and he cured and saved an innumerable number of people. This is just a broad outline of his relief activities during such an emergency.

Later on, as the *dojo*[1] became too small, in February of the fourteenth year (AD 1925) the new suburban house was built at Nakano according to divination. Due to his respected and far-reaching reputation many people from local districts wished to invite him. Sensei, accepting the invitations, went to Kure and then to Hiroshima and Saga, and reached Fukuyama. Unexpectedly he became ill and passed away there. It was 9 March of the fifteenth year of *Taisho* (AD 1926), aged 62.

His spouse was Suzuki, and was called Sadako. One boy and one girl were born. The boy was named Fuji and he succeeded to the family. Sensei's personality was gentle and modest and he never behaved ostentatiously. His physique was large and sturdy. He always wore a contented smile. He was stout-hearted, tolerant and very prudent upon undertaking a task. He was by nature versatile and loved to read books. He engaged himself in history books, medical books, Buddhist scriptures, Christian scriptures and was well versed in psychology, Taoism, even in the art of divination, incantation, and physiognomy. Presumably Sensei's background in the arts and sciences afforded him nourishment for his cultivation and discipline,

---

[1] *Dojo* is a place of the path.

and it was very obvious that it was this cultivation and discipline that became the key to the creation of Reiho (Reiki Ryoho).

On reflection, Reiho puts special emphasis not just on curing diseases but also on enjoying well-being in life with correcting the mind and making the body healthy with the use of an innate healing ability. Thus, before teaching, the *Ikun*[2] (admonition) of the Meiji Emperor should reverently be read and Five Precepts be chanted and kept in mind mornings and evenings.

First it reads, 'Today do not anger', second it reads, 'Do not worry', third it reads 'Be thankful', fourth it reads, 'Work with diligence', fifth it reads, 'be kind to others'.

These are truly great teachings for cultivation and discipline that agree with those great teachings of the ancient sages and the wise. Sensei named these teachings 'Secret Method to Invite Happiness' and 'Miraculous Medicine to Cure All Diseases'; notice the outstanding features of the teachings. Furthermore, when it comes to teaching, it should be as easy and common as possible, nothing lofty. Another noted feature is that during sitting in silent meditation with *Gassho* and reciting the Five Precepts mornings and evenings, the pure and healthy minds can be cultivated and put into practice in one's daily routine. This is the reason why Reiho is easily obtained by anyone.

Recently the course of the world has shifted and a great change in thought has taken place. Fortunately with the spread of this Reiho, there will be many that supplement the way of the world and the minds of people. How can it be for just the benefit of curing chronic diseases and longstanding complaints?

A little more than 2000 people became students of Sensei. Those senior disciples living in Tokyo gathered at the *dojo* and carried on the work (of the late Sensei) and those who lived in local districts also spread the teachings. Although Sensei is gone, Reiho should still be widely propagated in the world for a long time. Ah, how prominent and great Sensei is that he offers the teachings to people out there after having been enlightened within!

Of late the fellow disciples consulted with each other about building the stone memorial in a graveyard at Saihoji Temple in Toyotama-gun so as to honour his merits and to make them

---

[2] The translator, Hyakuten Inamoto, states that '*ikun*' means *waka*.

immortalized and I was asked to write it. As I deeply submit to Sensei's greatness and am happy for the very friendly teacher/disciple relationships among fellow students, I could not decline the request, and I wrote a summary in the hope that people in the future shall be reminded to look up at him in reverence.

February, the second year of *Showa* (AD 1927)
Composed by: *Ju-sanmi* (subordinate third rank),
Kun-santo (the Third Order of Merit)
Doctor of Literature Okada Masayuki

Calligraphy by: Navy Rear Admiral,
Ju-yonmi (subordinate fourth rank), *Kun-santo* (the Third Order of Merit),
Ko-yonkyu (the distinguished service fourth class)
Ushida Juzaburo

Translated by Hyakuten Inamoto
© Copyright Hyakuten Inamoto 2003

Appendix C
Zazen Shikan Taza

Tendai Ceasing and Contemplation Meditation

Mikao Usui is said to have studied this particular Tendai meditation when meditating on *kurama yama* for 21 days.

The following meditative practice is offered as a means of providing aspirants with a concrete, usable component of authentic Tendai Ceasing and Contemplation Meditation.

A. OUTSIDE THE MEDITATION HALL OR SPIRITUAL PRACTICE AREA

1. *Shikan Zen Yo No Ichi Ge* (The Verse Displaying the Main Point of Samatha-Vipasyana Meditation)

Recite once:

In the genuine practice of entering Nirvana, apparently there are a multitude of roads. But if we think about only the most vital necessities, two methods stand out. The first, *Samatha*, quiets one's evil passions, and the second, *Vipasyana*, further leads one to deny unwholesome desires. When *Samatha* (stopping) results in one's winning entry into *Dhyana-Samadhi* (meditation trance), then Vipasyana (insight) becomes the foundation of *Prajna* (wisdom). When both *Samatha* and *Vipasyana* are successfully practiced, the meditator enters *Samadhi* and receives *Prajna*. In that state, the Dharma's altruistic goal of helping both self and others is fully completed.

2. *Kokoro No Ryo* (Verse on Food for the Heart/Mind)

Recite once each:

Practicing the Dharma includes food and clothes, but in food and clothes the practice of Dharma is not found.
Monetary wealth is not a national treasure; a person who brightens a single corner is a national treasure.
The height of compassion is to welcome evil onto myself while giving good deeds to other people, and to forget myself while doing good for others.
By holding grudges and repaying with hatred, hatred never ends; but by repaying with virtue, hatred is completely exhausted. Rather than bearing grudges about the things happening in this long night's dream called the world, cross the boundary into the Dharma realm of the true Buddha.

3. Method of Entering the Hall

Line up outside the Hall. Recite the *Sange Mon* (Repentance Verse) once:
Ga Shaku Sho Zo Sho Aku Go, Kai Yu Mu Shi Ton Jin Chi, Ju Shin Go I Shi Sho Sho, Issai Ga Kon Kai Sange
From beginningless time I have generated negative karma through my misdirected thoughts, words and deeds. I wish to acknowledge and atone for all.

Enter the hall.

B. WITHIN THE MEDITATION HALL OR SPIRITUAL PRACTICE AREA

4. *San Rai* (Three Prostrations)

Recite three times, each time performing a Grand Prostration:
Isshin Chorai Jippo Hokai Joju Sanbo

5. Ten Non-Virtuous States of Mind (The Recitation on Self Discipline)

This is done individually. Contemplate:
Reflecting on my own life, I should abandon those heart-states in which bad actions accumulate, namely the realms of hells, animals, hungry ghosts, fighting entities, mundane life, heavens, evil spirits, Hinayana followers, professional priests and conflicting emotions.

6. *Godai Gan* (Five Great Vows)

Shujo Muhen Segan Do
Fukuchi Muhen Segan Shu
Homon Muhen Segan Gaku
Nyorai Muhen Segan Ji
Mujo Bodai Segan Jo
Goji Busshi Jodaigan

Sentient Beings are limitless; I vow to save them all.
Knowledge and wisdom are limitless; I vow to accumulate them all.
The Dharmas are infinite; I vow to study them all.
The Tathagatas are endless; I vow to serve them all.
Supreme Enlightenment is unsurpassed; I vow to attain it.
May this seeker of enlightenment fulfil these vows.
Take your seat for meditation.

7. Entering *Samadhi*

First, check one's posture. If sitting in the half-lotus position, place the left leg over the right leg. Pull it close to the body, with the left toes and the right heel equally spaced. Loosen the belt and arrange the clothes neatly so as to cover the legs. Form the meditation mudra with the hands in the lap, right palm on top of the left palm, with the tips of the thumbs lightly touching, pulled close under the stomach. Twist the body left and right a number of times, coming to rest in a correct, straight posture. The backbone should not be curved, and the shoulders are thrown back. If the posture should relax, without hurrying, quickly correct it.

Clear the air passages, expelling muddy spirits. Exhale with the mouth open, releasing the stagnant air slowly while leaning slightly forward. Don't exhale quickly or slowly, but continue until you are satisfied. Breathe all defects out during exhalation, completely exhausting them. Then straighten up again, and through the nose breathe in endless, pure spirit. Imagine it entering through the top of the head, in and out three times. Then with the torso straight and relaxed, allow the diaphragm to move in tandem with the movement of air through the nose. Close the mouth, teeth lightly together, tongue against the upper palate. With the eyes half-closed to reduce the brightness of the outside light, let the line of sight fall about six feet in front. Second, check the breathing. Listening to the sound of the in and out breaths, it should not be loud, not gasping or sucking in air, not jerky, puckering or sliding. Allow the breathing to remain in a natural state, as if in a closed system. Third, check the activity of the thoughts. Separate the attention from the breathing and concentrate it at the red field. Abandon those thoughts outside the practice, such as gross thoughts, random thoughts, daydreaming, thoughts about emotional ups and downs, or relaxed and uptight states.

8. Dwelling in *Samadhi*

Observe the harmony of the Three Mysteries of the body, the breath and the thoughts. Note when the three are not in harmony, and continually apply mindfulness and recollection to again produce unity and harmony of the body, breath and thoughts. Rely on this practice to cross over. One sits single-pointedly, not being shaken by thoughts or activities of daily life, not even if enveloped in raging flames.

9. Exiting *Samadhi*

First, release the mind from *Samadhi*, and establish connections and relations. Next, open the mouth and breathe deeply so as to release the spirit. Next, move the body very slightly. Then move the hands, arms, elbows, shoulders, neck and head. Next, rub the pores of the whole body, then rub the palms together, using the warmth to cover the eyes. Next, open the eyes behind the palms. Finally, light incense or recite sutras depending on the time.

10. Method for Leaving the Hall

If there is time, recite sutras. This can be the Heart Sutra, the Ten-Verse Kannon Sutra, portions of the Lotus Sutra, the Sutra of Saintly Fudo or any other sutra you choose. You may also chant the *Nembutsu* and dedicate merit.

Finally, recite the *San Rai* (Three Prostrations) again, three times, each time performing a Grand Prostration.

Isshin Chorai Jippo Hokai Joju Sanbo

Depart the hall.

From the Mount Hiei Summer Ango
Translated by Keisho, compiled by Jiho
Edited from the original by Jion
© Tendai Lotus Teachings

Appendix D
Imperial Rescript on Education

It has been suggested that Mikao Usui taught the Imperial Rescript on Education to his students. Some suggestions have also been that the five precepts are based on the rescript.

> Copies of this rescript were distributed to every school in Japan and hung alongside the Emperor's portrait, where all made obeisance to them. In such awe were they held that on occasion teachers and principals risked their lives to rescue them from burning buildings. All moral and civic instruction after 1890 was based on the principles –largely Confucian – set forth here. Issuance of the rescript at that time reflected a powerful reaction to the Westernizing tendencies of the early Meiji Period, yet there can be no doubt that this type of thinking was already strongly prevalent and only reinforced by the indoctrination of the new public schools. This rescript was the work of many hands, as were most of Emperor Meiji's pronouncements, but principally those of Inoue Kowashi, a Kumamoto *Samurai* known for his Chinese learning and later minister of education.

> (This commentary is from a book entitled *Japanese Education*, by a scholar named Kikuchi. It is found in *Tsunoda and Debary, Sources of Japanese Tradition*, p. 139.)

We have here two versions of the Rescript: one, in ornate vocabulary, captures the difficult style of the original. The second is in more standard modern English and both are printed with permission from Andrew Gordon's book, *A Modern History of Japan*.

1. Imperial Rescript on Education

October 30, 1890 (twenty-third year of the Meiji Era)

Know ye, Our subjects:
Our Imperial Ancestors have founded Our Empire on a basis broad and everlasting, and have deeply and firmly implanted virtue; Our subjects ever united in loyalty and filial piety have from generation to generation illustrated the beauty thereof.

This is the glory of the fundamental character of Our Empire, and herein also lies the source of Our education. Ye, Our subjects, be filial to your parents, affectionate to your brothers and sisters; as husbands and wives be harmonious, as friends true; bear yourselves in modesty and moderation; extend your benevolence to all; pursue learning and cultivate arts, and thereby develop intellectual faculties and perfect moral powers; furthermore, advance public good and promote common interests; always respect the Constitution and observe the law; should emergency arise, offer yourselves courageously to the State; and thus guard and maintain the prosperity of Our Imperial Throne coeval with heaven and earth.

So shall ye not only be Our good and faithful subjects, but render illustrious the best traditions of your forefathers.

The way set forth here is indeed the teaching bequeathed by Our Imperial Ancestors, to be observed alike by Their Descendants and the subjects, infallible for all ages and true in all places. It is our wish to lay it to heart in all reverence, in common with you, Our subjects, that we may all attain to the same virtue.

2. Imperial Rescript on Education

October 30, 1890 (twenty-third year of the Meiji Era)

I, the Emperor, think that my ancestors and their religion founded my nation a very long time ago. With its development a profound and steady morality was established. The fact that my subjects show their loyalty to me and show filial love to their parents in their millions of hearts all in unison, thus accumulating virtue generation after generation is indeed the pride of my nation, and is a profound idea and the basis of our education.

You, my subjects form full personalities by showing filial love to your parents, by making good terms with your brothers and sisters, by being intimate with your friends, by making couples who love each other, by trusting your friends, by reflecting upon yourselves, by conveying a spirit of philanthropy to other people and by studying to acquire knowledge and wisdom.

Thus, please obey always the constitution and other laws of my nation in your profession in order to spread the common good in my nation. If an emergency may happen, please do your best for Our nation in order to support the eternal fate and future of my nation. In this way, you are my good and faithful subjects, and you come to appreciate good social customs inherited from your ancestors. The way of doing this is a good lesson inherited from my ancestors and religion which you subjects should observe well together with your offspring.

These ideas hold true for both the present and the past, and may be propagated in this nation as well as in the other countries. I would like to understand all of this with, Our subjects, and hope sincerely that all the mentioned virtues will be carried out in harmony by all of you subjects.

Bibliography

Abé, Ryûichi. *The Weaving of Mantra*, Columbia University Press, New York, 1999.

Arnold, Larry and Nevius, Sandy. *The Reiki Handbook*, Psi, Oregon, 1992.

Ashton, W. G. (translated by) *The Nihongi*, 1896.

Barnett, Libby. *Reiki Energy Medicine: Bringing the Healing Touch into Home, Hospital and Hospice*, Healing Arts Press, Vermont, 1996.

Benor, Daniel, J. MD. *Spiritual Healing*, Vision Publications, Michigan, 2001.

Borang, Kasja Krishni. *Principles of Reiki*, HarperCollins, New York, 1997.

Bracy, John and Liu Xing-Han. *Ba Gua – Hidden Knowledge in the Taoist Internal Martial Art*, North Atlantic Books, Berkeley, 1998.

Brennan, Barbara Ann. *Hands Of Light*, Bantam Books, New York, 1988.

Brennan, Barbara Ann. *Light Emerging*, Bantam Books, New York, 1993.

Breen, John and Teeuwen, Mark. *Shintô in History – Ways of the Kami*, Curzon Press, Surrey, 2000.

Brown, Fran. *Living Reiki – Takata's Teachings*, Life Rhythm, California, 1992.

Chadwick, David. *Thank You and Ok! An American Zen Failure in Japan*, Penguin Books, London, 1994.

Chadwick, David. *The Life and Zen Teachings of Shunryu Suzuki*, Thorsons, London, 1999.

Chia, Mantak. *Awaken Healing Energy Through the Tao*, Aurora Press, Santa Fe, 1983.

Cleary, Thomas. *The Japanese Art of War – Understanding the Culture of Strategy*, Shambhala Publications, Boston, 1991.

Cohen, Kenneth S. *The Way of Qi Gong*, Ballantine Books, New York, 1997.

Dalai Lama. *The Power Of Compassion*, HarperCollins Publishers India Pvt Ltd, New Delhi, 1995.

Dalai Lama and Cutler, Howard C. *The Art of Happiness*, Hodder Headline Australia Pty Limited, Sydney 1998.

David-Neel, Alexandra. *Initiations and Initiates in Tibet*, Rider and Company, London, 1970.

Doi, Hiroshi. *Modern Reiki Method for Healing*, Fraser Journal Publishing, British Columbia, 2000.

Donden, Dr Yeshi. *Health Through Balance – An Introduction To Tibetan Medicine*, Snow Lion Publications, Ithaca, 1986.

Drury, Nevill. *The Elements of Shamanism*, Element Books, Massachusetts, 1989.

Ellis, Richard. *Practical Reiki – Focus Your Body's Energy for Deep Relaxation and Inner Peace*, Sterling Publishing Company, New York, 1999.

Floyd, H. Ross. *Shintô: The Way of Japan*, Greenwood Publishing Group, Westport, 1965.

Funakoshi, Gichin. *Karate-dô – My Way of Life*, Kodansha America Inc., New York, 1975.

Gaia, Laurelle Shanti. *The Book on Karuna Reiki – Advanced Healing Energy for Our Evolving World*, Infinite Light Healing Studies Center, Colorado, 2001.

Gleinsner, Earlene F. *Reiki in Everyday Living*, Jaico Publishing House, Delhi, 1997.

Gordon, Andrew. *A Modern History of Japan: From Tokugawa Times to the Present*, Oxford University Press, Oxford, 2002.

Gray, John Harvey and Lourdes. *Hand to Hand*, Xlibris Corporation, 2002.

Groner, Paul. *Saicho – The Establishment of the Japanese Tendai School*, University of Hawaii Press, Honolulu, 2000.

Haberly, Helen J. *Reiki – Hawayo Takata's Story*, Archedigm Publications, Maryland, 2000.

Hadamitzky, Wolfgang and Spahn, Mark. *Kanji & Kana – A Handbook and Dictionary of the Japanese Writing System*, Charles E. Tuttle Co. Inc, Boston, 1981.

Hall, Mari. *Practical Reiki – A Practical Step by Step Guide to this Ancient Healing Art*, Thorsons, London, 1997.

Hall, Mari. *Reiki for Common Ailments – A Practical Guide to Healing*, Piatkus Books, London, 1999.

Hayashi, Chûjirô. *Ryôhô Shishin*, Japan.

Hensel, Thomas A. and Emery, Kevin Ross. *The Lost Steps of Reiki – The Channeled Teachings of Wei Chi*, Lightlines Publishing, Portsmouth, 1997.

Hérail, Francine. *Histoire du Japon – des origines À la fin de Meiji*, Publications Orientalistes de France, Aurillac, 1986.

Hirschi, Gertrude. *Mudras – Yoga in your Hands*, Samuel Weiser Inc., York Beach, 2000.

Honervogt, Tanmaya. *The Power of Reiki – An Ancient Hands-On Healing System*, Henry Holt and Company, Inc. New York, 1998.

Honna, Nobuyuki and Hoffer, Bates. *An English Dictionary of Japanese Culture*, Yuhikaku Publishing Co. Ltd. Tôkyô, 1986.

Horan, Paula. *Empowerment Through Reiki*, Lotus Press, Twin Lakes, 1998.

Horan, Paula. *Core Empowerment*, Full Circle, Delhi, 1998.

Horan, Paula. *108 Questions & Answers*, Full Circle, Delhi, 1998.

Horan, Paula. *Abundance Through Reiki*, Windpferd, Aitrang, 1990.

Ikeda, Mitsuru (translated by Andrew Driver). *The World of the Hotsuma Legends*, Japan Translation Center, Tôkyô 1996.

Irie, Taikichi and Aoyama, Shigery (translated by Thomas I. Elliott). *Buddhist Images*, Hoikusha Publishing Co Ltd., Osaka, 1999.

Japan, seventh edition, Lonely Planet Publications, Melbourne, October 2000.

Jarell, David G. *Reiki Plus Natural Healing*, Reiki Plus, Key Largo, 1997.

Jung, C.G. (edited by Jolande Jacobi). *C.G. Jung – Psychological reflections – an anthology of his writings 1905–1961*, Ark Paperbacks, London, 1989.

Kelly, Maureen J. *Reiki and the Healing Buddha*, Lotus Press, Twin Lakes, 2000.

Keene, Donald. *Emperor of Japan – Meiji and His World, 1852–1912*, Columbia University Press, New York, 2002.

Klinger-Omenka, Ursula. *Reiki with Gemstones*, Motilal Banarsidass Publishers, Delhi, 1999.

Koans – The Lessons of Zen, Hyperion, New York, 1997.

Lewis, Dennis. *The Tao of Natural Breathing*, Full Circle, Delhi, 1998.

Lubeck, Walter. *Rainbow Reiki*, Lotus Light Publications, Twin Lakes, Wisconsin, 1997.

Lubeck, Walter. *Reiki Way of the Heart*, Motilal Banarsidass Publishers, Delhi, 1999.

Lubeck, Walter. *The Complete Reiki Handbook*, Windpferd, Aitrang, 1990.

Lubeck, Walter and Petter, Frank Arjava and Rand, William Lee. *The Spirit of Reiki*, Lotus Press, Twin Lakes, Wisconsin, 2001.

Lugenbeel, Barbara. *Virginia Samdahl – Reiki Master Healer*, Grunwald and Radcliff, Virginia Beach, 1984.

Matthiessen, Peter. *Nine-Headed Dragon River*, Shambhala Publications, Boston, 1986.

McCarthy, Patrick and Yukio. *Funakoshi Gichin's Tanpenshu*, International Ryukyu Karate Research Society, Brisbane, 2002.

Milner, Kathleen. *Reiki & Other Rays of Touch Healing*, 1994.

Maruyana, Koretsohi. *Aikidô with Ki*, Ki-no-Kenkyûkai, Tôkyô, 1984.

Matsumoto, Yoshinosuke (translated by Andrew Driver). *An Unknown History of Ancient Japan, The Hotsuma Legends – Paths of the Ancestors*, Japan Translation Center, Tôkyô, 1999.

Mitchell, Paul David. *Reiki – The Usui System of Natural Healing (The Blue Book)*, Mitchel, Paul David, Idaho, 1985.

Mizutani, Osamu and Nobuku. *An Introduction to Modern Japanese*, Japan Times Ltd., Tôkyô, 1977.

Mochizuki, Toshitaka. *Iyashi No Te*, Tama Shuppan, Tôkyô, 1995.

Mochizuki, Toshitaka. *Chô Kantan Iyashi No Te*, Tama Shuppan, Tôkyô, 2001.

Murumoto, Wayne. 'What is a Ryu?' Issue 8, *Furyu – The Budo Journal*, Tengu Press, Hawaii.

Musashi, Miyamoto (translated by Thomas Cleary). *The Book of Five Rings*, Shambhala Publications, Boston, 1999.

Myss, Caroline. *Anatomy of the Spirit*, Random House, New York, 1997.

Myss, Caroline. *Sacred Contracts*, Bantam Books, New York, 2001.

Nelson, Andrew N. *The Modern Reader's Japanese-English Character Dictionary*, Charles E. Tuttle Co. Inc., Boston, 1962.

Oda, Ryuko. *Kaji – Empowerment and Healing in Esoteric Buddhism*, Kineizan Shinjao-in Mitsumonkai, Japan, 1992.

Papinot, Edmond. *Historical and Geographical Dictionary of Japan*, Charles E. Tuttle Co. Inc. Boston, 1972.

Petter, Frank Arjava. *Reiki Fire*, Lotus Press, Twin Lakes, 1998.

Petter, Frank Arjava. *The Original Reiki Handbook of Dr. Mikao Usui*, Lotus Press, Twin Lakes, 1999.

Petter, Frank Arjava. *Reiki – The Legacy of Dr. Usui*, Lotus Light Publications, Twin Lakes, 1998.

Rand, William Lee. *Reiki – The Healing Touch, First and Second Degree Manual*, Vision Publications, Michigan 1990.

Rand, William Lee. *Reiki for a New Millennium*, Vision Publications, Michigan, 1998.

Ray, Barbara Weber. *The Reiki Factor – First Edition*, Exposition Press, New York, 1983.

Reed, William. *Ki – A Practical Guide for Westerners*, Japan Publications Inc., Tôkyô, 1986.

Reid, Daniel. *Chi-gung: Harnessing the Power of the Universe*, Simon & Schuster, London, 1998.

Reiki Ryôhô Hikkei, Usui Reiki Ryôhô Gakkai, Japan.

Rowland, Amy Z. *Traditional Reiki for our Times – Practical Methods for Personal and Planetary Healing*, Healing Arts Press, Vermont, 1998.

Saso, Michael. *Tantric Art and Meditation*, Tendai Education Foundation, Honolulu, 1990.

Shaw, Scott. *The Warrior is Silent*, Inner Traditions International, Rochester, 1998.

Shewmaker, Diane Ruth. *All Love – A Guidebook to Healing with Sekhem-Seichim Reiki and SKHM*, Celestial Wellspring, Olympia, 1999.

Simon, David. *The Wisdom of Healing – A Comprehensive Guide to Ayurvedic Mind-Body Medicine*, Random House, London, 1997.

Stein, Diane. *Essential Reiki – A Complete Guide to an Ancient Healing Art*, Crossing Press, Berkeley, 1995.

Stevens, John. *Sacred Calligraphy of the East*, Shambhala Publications, Boston, 1996.

Stevens, John. *The Art of Peace*, Shambhala Publications, Boston, 1992.

Stevens, John. *Three Budo Masters*, Kodansha International Ltd, New York, 1995.

Sogyal Rinpoche. *The Tibetan Book Of Living And Dying*, Harper, San Francisco, 1994.

Suzuki, D. T. *Buddha of Infinite Light – The Teachings of Shin Buddhism, The Japanese Way of Wisdom and Compassion*, Shambhala Publications, Boston, 1998.

Suzuki, Shunryu. *Zen Mind, Beginners Mind*, Weatherhill, New York, 1970.

Suzuki, Shunryu. *Branching Streams Flow in the Darkness: Lectures on the Sandokai*, University of California Press, Berkeley, 1999.

Takata Furumoto, Alice. *The Gray Book*, Takata Furumoto, Alice, 1982.

The Encyclopedia of Eastern Philosophy and Religion, Shambhala Publications, Boston, 1994.

Thondup, Tulku. *The Healing Power of Mind*, Penguin Books, Victoria, 1997.

Tohei, Koichi. *Ki in Daily Life*, Ki-no-Kenkyûkai, Tôkyô, 1980.

Tohei, Koichi. *Book of Ki – Coordinating Mind and Body in Daily Life*, Japan Publications Inc, Tôkyô, 1976.

Tolle, Eckhart. *The Power of NOW*, Hodder Headline Australia PTY LTD, Sydney, 2000.

Tomita, Kaiji. *Reiki To Jinjutsu – Tomita Ryû Teate Ryôhô*, BAB Japan, Tôkyô, 1999.

Trungpa, Chogyam. *Cutting Through Spiritual Materialism*, Shambhala Publications, Boston, 1987.

Tzu, Sun (translated by Thomas Cleary). *The Art of War*, Shambhala Publications, Boston, 1999.

Unno, Taitetsu. *River of Fire – River of Water – An Introduction to the Pure Land Tradition of Shin Buddhism*, Doubleday, New York, 1998.

Walshe, Neale Donald, *Conversations with God, 1, 2 and 3*, G.P. Putnam's Sons, New York, 1995.

Watson, Brian N. *The Father Of Jûdô – A Biography of Jigorô Kanô*, Kodansha America, Inc., New York, 2000.

Wilhelm, Richard (translated and explained by). *The Secret of the Golden Flower*, Harcourt Brace & Company, New York, 1962.

Wu, John C. H. *The Golden Age of Zen*, Doubleday, New York, 1996.

Yamaguchi, Tadao and Petter, Arjava Frank. *Die Reiki-Techniken des Dr. Hayashi*, Windpferd, Aitrang, 2003

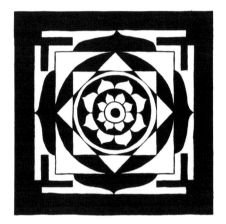

Index